To a stimulating teacher

(Stanley S. Schocket M.D)

many thanks for all that
you have taught me but
most of all for stimulating
me / to look beyond
the obvious

Warm Regards

Bill.

AN ANTHOLOGY OF
OPHTHALMIC CLASSICS

AN ANTHOLOGY OF
OPHTHALMIC CLASSICS

Edited, with comments, biographical notes, and portrait illustrations

JAMES E. LEBENSOHN, M.D., Ph.D.

Emeritus Associate Professor of Ophthalmology, Northwestern University;
Associate Editor, American Journal of Ophthalmology;
Former Section Editor, Survey of Ophthamology

FOREWORD BY
C. WILBUR RUCKER, M.D.

Emeritus Professor of Ophthalmology, Mayo Foundation, University of Minnesota;
Consulting Ophthalmologist, Mayo Clinic

The Williams & Wilkins Co./Baltimore 1969

Library of Congress
Catalog Card Number 76-94010

Composed and printed at the
Waverly Press, Inc.
Mt. Royal and Guilford Aves.
Baltimore, Md. 21202, U.S.A.

Foreword

In this book are reproduced some of the epoch-making contributions to ophthalmology, fundamentals upon which subsequent progress has been built. Great as they are, most of them have as their basis a series of preceding lesser contributions, without which they could not have been constructed. Some are splendid examples of imaginative thinking; others resulted from the authors' perseverence in developing ideas beyond the perception of their predecessors. Many are inspiring demonstrations of clear minds at work on problems still confronting us today.

Few of the original publications reproduced here are rapidly available except in large medical libraries. All have appeared since 1956 in the *Survey of Ophthalmology*, one at a time, under the heading "Classics of Ophthalmology". Each is accompanied by pertinent historical notes and by a short biography of the author, often with his portrait. Assembled now in a single volume, they can provide fascinating reading for anyone with a bit of curiosity about the past.

Responsible for selecting these classics, and for writing the comments and biographical notes, is Dr. James E. Lebensohn, now an emeritus associate professor of Ophthalmology at Northwestern University, where he taught optics and physiology of the eye. His long time interest in medical history, his remarkable erudition, and his unusual effectiveness and popularity as a teacher superbly qualify him for the task. Ophthalmologists probably have as full an appreciation and knowledge of the builders of their specialty as have members of other specialties, but that is not enough. Perhaps this book will intensify their interest and their awareness of the remarkable men who preceded them.

C. WILBUR RUCKER, M.D.
Mayo Clinic.

Introduction

Compilations of classic contributions in the basic sciences, internal medicine and various other specialties have appeared but none in ophthalmology prior to the present undertaking. Because of space limitation, the scope of contributors is far from complete though restricted to non-living authors. My choice was based on the availability of articles, intrinsic historical importance and current progress in the subject treated. The Classics are entirely in the words of the author or translator; but for the sake of brevity and clarity, non-essential material was deleted.

On embarking in ophthalmology, my beloved uncle, an ophthalmologist with a love of history, presented me with the American Encyclopedia of Ophthalmology and Garrison's History of Medicine, both of which have been a source of continual inspiration. Upon my return from World War II, Dr. Derrick T. Vail, who was acquainted with my previous historical papers, appointed me Associate Editor of the American Journal of Ophthalmology and at his suggestion I contributed a historical editorial annually from 1946 to 1967. In seeking original data, I corresponded with ophthalmologists in Great Britain and Ireland, France, Germany, Switzerland, Spain, Italy, Norway, Israel, Iraq and Brazil, as well as many in America, and was delighted with their friendly collaboration. I am indebted to these correspondents for portraits and biographical facts regarding Ferrall, Wolfe and Elliot, Schiotz, Holth and Raeder, Javal and Kalt and for the imaginative sketches of Daviel and Helmholtz.

When Dr. Frank W. Newell became editor of the newly launched Survey of Ophthalmology, he knew of my plans for a prospective Classics of Ophthalmology and proposed a section in the bi-monthly for their publication. Thanks to the continued interest of successive editors of the Survey, Dr. Irving H. Leopold, Dr. James H. Allen and Dr. Bernard Schwartz, the Classics have been published regularly till 1969 when I felt it was time to assemble them in book form.

"Un livre est toujours un moyen de faire un meilleur livre" (Michelet). As the years pass and our present leaders in ophthalmology become history, I hope that some young confrere will complete another volume of Classics that will record their achievements and rectify my unavoidable omissions.

JAMES E. LEBENSOHN

Contents

Four. Physiologic Optics

Five. Anatomy

Six. Cataract

Ten. Ocular Motor Disorders

Eleven. Diverse Surgical Innovations

Twelve. Neuro-ophthalmology

Thirteen. Comparative Ophthalmology

Fourteen. Environmental Adjustment

Author Contents

Part One

Casualties of Newborn

The Prophylactic Treatment of Ophthalmia Neonatorum*

CARL SIEGMUND FRANZ CREDE

Leipsig, Germany

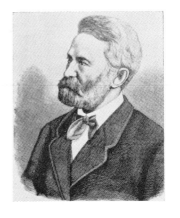

Again I expressly point out, that all the other usual eyesicknesses of children, which formerly could be observed rather frequently along with blennorrhea in the first days after birth, and which are not dangerous but annoying nevertheless, have all as good as disappeared since the introduction of my prophylaxis.

To prevent any misunderstandings, I shall describe exactly how the process was used in the Leipsig Institute.

After the ligature and division of the umbilical cord we first removed from the children in the usual manner the sebacious matter, blood and mucus which clung to them; then they were brought to the bath and there their eyes were cleansed on the outside, not with the bath water but with other clean water by means of a clean linen cloth or better still with prepared cotton. The eyelids and the portions surrounding the eyes were scrupulously cleansed by means of cotton soaked in simple hydrant-water, and especially all the smegma was removed. Then, on the table, before clothes are put on the child, each eye is opened by

* Based on the translation by Herbert Thoms, M.D., New Haven, Conn. Excerpt from *Die Verhütung der Augenentzündung bei Neugeborenen, der haüfigsten und wichtigsten Ursache der Blindheit,* 63 pp. A. Hirschwald, Berlin, 1884.

1

two fingers and a single drop of a 2 per cent solution of silver nitrate hanging on a little glass rod is brought close to the cornea until it touches it, and is dropped on the middle of it. No further care is given to the eyes. In the next 36 hours, in case a slight reddening or swelling of the lids with secretion of mucus should follow, the instillation should not be repeated.

The solution of silver nitrate is contained in a bottle of dark glass with a glass stopper. The glass-rod used is 15 cm. long, 3 mm. thick and rounded at both ends. The little bottle and rod are kept in a small drawer in the swaddling-table. The solution is renewed about every six weeks, but can be used much longer without damaging its effects.

Rinsing of the female genitalia is performed for the sake of cleanliness, but it has no influence on the treatment of the infection, even if sterilized water or antiseptic solutions are chosen. The catarrhal secretion of the genital organs, so frequently met with, cannot produce a specific infection of the eyes, but only a catarrh. Only the virus of gonorrhea can produce the blennorrhea of the newborn, and nitrate of silver is a specific against the gonococcus.

In the Leipsig Lying-in Hospital, the instillations were made by the head-midwife. A student-midwife delicately draws apart a little the child's eyelids with the fingers of one hand. By this assistance all the students are trained, and soon carry out the process themselves.

Within a period of almost three years, there occurred in 1160 children only one case of blennorrhea. Individual illnesses, in which the blame must be placed on omission or a false execution of the prophylactic process, will never be able to be completely checked. The same percentage has continued to hold good from the conclusion of my third report up to end of March 1884, thus for one more whole year. The percentage of blennorrhea of the newborn was thus reduced from 10 per cent to less than 0.1 per cent.

Comment: Conjunctivitis in the newborn may stem from gonorrhea, staphylococcic infection, inclusion blennorrhea or from chemical reaction to silver nitrate prophylaxis. Infants are especially susceptible to microbic infection because of the absence at birth of tears and of subconjunctival lymphoid tissue. Premature infants are exposed to even greater hazard due to their anemic status. The commonest and most virulent form of ophthalmia neonatorum is that due to gonorrhea, and almost all cases in full-term infants that result in destruction of sight are due to this infection. Both eyes are usually involved. Serous discharge and edema of the lids appear about 24 hours after birth. In a day or two the discharge becomes copious and purulent. Before the advent of antibiotic therapy, corneal ulceration occurred in 27 per cent of cases. As traumatism may be a precipitating factor, the baby's arms should be confined so that they cannot reach his eyes and vigorous syringing should be avoided. The corneal ulcer may leave a scar or perforate, then causing adherent leukoma, anterior polar cataract, anterior staphyloma, panophthalmitis or phthisis bulbi. The causative organism is a Gram-negative diplococcus with its flattened concave surfaces in apposition, discovered by Neisser in 1879. A prompt diagnosis can be made by examining scrapings from the retrotarsal fold. Gonorrheal infection is a specific human disease and is not transmissable to animals.

Previous to Credé's prophylaxis, the development of blindness during the first days of life was a tragedy too well known. In 1881, when Credé initiated his method, 35 per cent of the pregnant women in public hospitals were infected with gonorrhea. Though the Credé method of prophylaxis received immediate widespread confirmation, the toll of unnecessary blindness from ophthalmia neonatorum continued. In 1887, Lucien Howe prompted the American Ophthalmological Society to recommend legislative measures making Credé prophylaxis obligatory. Yet in 1907, 20 years later, ophthalmia neonatorum was responsible for one quarter of children in schools for the blind and for 10 per cent of the total blind population. By 1917 the Credé method was compulsory in only 6 states, though 30 states required the immediate reporting of cases of ophthalmia neonatorum. More aggressive methods were evidently required. A report to the State of New York submitted by E. Park Lewis was read by Miss Schuyler of the Russell Sage Foundation. A New York foundation to campaign for the prevention of such unnecessary blindness was started with a grant of $5000. Eventually this movement was extended to the entire country and became the National Society for the Prevention of Blindness.

Credé advocated the instillation of 2 per cent silver nitrate, but since this excited excessive reaction, the 1 per cent solution, which is equally effective, is now in general use. This method has been used continuously in the Sloane Hospital for Women for a quarter century and has reduced the incidence of gonorrheal ophthalmia neonatorum to 0.013 per cent. In view of the long effective record of Credé prophylaxis, it has been considered unwise to substitute antibiotic prophylaxis. Though antibiotics have no irritant cytologic effect, they must be kept refrigerated, the expiration date must be kept in mind and they may induce allergy and resistant strains. Moreover, repeated use probably is required to be entirely effective. Antibiotics are best reserved for treatment. Penicillin ointment, 100,000 units per gm., should be instilled hourly; and intramuscular injections of 100,000 units of crystalline penicilline, 300,000 units of procaine penicillin should be given every 12 hours, until two negative smears are obtained at an interval of 48 hours.

Reference

Norn, M. S.: Cytology of conjunctival fluid in newborn with reference to Credé's prophylaxis. Acta ophth., *38:* 491–495, 1960.

Biographical Note

Karl Siegmund Franz Credé (1819–1892) was born in Berlin, where he was educated, graduating in medicine in 1842. After five years of postgraduate study, he joined the staff of the Obstetrical Clinic in Berlin, and in 1850 became privat-docent. Six years later he was appointed Professor of Obstetrics at Leipsig and Director of the Leipsig Lying-in Institution. He

4

will be remembered for two discoveries of the greatest importance—the method of removing the placenta by external manual expression, and the prevention of infantile gonorrheal conjunctivitis by instillation of silver nitrate. He contributed several notable texts in obstetrics and was editor of the Monatsschrift für Geburtskunde (1853–69) and of the Archiv für Gynäkologie (1870–92). After his death the grateful citizens of his adopted city placed a memorial bust of the great man in the Leipsig University Frauenklinik.

Reference

Rosenberg, J.: Obituary. Am. J. Obst., *25:* 780–782, 1892.

Congenital Cataract Following German Measles in the Mother

NORMAN McALISTER GREGG, M.D.

Sydney, Australia

Trans. Ophthal. Soc. Aust., *3:* 35–45, 1941

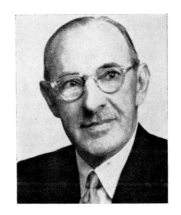

In the first half of the year 1941 an unusual number of cases of congenital cataract made their appearance in Sydney. Their frequency, unusual characteristics and wide distribution warranted closer investigation, and this report brings to notice some of the more important features. The number of cases included in this review is seventy-eight.

General Description and Special Features

The first striking factor is that the cataracts, usually bilateral, were obvious from birth as dense white opacities completely occupying the pupillary area. Most of the babies were of small size, ill nourished and difficult to feed. Many of them were found to be suffering from a congenital defect of the heart. The pupillary reaction to light was weak and sluggish; in some cases the irides had a somewhat atrophic appearance. This was more noticeable after mydriasis when the pupillary border appeared as a flat dark band seemingly devoid of any iris stroma.

Full mydriasis was difficult to obtain; moreover, an unusual number showed intolerance to atropine, and one was forced to rely upon repeated instillations of homatropine.

Cataract. After dilatation the opacities appeared densely white— sometimes quite pearly—in the central area with a small, clear zone between this and the pupillary border. Closer examination revealed in this zone a less dense opacity of smoky appearance, and outside this a narrow ring through which a red reflex could be obtained. Although the general appearance was much the same in all cases, two main types were noticed. In one the contrast between the larger dense white central area and the smaller cloudy peripheral zone was very marked. In the other the density of the cataract was more uniform throughout. In my opinion the apparent differences are due to a variation in intensity and duration of the noxious factor.

The appearance of the cataract does not correspond to any of the large number of morphological types of congenital lenticular opacities that have been described. In sixteen cases of the series the cataract was unilateral. In all cases the babies appeared to follow readily any movement of the light stimulus.

Nystagmus. In the very young patients nystagmus was not noted, but in the older babies it was present. It was a searching movement of the eyeballs and indicated the absence of any development of fixation. It was always present beyond the age of three months.

Variations. One case was referred to me at the age of three weeks. The corneae were quite white at birth. I noted a corneal haze, denser in the center than in the periphery. The iris was just visible in the peripheral zone. The tension was normal. Two weeks later the corneae had cleared and the typical white cataracts were seen in the pupillary area. Two other cases with similar corneal involvement have been noted. There had apparently been some temporary interference with the nutrition of the cornea.

Monocular cases. Sixteen of these have been reported. In my cases the affected eye was definitely *microphthalmic,* and examination of the other eye under mydriasis revealed a large pale area with some scattered pigmentation. The microphthalmia suggests an inhibitory effect on the development of the eye generally.

Heart. An extremely high percentage of these babies had a congenital defect of the heart. In the series it has been present in 44 cases. Autopsy revealed a wide patency of the ductus arteriosus. Fifteen deaths have been recorded.

Etiology

The remarkable similarity of the opacities in the lens, the frequency of an accompanying affection of the heart and the widespread geographical incidence suggested some common factor of infective nature rather than a purely developmental defect. The question arose whether this factor could have been some infection occurring in the mother during pregnancy which had interfered with the developing cells of the lens. From the date of the birth of the baby it was estimated that the early period of pregnancy corresponded with the period of the widespread and severe epidemic in 1940 of German measles. In each new case the mother had suffered from that disease early in pregnancy, most frequently in the first or second month. The health of the mother during the remainder of pregnancy was described as good. Ida Mann has demonstrated that the exanthemata are known to be transmissible trans-placentally.

Whatever the disturbing factor may be, it is fair to assume that the earlier it acts, the more will the central portion of the lens suffer. In the developing lens, in the 26 mm. stage of the embryo, the original central primitive fibers have completed their growth. In the cases under review the cataractous process has involved these early fibers. Can we not fairly assume that the morbid influence began early? As successive layers of fibers were also affected, this noxious factor must have persisted in diminishing strength until with its disappearance some normal fibers were formed. The remarkable frequency of the accompanying congenital defect of the heart and the apparent constancy in type of this defect seem to indicate a common causative factor.

Incidence of German Measles in This Series

In all but 10 cases in this series the history of German measles infection is present. In two the report is negative; in the remaining cases the report is "not known." The majority of these were cases before a possible association between German measles and congenital cataracts was promulgated. In the vast majority of the cases infection occurred either in the first or second month of pregnancy. In a few cases it was during the third month. Out of 35 cases in which the record is available, the affected baby was the first child in 26 instances. It was this young adult group which was particularly affected by this epidemic of German measles.

Nature of Epidemic

I have not previously seen German measles of such severity and accompanied by such severe complications as occurred during this epidemic in 1940. The average stay in hospital was eight days as against four days in previous years.

Operation

Discission has frequently proved difficult. The anterior chamber is particularly shallow, and in many the dense central portion of the lens has proved very resistant to the needle. Absorption has been slower than that of ordinary lamellar cataracts.

Prognosis

It is difficult to forecast the future for these unfortunate babies. We cannot be sure that there are not other defects which are not evident

8

now. The prognosis for vision depends on the presence or absence of nystagmus and on the condition of the retina.

The only sure treatment available is that of prophylaxis. We must recognize and teach the potential dangers of such an epidemic or, I think, any other exanthem, and do all in our power to guard the young married woman from the risk of infection.

Comment: Gregg was the first to prove that congenital deformities may arise from maternal infection at a critical stage of gestation. Rubella is definitely incriminated, but the occurrence of congenital deformities from other maternal diseases, although likely, is yet unproven. In the 125 years that rubella was known before Gregg's publication the congenital rubella syndrome was not identified but instead mistakenly attributed to genetic abnormalities. Charcot said appropriately, "Disease is old and nothing about it has changed. It is we who change as we learn to recognize what was formerly imperceptible."

The manifestations of rubella embryopathy depend on the date of embryonal infection. Since each organ during embryogenesis has a phase of particular sensitivity, an embryopathic calendar may be established. Maternal rubella before the fifth week of gestation, while the primary lens fibers are forming, results in cataracts. The lens capsule, developed during the fifth week, probably acts as a barrier later to the rubella virus. Cardiac defects occur at about the same time as cataracts. Maternal infection at the eighth week, when the organ of Corti undergoes differentiation produces deafness; also at this time infection of the central nervous system determines psychomotor retardation.

When the rubella infection assails the mother in the first month of gestation, the frequency of congenital malformations is about 50 per cent; in the second month, 22 per cent; in the third month, 6 per cent; and after the fourth month no embryopathic defects ensue. In affected offspring ocular involvement and cardiac defects occur in about 60 per cent; complete or partial deafness in 50 per cent; psychomotor retardation in 40 per cent, and dental anomalies in 3 per cent. The Perkins School for the Blind finds that combined blindness and deafness from the rubella syndrome is more common than blindness alone. The birth weight of the infected infant is low, under 6 pounds, and postnatal growth is retarded. The deposition of fat is minimal, causing the appearance of deeply set eyes in a small head.

In 1962 Parkman and co-workers and Weller and Neva announced simultaneously isolation of the rubella virus. Previous attempts using eggs and animals had failed, but success was achieved with a new virological technique based on the demonstration that a single layer of cells growing on the inner surface of a test tube could serve as a host. After these cell cultures were inoculated with rubella virus, virus infection was not apparent but the infected cells resisted superinfection by viruses that destroyed control cell cultures. Using this indirect technique, the investigators identified and propagated the rubella virus.

This accomplishment and the ability to test for neutralizing antibody in the serum led to a greater understanding of the congenital rubella syndrome and a full explanation of the marked contrast between congenital and acquired rubella. Serological tests of pregnant women in continental United States revealed that about 25 per cent were without antibody to rubella.

Rubella infection *in utero* extends to all organs. The virus is present in cataractous lenses and remains longer there than in other tissues. It has been isolated from the cataractous material in a child operated on at the age of 2 years, 11 months, but this finding is exceptional in duration. Infection of the central nervous system is disclosed in the spinal fluid by the presence of rubella virus, elevated protein and pleocytosis. Among transient abnormalities are thrombocytopenic purpura, radiolucense in the metaphyseal portion of the long bones, hepatosplenomegaly, hepatitis, hemolytic anemia and bulging anterior fontanelle.

At autopsy the virus has been obtained from kidneys, lungs, spleen, adrenals and thymus. This virus is not cytolytic and during cell division in the tissues is passed on to the daughter cells. Viral persistence despite the presence of circulatory antibodies is due to its protective intracellular position. The virus is excreted in the nasopharyngeal mucus and the urine, feces, spinal fluid, bone marrow and aqueous. The most frequent source of positive cultures comes from the throat. While shedding virus, infants are potential hazards to their contacts, and nonimmune nurses have been infected with rubella. The excretion rate steadily declines and at 18 months of age only 5 per cent of infants were shedding virus. When shedding ceases, virus may still be in the lens for 9 months or longer.

The most obvious ocular abnormality is a sharply demarcated, pearly nuclear cataract, unilateral or bilateral. The cataract may be partial at birth and almost total a few months later. The rapid increase in size and density of rubella cataracts differentiates them from the usual congenital forms. The rubella cataract is associated with a relative microphthalmos, iris hypoplasia and incomplete development of the chamber angle consequent to a retardation of ocular development, effected by the virus infection. In bilateral cataracts a searching nystagmus appears a few months after birth that is lessened but not eliminated by cataract extractions and corrective lenses.

Pathological studies find the lens capsule normal and the fibers at the equatorial rim relatively normal. The perinuclear area shows a variable degree of liquefaction. Pathognomonic of rubella cataract are pyknotic nuclei in the cells of the lens nucleus. Of infants with rubella cataracts 35 per cent have convergent strabismus before 6 months and 60 per cent at 18 months. Correction of the strabismus should be attempted only after successful cataract surgery, lens correction and judicious patching of the fixing eye. Operations on rubella cataracts are attended with frequent complications. The surgical trauma excites a severe and prolonged iridocyclitis, probably activated by the release of virus, that often leads to pupillary and cyclitic membranes and atrophy bulbi. Intervention should be deferred until the infection has apparently abated. Of 48 eyes operated on by Scheie only three maintained adequate pupillary openings.

Consistently present are iridocyclitis and its sequelae: stromal atrophy, hypoplasia of the dilator and sphincter muscles, focal necrosis of the pigment epithelium of the ciliary body and incomplete development of the chamber angle. The incidence of glaucoma is 10 per cent and is indistinguishable from the hereditary infantile type. A transient opacity of the cornea may occur, variously attributed to viral infection of the endothelium with recovery, temporary glaucoma abated by progressive differentiation of the chamber angle or a transitory interference with corneal nutrition. Impatency of the lacrimal passages occasionally occurs, but the absence of other congenital eye defects such as colobomata, retinal dysplasia, extreme microphthalmos and anophthalmos is notable.

A pigmentary dystrophy is present in the retina in 45 per cent of rubella infants in whom fundus observation is possible. The abnormality is first seen a few months after birth, remains stable and does not affect visual functions. The pigmentation is patchy, variable in amount and location and more frequent about the posterior pole than in the periphery. The escape of retinal functions from damage is due to the late differentiation of the retina, which begins during the fourth month of gestation. François examined 76 patients with Amalric's syndrome (congenital deaf mutism with pigment displacement in the macular area, irregular dissemination of pigment spots and pigment dust in the rest of the fundus). He found that 23 were definitely the result of maternal rubella infection.

An effective attenuated live virus, developed by Parkman in 1966, has passed thorough investigation. Since this became available for the systematic immunization of susceptible pregnant women, the eradication of congenital rubella can be confidently anticipated, and one more source of infant blindness will be relegated to the limbo occupied by smallpox, ophthalmia neonatorum and the retinopathy of prematurity.

References

Rubella Symposium. Arch. Ophthal. (Chicago), 77: 425–473, 1967.
Zimmerman, L. E.: The histopathologic basis for the ocular manifestations of the congenital rubella syndrome. Amer. J. Ophthal., 65: 837–862, 1968.

Biographical Note

Norman McAlister Gregg (1892–1966) graduated with first class honors from the University of Sydney Medical School in 1915, and left immediately for the British Expeditionary Forces in France where he served 3 years and was awarded the Military Cross. On returning to Sydney he joined the staff of the Royal Prince Alfred Hospital and in time was appointed senior ophthalmic surgeon. In addition, he attended the Royal Alexandria Hospital for Children as honorary ophthalmic surgeon, an appointment that led to his brilliant discovery of the relationship of maternal rubella to congenital cataract.

In early 1941 two mothers in succession brought babies with cataracts for his attention. On questioning the mothers about their health throughout pregnancy he learned that both had suffered with rubella in the first trimester. Suspecting a correlation, Gregg embarked forthwith on clinical research that established definitely the relationship of maternal rubella to cataracts in the offspring. His epochal contribution was soon confirmed by his Australian colleagues and subsequently by reports from abroad.

In 1951 the University of Toronto honored him with the Mickle award. Other honors included the Britannica Australia Award and the Cook and Addington Medals. He received honorary doctorates from the Universities of Sydney and Melbourne and the Australian National University, and was elected Fellow of the Royal Australian College of Physicians. The Gregg Prize was established by the Ophthalmological Society of New South Wales in his honor, and in 1953 he was knighted by the queen.

Sir Norman permanently influenced both Australian and international ophthalmology. Of many sided interests, Gregg helped found the Ophthalmic Research Institute of Australia, officiated as president of the Royal Sydney Golf Club and was an active leader in all projects for community welfare.

Reference

Ryan, H.: Obituary. Amer. J. Ophthal., *63:* 180–181, 1967.

Extreme Prematurity and Fibroblastic Overgrowth of Persistent Vascular Sheath Behind Each Crystalline Lens

T. L. TERRY, M.D.

Boston, Massachusetts

Am. J. Ophth., 1942, *25:* 203–204.

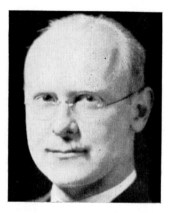

A six-month-old infant, one of twins born about two months prematurely, was found to have a grayish-white, opaque membrane behind each crystalline lens. The pupillary responses were normal and the eyes transilluminated clearly. A jerky, irregular, and somewhat searching nystagmus was present. The membrane did not cover the entire posterior surface of the lens. Below at the extreme periphery, a clear fundus reflex could be obtained when the pupils were fully dilated. In this region thin dentate processes extended from the membrane peripherally as if they were attached to the ciliary processes. The membrane was apparently what is commonly, but perhaps erroneously, called persistent tunica vasculosa lentis. One of the consultants, Dr. Paul A. Chandler, has a case almost identical in appearance in an infant also born very prematurely. Both of these infants were under the care of Dr. Stewart Clifford who discovered the ocular pathology. Recently, three other cases have been seen in the clinic of the Massachusetts Eye and Ear Infirmary. The findings are quite similar to those mentioned, even to the dentate periphery. All of these infants were premature, all weighed three pounds or less at birth, and no evidence of hereditary factors has been found.

It has not been determined whether this abnormal tissue is a persistence of the entire vascular structure of the fetal vitreous or a fibroplastic overgrowth of the persistent tunica vasculosa lentis. Since the hyaloid artery does not close normally until about four to six weeks before full-term development, prematurity could be an important factor not only in preventing normal involution but also in producing an overgrowth of supporting tissue. In all probability this abnormal membrane does grow after birth since it has no exact counterpart in the normal fetal development of the eye. The sporadic persistence of tunica vasculosa lentis in full-term infants is usually limited to one eye as if the lack of involution were a purely local disturbance.

Correspondence with ophthalmologists in many medical centers and review of the literature indicate that this condition has not been encountered generally and that no really satisfactory therapy has been devised. Treatment of these infants, so far, has been along three lines. In some cases it was decided to temporize, awaiting delayed involutional processes. Another patient was given X-ray therapy to see if irradiation would close the embryonic vessels supplying the membrane or have any specific lytic effect on the differentiating mesenchyme that is presumed to make up the membrane. In another case an attempt was made to close the hyaloid artery behind the membrane by diathermy. Such bold surgery was used because a spontaneous hemorrhage in the membrane, increasing in amount, was threatening to become disastrous. Although all of these treatments seem of some benefit, insufficient time has elapsed to evaluate them. From laboratory specimens in unilateral cases, unrelated to prematurity, it is evident that bold removal of the membrane following eradication of the lens is dangerous. Removal of portions of the ciliary processes and retina with the membrane has occurred.

In view of these findings perhaps this complication should be expected in a certain percentage of premature infants. If so, some new factor has arisen in extreme prematurity to produce such a condition. Should this group of cases be not a most unusual coincidence, but a complication in extreme prematurity, then it is important not only to establish the frequency but also to work out promptly the most satisfactory therapy.

A careful study of all cases and pathologic material is being made and an intensive experimental investigation has been started. A complete report will be published later. The purpose of this preliminary report is to bring this condition to the attention of the profession. Other ophthalmologists having similar cases may become interested in the problem so that the frequency, the cause, and the full nature may be determined. Not only might extremely premature infants receive whatever prophylactic treatment proves most effective but also the discovery of an effective therapy might come soon enough to prevent the infants now being observed from developing amblyopia ex anopsia.

Comment: Retinopathy of prematures (retrolental fibroplasia) occurs predominantly in prematures weighing less than 4 pounds. Since the disease is post-natal it was suspected early that some exogenous factor caused this pathologic response. The active phase comprises five stages: (1) Dilation and tortuosity of retinal vessels (this first stage is usually perceptible between the third and sixth week); (2) retinal hemorrhages, with neovascularization and clouding of the peripheral retina; (3) peripheral localized retinal detachment; (4) annular or hemispheric detachment; and (5) complete retinal detachment. Spontaneous regression may occur in the first two stages, and may be expected if the morbid process does not advance for 15 days. On the other hand, poor pupillary dilation with homatropine is a bad prognostic sign. The cicatricial results of the disease likewise are divisible into five stages: (1) The periphery of the fundus shows some opaque tissue without visible retinal detachment. (2) The peripheral fundus shows a larger cicatricial plaque, usually temporal, with some localized retinal detachment. (3) The opaque tissue incorporates a retinal fold which extends to the disk. At this stage the visual acuity varies from 20/50 to 5/200. (4) The pupillary area is partly obstructed by retrolental tissue, allowing still a red reflex over a sector of the fundus. (5) The pupillary area is entirely obstructed and no fundus reflex is obtainable. The cicatricial phase occurs about 14 weeks after the first evidence of the disease. Secondary developments of the final stages are vascularization and atrophy of the iris, posterior synechias, seclusion of the pupil, flattening of the anterior chamber, chronic glaucoma and eventually microphthalmos and enophthalmos.

Controlled clinical studies and animal experiments have established the over use of oxygen as the principal factor in the production of the retinopathy of prematures. The puppy, kitten and mouse have a retinal vasculature at birth that approximates the complete retinal vasculature of human prematures. When these animals were exposed from birth to 60 to 80 per cent oxygen concentration for 4 days or longer, the characteristic pathologic and clinical changes of human retrolental fibroplasia were produced. On an immature retinal vasculature excessive oxygen effects initially a vasoconstriction followed by a secondary vasoproliferative phase. This vasoconstrictive effect of oxygen is limited to an immature retinal vasculature and is confined to the retinal vessels predominantly.

References

Reese, A. B., King, M. J. and Owens, W. C.: A classification of retrolental fibroplasia. Am. J. Ophth., *36:* 1333–1335, 1953.
Patz, A.: Oxygen studies in retrolental fibroplasia. Am. J. Ophth., *38:* 291–308, 1954.

Biographical Note

Theodore Lasater Terry (1899–1946) was born at Ennis, Texas and studied both medicine and postgraduate pathology at the University of Texas Medical School, where he taught for some years. After completing an ophthalmic residency at the Massachusetts Eye and Ear Infirmary he was appointed to its staff as a half-time ophthalmic pathologist under Frederick, H. Verhoeff. He also served ophthalmology at the Harvard Medical School and became acting head of the department during World War II. Terry was the first to recognize the entity which he called "retrolental fibroplasia" as a new and increasing cause of infant blindness. He perceived the complexity of the problem, organized "The Foundation for Vision" for which he secured powerful financial support and directed the effort at its solution from every angle. In 1942 he was awarded the certificate of merit from the American Academy of Ophthalmology and Otolaryngology for his initial researches on this disease. Continued research after his death revealed that the designation he coined, "retrolental fibroplasia," was based on a misconception of the true nature of the disease. Though this term is still the most widely used, many would substitute for it the more accurate descriptive phrase, "the retinopathy of prematures," particularly since a true retrolental fibroplasia does occur as a monocular congenital abnormality in full term infants.

Reference

Lancaster, W. B.: Obituary. Am. J. Ophth., *30:* 498–501, 1947.

Part Two
Genetic Abnormalities

Extraordinary Facts Relating to the Vision of Colors

JOHN DALTON

MEMOIRS OF THE LITERARY AND PHILOSOPHICAL SOCIETY OF MANCHESTER, 1798, 5(*pt. 1*): 28*

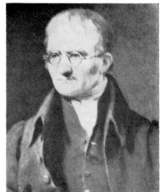

It will scarcely be supposed, that any two objects, which are every day before us, should appear hardly distinguishable to one person, and very different to another, without the circumstance immediately suggesting a difference in their faculties of vision; yet such is the fact, not only with regard to myself, but to many others also, as will appear in the following account.

I was always of the opinion, though I might not often mention it, that several colors were injudiciously named. The term pink, in reference to the flower of that name, seemed proper enough; but when the term red was substituted for pink, I thought it highly improper; it should have been blue, in my apprehension, as pink and blue appear to me very nearly allied; whilst pink and red have scarcely any relation.

In the course of my application to the sciences, that of optics necessarily claimed attention; and I became pretty well acquainted with the theory of light and colours before I was apprized of any peculiarity in my vision. I had not, however, attended much to the practical discrimi-

* Read October 31st, 1794.

nation of colours, owing, in some degree, to what I conceived to be a perplexity in their nomenclature. Since the year 1790, the occasional study of botany obligated me to attend more to colours than before. With respect to colours that were white, yellow, or green, I readily assented to the appropriate term. Blue, purple, pink, and crimson appeared rather less distinguishable; being, according to my idea, all referable to blue. I have often seriously asked a person whether a flower was blue or pink, but was generally considered to be in jest. Notwithstanding this, I was never convinced of a peculiarity in my vision, till I accidentally observed the colour of the flower of the Geranium zonale by candle-light, in the Autumn of 1792. The flower was pink, but it appeared to me almost an exact sky-blue by day; in candle-light, however, it was astonishingly changed, not having then any blue in it, but being what I called red, a colour which forms a striking contrast to blue. Not then doubting but that the change of colour would be equal to all, I requested some of my friends to observe the phaenomenon; when I was surprised to find they all agreed, that the colour was not materially different from what it was by day-light, except my brother who saw it in the same light as myself. This observation clearly proved, that my vision was not like that of other persons; and, at the same time, that the difference between day-light and candle-light, on some colours, was indefinitely more perceptible to me than to others. It was nearly two years after that time, when I entered upon an investigation of the subject, having procured the assistance of a friend, who, to his acquaintance with the theory of colours, joins a practical knowledge of their names and constitutions. I shall now proceed to state the facts ascertained under the three following heads:

  I. An account of my own vision.
  II. An account of others whose vision has been found similar to mine.
  III. Observations on the probable cause of our anomalous vision.

I. Of My Own Vision

It may be proper to observe, that I am shortsighted. Concave glasses of about five inches focus suit me best. I can see distinctly at a proper distance; and am seldom hurt by too much or too little light; nor yet with long application.

My observations began with the solar spectrum, or coloured image of the sun, exhibited in a dark room by means of a glass prism. I found that persons in general distinguish six kinds of colour in the solar image; namely, red, orange, yellow, green, blue, and purple. Newton, indeed, divides the purple into indigo and violet; but the difference between him and others is merely nominal. To me it is quite otherwise;

I see only or at most three distinctions. These I should call yellow and blue; or yellow, blue, and purple. My yellow comprehends the red, orange, yellow, and green of others; and my blue and purple coincide with theirs. That part of the image which others call red, appears to me little more than a shade, or defect of light; after that the orange, yellow, and green seem one colour, which descends pretty uniformly from an intense to a rare yellow, making what I should call different shades of yellow. The difference between the green part and the blue part is very striking to my eye: they seem to be strongly contrasted. That between the blue and purple is much less so. The purple appears to be blue, much darkened and condensed. In viewing the flame of a candle by night through the prism, the appearances are pretty much the same, except that the red extremity of the image appears more vivid than that of the solar image.

I now proceed to state the results of my observations on the colours of bodies in general, whether natural or artificial, both by day-light and candle-light. I mostly used ribbands for the artificial colours.

Red (By day-light). Under this head I include crimson, scarlet, red, and pink. All crimsons appear to me to consist chiefly of dark blue; but many of them seem to have a strong tinge of dark brown. I have seen specimens of crimson, claret, and mud, which were very nearly alike. Crimson has a grave appearance, being the reverse of every shewy and splendid colour. Woollen yarn dyed crimson or dark blue is the same to me. Pink seems to be composed of nine parts of light blue, and one of red, or some colour which has no other effect than to make the light blue appear dull and faded a little. Pink and light blue therefore compared together, are to be distinguished no otherwise than as a splendid colour from one that has lost a little of its splendour. Besides the pinks, roses, &c. of the gardens, the following British flora appear to me blue; namely, Statice Armeria, Trifolium pratense, Lychnis Flos-cuculi, Lychnis dioica, and many of the Gerania. The colour of a florid complexion appears to me that of a dull, opake, blackish blue, upon a white ground. A solution of sulphate of iron in the tincture of galls (that is, dilute black ink) upon white paper, gives a colour much resembling that of a florid complexion. It has no resemblance of the colour of blood. Red and scarlet form a genus with me totally different from pink. My idea of red I obtain from vermilion, minium, sealing wax, wafers, a soldier's uniform, &c. These seem to have no blue whatever in them. Scarlet has a more splendid appearance than red. Blood appears to me red; but it differs much from the articles mentioned above. It is much more dull, and to me is not unlike that colour called bottle-green. Stockings spotted with blood or with dirt would scarcely be distinguishable.

Red (By candle-light). Red and scarlet appear much more vivid than by day. Crimson loses its blue and becomes yellowish red. Pink is by far the most changed; indeed it forms an excellent contrast to what it is by day. No blue now appears; yellow has taken its place. Pink by candle-light seems to be three parts yellow and one red, or a reddish yellow. The blue, however, is less mixed by day than the yellow by night. Red, and particularly scarlet, is a superb color by candle-light; but by day some reds are the least shewy imaginable; I should call them dark drabs.

Orange and Yellow (By day-light and candle-light). I do not find that I differ materially from other persons in regard to these colours. I have sometimes seen persons hesitate whether a thing was white or yellow by candle-light, when to me there was no doubt at all.

Green (By day-light). I take my standard idea from grass. This appears to me very little different from red. The face of a laurel-leaf (Prunus Lauro-cerasus) is a good match to a stick of red sealing-wax; and the back of the leaf answers to the lighter red of wafers. Hence it will be immediately concluded, that I see either red or green, or both, different from other people. The fact is, I believe that they both appear different to me from what they do to others. Green and orange have much affinity also. Apple green is the most pleasing kind to me; and any other that has a tinge of yellow appears to advantage. I can distinguish the different vegetable greens one from another as well as most people; and those which are nearly alike or very unlike to others are so to me. A decoction of bohea tea, a solution of liver of sulphur, ale, &c. &c. which others call brown, appear to me green. Green woollen cloth, such as is used to cover tables, appears to me a dull, dark, brownish red colour. A mixture of two parts mud and one red would come near it. It resembles a red soil just turned up by the plough. When this kind of cloth loses its colour, as other people say, and turns yellow, then it appears to me a pleasant green. Very light green paper, silk, &c. is white to me.

Green (By candle-light). I agree with others, that it is difficult to distinguish greens from blues by candle-light; but, with me, the greens only are altered and made to approach the blues. It is the real greens only that are altered in my eye; and not such as I confound with them by day-light, as the brown liquids above mentioned, which are not at all tinged with blue by candle-light, but are the same as by day, except that they are paler.

Blue (By day-light and candle-light). I apprehend this colour appears very nearly the same to me as to other people, both by day-light and candle-light.

Purple (By day-light and candle-light). This seems to me a slight modification of blue. I seldom fail to distinguish purple from blue; but should hardly suspect purple to be a compound of blue and red. The difference between day-light and candle-light is not material.

Miscellaneous Observations. Colours appear to me much the same by moon-light as they do by candle-light. Mr. Boyle observed colours by moon-light to differ from those by day-light.

Colours viewed by lightning appear the same as by day-light; but whether exactly so, I have not ascertained.

Colours viewed through a transparent sky-blue liquid, by candle-light, appear to me as well as to others the same as by day-light.

Most of the colours called drabs appear to me the same by day-light and candle-light.

A light drab woolen cloth seems to me to resemble a light green by day. These colours are, however, easily distinguished by candle-light, as the latter becomes tinged with blue, which the former does not. I have frequently seen colours of the drab kind, said to be nearly alike, which appeared to me very different.

My idea of brown I obtain from a piece of white paper heated almost to ignition. This colour by day-light seems to have a great affinity to green, as may be imagined from what I have said of greens. Browns seem to me very diversified; some I should call red; dark brown woollen cloth I should call black.

The light of the rising or setting sun has no particular effect; neither has a strong or weak light. Pink appears rather duller, all other circumstances alike, in a cloudy day.

All common combustible substances exhibit colours to me in the same light; namely, tallow, oil, wax, pit-coal.

My vision has always been as it is now.

II. An Account of Others Whose Vision Has Been Found Similar to Mine

It has been already observed that my brother perceived the change in the colour of the geranium such as myself. Since that time having made a great number of observations on colours, by comparing their similarities, &c. by day-light and candle-light, in conjunction with him, I find that we see as nearly alike as any other persons do. He is shorter sighted than myself.

As soon as these facts were ascertained, I conceived the design of laying our case of vision before the public, apprehending it to be a singular one. I remembered, indeed, to have read in the Philosophical Transactions for 1777, an account of Mr. Harris of Maryport in Cumberland, who, it was said, "could not distinguish colours;" but his case appeared to be different from ours. Considering, however, that one anomaly in vision may tend to illustrate another, I reperused the account; when it appeared extremely probable that if his vision had been fully investigated, and a relation of it given in the first person, he would have agreed with me. There were four brothers in the same predicament, one of whom is now living. Having an acquaintance in Maryport, I solicited him to propose a few queries to the survivor, which he readily did (in conjunction with another brother, whose vision has nothing peculiar), and from the answers transmitted to me, I could no longer doubt of the similarity of our cases. To render it still more circumstantial, I sent about twenty specimens of different coloured ribbands, with directions to make observations upon them by day-light and candle-light; the result was exactly conformable to my expectation.

It then appeared to me probable, that a considerable number of individuals might be found whose vision differed from that of the generality, but at the same time agreed with my own. Accordingly I have since taken every opportunity to explain the circumstances amongst my acquaintance, and have found several in the same predicament. Only one or two I have heard of who differ from the generality and from us also. It is remarkable that, out of twenty-five pupils I once had, to whom I explained this subject, two were found to agree with me; and, on another similar occasion, one. Like myself, they could see no material difference betwixt pink and light blue by day, but a striking contrast by candle-light. And, on a fuller investigation, I could not perceive they differed from me materially in other colours. They, like all the rest of us, were not aware of their actually seeing colours different from other people; but imagined there was great perplexity in the names ascribed to particular colours. I think I have been informed already of nearly twenty persons whose vision is like mine. The family at Maryport consisted of six sons and one daughter; four of the sons were in the predicament in question. Our family consisted of three sons and one daughter who arrived at maturity; of whom two sons are circumstanced as I have described. The others are mostly individuals in families, some of which are numerous. I do not find that the parents or children in any of the instances have been so, unless in one case. Nor have I been able to discover any physical cause whatever for it. Our vision, except as to colours, is as clear and distinct as that of other persons. Only two or three are short sighted. It is remarkable that I have not heard of one female subject to this peculiarity.

From a great variety of observations made with many of the above mentioned persons, it does not appear to me that we differ more from one another than persons in general do. We certainly agree in the principal facts which characterize our vision, and which I have attempted to point out below. It is but justice to observe here, that several of the resemblances and comparisons mentioned in the preceding part of this paper were first suggested to me by one or other of the parties, and found to accord with my own ideas.

Characteristic Facts of Our Vision. (1) In the solar spectrum three colours appear, yellow, blue, and purple. The two former make a contrast; the two latter seem to differ more in degree than in kind.

(2) Pink appears, by day-light, to be sky-blue a little faded; by candle-light it assumes an orange or yellowish appearance, which forms a strong contrast to blue.

(3) Crimson appears a muddy blue by day; and crimson woollen yarn is much the same as dark blue.

(4) Red and Scarlet have a more vivid and flaming appearance by candle-light than by day-light.

(5) There is not much difference in colour between a stick of red sealing wax and grass, by day.

(6) Dark green woollen cloth seems a muddy red, much darker than grass, and of a very different colour.

(7) The colour of a florid complexion is dusky blue.

(8) Coats, gowns, &c. appear to us frequently to be badly matched with linings, when others say they are not. On the other hand, we should match crimsons with claret or mud; pinks with light blues; browns with reds; and drabs with greens.

(9) In all points where we differ from other persons, the difference is much less by candle-light than by day-light.

III. Observations Tending to Point Out the Cause of Our Anomalous Vision

Reflecting upon these facts, I was led to conjecture that one of the humours of my eye must be a transparent, but coloured, medium, so constituted as to absorb red and green rays principally, because I obtain no proper ideas of these in the solar spectrum; and to transmit blue and other colours more perfectly. Our type of eyes admit blue rays in greater proportion than those of other people; therefore when any kind of light is less abundant in blue, as is the case of candle-light compared to day-light, such eyes serve in some degree to temper that light, so as to reduce it nearly to the common standard. This seems to be the reason why colours appear to me by candle-light, almost as they do to others by day-light.

Comment: Dalton was the very first to record an account of congenital color-blindness. He was a devout Quaker and on one occasion outraged a religious meeting by appearing in a pair of flaming red colored stockings. When he was invested with the scarlet gown of the University, the color seemed to him similar to that of trees. In 1854 Wilson of Edinburgh was led to appreciate the practical importance of color blindness when he discovered that some of his students were unable to judge correctly the colors of chemical precipitates. He made the first suggestion that the color-blind are unfit to become painters, dyers, tailors, chemists, botanists, geologists, physicians, seamen or railroad employees. In the investigation of a serious railway accident in Sweden in 1875 it seemed that color blindness was the probable cause of the diseaster. Through the efforts of Holmgren a rule was adopted the following year that only persons with normal color vision were to be employed in the Swedish railroad service; a procedure that has been followed since throughout the world.

Biographical Note

John Dalton (1766–1844) was born in England and spent most of his life as a simple schoolmaster. His only university degree was an honorary LL.D. conferred by the University of Edinburgh when he was 68. At the age of 36 he proposed the atomic hypothesis which was supported by the elaborate experiments of Berzelius eight years later. Before Dalton's interests became dominated by chemistry he had written on English grammar, meteorologic observations, and his own color-blindness. A bust in his honor, which cost $10,000, is placed in the entrance hall of the Manchester Royal Institution, a fitting memorial to one of the world's great scientists.

As a son of a poor weaver, he learned to rely on his own resources from earliest youth. He started teaching at his village school at the age of 12. Every free hour of his life was henceforth devoted to intellectual pursuits. Always financially poor, his crude experiments with crude apparatus eventually led to the discovery of several basic laws of science. His first scientific paper, inspired by his own extreme color-blindness, was the first systematic presentation of congenital color-blindness. He next turned to meterology and came to the conclusion that the different size of oxygen and nitrogen particles was an important factor in the stable composition of air. This led to the investigation of the number and weight of the chemical elementary principles which enter into any sort of combination, and then in 1808 to the announcement of his atomic theory. Dr. William Prout, an English physician who ardently espoused Dalton's theory, proposed in 1815 the hypothesis that hydrogen was the universal substance, and that the atoms of other elements were really aggregates of hydrogen atoms.

References

Jaffe, B.: Crucibles. New York, Tudor Pub. Co., 1934.
Moore, F. J.: A History of Chemistry. 3rd ed. New York, McGraw-Hill, 1939.
Lebensohn, J. E.: Dalton bicentenary. Am. J. Ophth. 62: 985–986, (Nov.) 1966.

On Some Hereditary Diseases of the Eye

EDWARD NETTLESHIP, M.D.

London, England

Tr. Ophth. Soc. U. Kingdom, *29:* 57–198, 1909

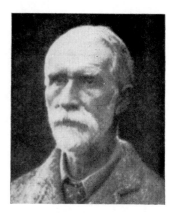

The Mendelian theory in its simple form is so precise, and in regard to a number of unit characters in certain plants and animals its expectation has been found to fit so nearly with experimental results, that no surprise can be felt at the attraction it has for workers in human heredity. Among normal human characters the color of the iris has been investigated and Hurst has shown that pigmentation is in Mendelian terms dominant to lack of pigment. In regard to human diseases and defects I consider that many pedigrees are, in their broad features, consistent with Mendelian theory.

I will refer next to the question of sex liability in some of the hereditary eye conditions. We have first the sex-limited group—ordinary color-blindness, Leber's disease of the optic nerves, and one form of congenital night-blindness. In these so large a majority of the affected persons are males that affected females are regarded as rare exceptions.

Next come diseases that have no special correlation with sex; the lump sum of males and females is about equal. The best examples are all forms of post-natal cataract, glaucoma, and a second form of congenital stationary night-blindness.

In the third group—containing all forms of congenital cataract, retinitis pigmentosa, albinism, and some of the less frequent affections, such as congenital day-blindness—we find a fairly uniform, though not extreme, preponderance of males—about 55 per cent males and 45 per cent females. The few facts now brought forward favor the view that, in man, the male is on the whole more liable than the female to many innate defects and diseases.

Albinism

What I have to say about albinism must be in connection with the incomplete or partial cases that have often hitherto been entered as hereditary nystagmus. The note of all these cases is the blue or gray iris, hair now brown, but with the history that it was very fair or even "white" in early childhood, and a more or less albinotic fundus; almost all have nystagmus and marked amblyopia; when sight is good and the eyes steady, we must suppose that the retinal epithelium, at least at the yellow-spot region, is sufficiently pigmented. The hypothesis is that the imperfect sight, and with it the nystagmus, is caused by deficiency of pigment in the retinal epithelium; that this want may vary in degree, and may even affect only the central region of the fundus. In albinism with quite translucent iris, *i.e.,* no pigment in the retinal layer, stroma pigment is occasionally present in sufficient quantity to give the iris an ordinary brown color. A great puzzle is the frequency and high grade of the ametropia and especially of astigmatism in nearly all recognized albinos, and the same problem meets us for these cases of blue-eyed nystagmus, and appears to furnish another link between the two groups.

We can seldom be sure of the precise date at which the nystagmus begins in albinos. In some albinos the oscillation has certainly not been noticed until the child was many weeks or even some months old, and the movements are slower and perhaps less rhythmical at first than they become afterwards. Albinotic infants not infrequently keep their eyelids closed for weeks after birth; but it has been found that, with the eyelids held open, they evidently perceived the difference between light and shade, and that the pupils responded to light. I have nine or ten pedigrees illustrating nystagmus by what I look upon as incomplete albinism limited to the eyes.

In their heredity these partial cases appear to be almost perfectly sex-limited; of 43 affected persons, 40 were males, and the descent was through the mother in every case; no affected male ever had an affected child. In these characters, the group I am calling incomplete ocular albinism differs from general albinism. It is true that in general albinism the descent is usually discontinuous, but the normal parent who acts as carrier is by no means always the mother. In general albinism consanguinity of parents is common. This fact together with the very great frequency of discontinuous descent in human albinism point to its being a Mendelian recessive. Clinically we all know that every degree of defective pigmentation occurs in skin or hair or eyes, or in all together, to which we cannot refuse the term "albinism", qualified when necessary by such terms as "partial" or "incomplete".

Comment: The special entity of "ocular albinism" as distinguished from generalized albinism was first described by Nettleship in 1909 in the above excerpt of his Bowman Lecture. Subsequently his data were included in a study of all phases of albinism in which over 700 genealogies were presented (Pearson, K., Nettleship, E., and Usher, C. H.: *A Monograph on*

Albinism. London, 1913). Toucaine suggests that translocation of the chromosomes is responsible for the sex-linked pedigrees of ocular albinism. Hereditary ocular albinism is a typical example of intermediate sex-linked transmission. In the carrier, visual functions are intact. A proved carrier can expect that approximately half of her sons will have ocular albinism and that approximately half of her daughters will be carriers. In recent years several observers have noted that the heterozygous female carrier may show attenuated findings in the fundus and iris. The macula retains its reflex but is more densely pigmented; the peripheral fundus is much lighter than the posterior segment and shows irregular areas of pigmentation and depigmentation; and dustlike pigment is scattered throughout. The iris may be diaphanous and transillumine. Gillespie and Covelli found that the carrier changes are more pronounced in the blonde than in the brunette. In their eight proven carriers, only six showed the characteristic fundus picture and in only two was iris transillumination positive.

Generalized albinism behaves as an autosomal recessive. Consanguinity figures prominently; the incidence of first cousin parents is 17 per cent. Incomplete generalized albinism (albinoidism) is more common than total albinism and is particularly frequent in Negroes. An inborn error of metabolism, the absence of intracellular tyrosinase, is responsible for albinism, since the action of this enzyme on colorless dihydroxyphenylalanine (dopa) is essential for the production of melanin. In ocular albinism, it is the deficiency of melanin in the hexagonal cells of the retinal pigment epithelium that causes the symptoms of defective vision, nystagmus, and intolerance of light. For outdoors, the refractive correction in very dark sunglasses with side pieces enhances the comfort of the albinotic patient. According to Fonda, contact lenses with opaque white sclera and blue iris are less effective. He finds that the subnormal vision is helped best by strong reading additions to conventional glasses that correct the marked refractive error generally present.

References

Gillespie, F. D., and Covelli, B.: Carriers of ocular albinism with and without ocular changes. Arch. Ophth., Chicago, *70:* 209–213, 1963.
Fonda, G.: Low vision corrections in albinism. Arch. Ophth., Chicago, *68:* 754–761, 1962.

Biographical Note

Edward Nettleship (1845–1913), the son of a solicitor, was born at Kettering, Northamptonshire. Because of his love of the outdoors, he intended originally to become an agriculturist, and after graduation from the Royal Agricultural College he joined its faculty and served for 1 year as professor of veterinary surgery. He then switched to medicine and obtained his medical degree from the London Hospital Medical School. In 1868 he and Waren Tay worked at Moorfields Eye Hospital as clinical assistants to Jonathan Hutchinson with whom he maintained a lifelong friendship and for some years was associated with Hutchinson in private practice. In 1870 Nettleship qualified as F.R.C.S., and in 1871 he was appointed Curator and Librarian to Moorfields and began to explore the pathology of eye disease. His most important hospital appointments at which his fame was established were Moorfields Eye Hospital, where he became assistant surgeon in 1882 and surgeon in 1887, and St. Thomas' Hospital and Medical

School. At the latter he succeeded Liebreich in 1878 as ophthalmic surgeon and lecturer, and was so highly esteemed that in 1888 he was appointed Dean of the medical school. In 1880 he helped to found the Ophthalmological Society of the United Kingdom and was its president from 1895 to 1897. In 1897, Nettleship was elected president of the ophthalmic section of the British Medical Association for the annual meeting held at Montreal. Meanwhile he wrote a popular textbook for students on Diseases of the Eye, which went through five editions. In 1901, at the height of his professional success, he retired from practice to devote himself wholly to the study of heredity in relation to diseases of the eye. During the following 10 years he accomplished a prodigious amount of work, the value of which was recognized by his election to Fellow of the Royal Society in 1902. At the occasion of his retirement, his friends and pupils honored him with a fund intrusted to the Ophthalmological Society of the United Kingdom for a triennial award of the Edward Nettleship Gold Medal for scientific ophthalmic work. In 1909 it was awarded to Nettleship himself in recognition of his significant researches.

Reference

Lawford, J. B.: British masters of ophthalmology: Edward Nettleship. Brit. J. Ophth., 7: 1–9, 1923.

On the Association of Extensive Hemangiomatosis Nevus of the Skin with Cerebral (Meningeal) Hemangioma

FREDERICK PARKES WEBER, M.D.

London, England

PROC. ROY. SOC. MED., *22(pt. 1)*: 431–442, 1928–1929

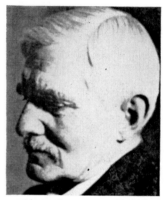

In patients in whom epilepsy, especially of the Jacksonian type, or spastic hemiplegia developed in early life, the hemangiomatous nature of the intracranial disease has been sometimes suggested by the presence of extensive hemangiomatous nevus of the skin, especially of the face (more or less trigeminal distribution) on the same side as the intracranial irritative or paralytic lesion.

I described the following case in 1922 (J. Neurology & Psychopathology, *3:* 314–319, 1922) when I wrote: "It is highly probable that the congenital cerebral disease is in some way connected with the presence of a vascular nevus of the meninges or brain on the left side—of the same nature as the extensive vascular nevus of the patient's body." I have since obtained better skiagrams of the patient's head and it may now be stated that the disease of the left side of the brain is of the nature of a diffuse meningeal angioma, comparable with the condition which was discovered post-mortem in Kalischer's case. This case of mine is the only one in which so great a difference between the two sides of the brain has been demonstrated by X-ray examination during life, without the aid of injection of air. The radiograms, in my paper of 1922, were the first reported of the kind. Similar unilateral cerebral changes have been demonstrated by radiograms in v. Dimitri's case (1923).

The patient, a woman now aged 28, is of a Hebrew family. The patient has very widespread capillary nevus, chiefly of the superficial "port-wine stain" type. On the back of the trunk this angioma is almost entirely limited by the median line to the left side; in front the distribution is more extensive on the left than on the right side. She has right-

sided spastic hemiplegia, apparently of congenital origin. There is a
condition of unilateral right-sided hypotrophy, as one would expect,
associated with the right-sided spastic hemiplegia.

In 1922, I wrote: "There is an absence of pubic and axillary hair, and
she has never menstruated; the sexual organs are probably infantile.
The left eyeball was larger than the right owing to congenital glaucoma
or buphthalmos. The right eye was normal but there was glaucomatous
excavation of the optic disk in the blind left eye. There was heterochromia iridis, the upper three-quarters of the left iris being brown, and
the whole of the iris of the right eye being gray-blue." In 1926, Dr.
Markus had to excise the left eye on account of purulent corneal ulceration and severe pain.

The patient seems not to be deficient in understanding simple
matters; she has never been to school, has not learned to read and write,
and on account of the paresis in her right upper extremity can do only
a little housework.

An X-ray of the head showed marked prognathism. The pituitary
fossa was infantile, a feature that might be considered in connection
with the patient's obesity and defective sexual development. The left
cerebral hemisphere was more opaque and gave a deeper shadow than
the right hemisphere. It seemed to occupy only two-thirds of the left
half of the cranial cavity and to be surrounded by cerebrospinal fluid
(external hydrocephalus). In skiagrams of the skull taken in June 1928,
the whole of the left side, excluding the cerebellum, appears to be small,
occupying only part of the cranial cavity, as if bound down by partially
calcified leptomeninges, the site of diffuse angiectatic hemangioma.
There is probably some calcareous deposit in the vessels of the meningeal angioma. The shadowing due to calcareous deposit does not extend
beyond the tentorium cerebelli, and there is no radiographic sign that
the cerebellum is affected.

In all cases of large facial hemangioma a radiogram of the brain
should be taken but in the interpretation it must be remembered that
deep facial as well as intracranial hemangiomata may be partially calcified. Unilateral congenital glaucoma on the side of the main capillary
nevus of the skin and the cerebral disease has been found. Unilateral
intracranial hemorrhage from blood-vessels connected with the meningeal angiomatous condition, occurring in early or in intra-uterine life,
may have been the original cause of the spastic hemiplagia and epileptic
fits in some of the cases.

In Lindau's disease hemangiomatous or hemangiomatous-cystic disease of the cerebellum is associated with capillary angioma of the retina
and sometimes with hemangiomatous lesions in other parts of the body.

The relation of retinal hemangiomatoses to Lindau's syndrome seems to me analogous to that of unilateral buphthalmos or congenital glaucoma to the syndrome which forms the subject of my present communication.

Comment: The association of buphthalmos with capillary nevi of the face, conjunctiva, mouth and pharynx was first noted by Schirmer (1860). The combination of a co-existing intracranial angiomatous condition was suggested by Sturge in 1879 and confirmed by Weber in 1929. Some factor is apparently involved that affects the area of distribution of one or more branches of the fifth nerve, for the meninges affected by angiomatous changes are likewise innervated by the trigeminal nerve. The Sturge-Weber disease has hence been called by Walsh "the vascular encephalo-trigeminal syndrome" and by Duke-Elder, "encephalofacial angiomatosis." After the syndrome was established, many reports followed, and by 1948 Larmande had collected more than 200 cases. The remarkable conjuncture of glaucoma with nervus of the face involving the eyelids (Naevus flammeus) suggests a cause and effect relationship. The glaucoma, like the angiomatous condition, is congenital; it is buphthalmic in about 70 per cent of cases and simulates chronic simple glaucoma with deep cupping of the disk in the remainder. It is generally unilateral. Other ocular changes include a dilatation of the vessels of the conjunctiva, sclera and iris, heterochromia, and frequently choroidal angioma and tortuous and dilated retinal vessels. Medical treatment of this glaucoma is ineffective, while surgical intervention is dangerous as disastrous hemorrhage may follow.

Reference

Duke-Elder, W. S.: *Textbook of ophthalmology,* Vol. V, pp. 5094–5095. C. V. Mosby Co., St. Louis, 1952.

Biographical Note

Frederick Parkes Weber (1863–1962) was the eldest son of Sir Hermann Weber, physician to Queen Victoria, who as a young man came to England from Germany. The younger Weber was educated at Cambridge and studied medicine at St. Bartholomew's Hospital, qualifying in 1889. He returned from extensive study abroad to attach himself to the German Hospital, where he was on active service for 50 years. Weber's voluminous writings, numbering over 1200, which included 20 books and monographs, began in 1890 with a paper on abnormal foramina in the heart and its valves, and continued to within weeks of his death in his 100th year. Weber was ever fascinated by unusual clinical manifestations such as green or blue urine, gynecomastia, changes in the fingernails, pigmentation of the mucous membranes, and vicarious menstruation. He described the trans-placental transmission of melanoma from mother to child. While investigating the causes of a large tongue, he became interested in primary amyloidosis, a condition to which he first called attention in England (1937). His name is attached to an unusual number of rare diseases, of which the best known are: (1) Sturge Weber's hemangiectatic nevus of the face and cerebral meninges; (2) Osler-Rendu-Weber's hereditary hemorrhagic telangiectasia; (3) Weber-Christian's relapsing febrile nodular non-suppurative panniculitis; (4) Weber-Klippel's hemangiectatic hypertrophy of the limbs; (5) Vaquez-Osler-Weber's polycythemia vera with spleno-megaly; and (6) Weber-Cockayne familial recurrent bullous eruption of the hands and feet. His passion for rare diseases is reflected in his books: *Rare Diseases and Debatable Subjects* (1947) and *Further Rare Diseases and Debatable Subjects* (1949).

His incomparable knowledge of rare diseases was perhaps related to his interest in rare objects. He was a fellow of the antiquarian societies of Cambridge and London, and of the Royal Numismatic Society. His valu-able collection of old coins, medals, vases and other rare antiques was finally distributed to the British, Bodleian and Fitzwilliam Museums, to the London Guildhall Library and to the Boston Medical Library.

Weber gave the first Michell Lecture of the Royal College of Physicians. He continued to attend meetings regularly, especially at the Royal Society of Medicine, until he had well passed the age of 90. Weber was admired the world over for his immense contributions to clinical medicine. When he finished a consultation, he had not finished with the patient; he would continue collecting facts as long as the patient lived. He treated patients with grave courtesy and listened attentively to everything they had to say. Before leaving he always said something encouraging and shook them earnestly by the hand.

References

McKusick, V. A.: Frederick Parker Weber. J. A. M. A., *183:* 45–49, 1963.
Obituary: Lancet, *1:* 1308–1309, 1962.

Part Three

Examination of the Eye

A New Discovery Touching Vision

PRIOR EDME MARIOTTE

Dijon, France

TRANSLATION BY JUSTEL, ROYAL SOC. OF LONDON, PHILOSOPHICAL TRANS., 1668, *3:* 668–671

Having often observed in anatomical dissections of men as well as brutes, that the optic nerve does never answer just to the middle of the bottom of the eye, i.e., to the place where is made the picture of the objects, we directly look on; and that in man it is somewhat higher, and on the side towards the nose; to make therefore the rays of an object to fall upon the optic nerve of my eye, and to find the consequence thereof, I made this experiment:

I fastened on an obscure wall about the height of my eye, a small round paper, to serve me for a fixed point of vision; and I fastened such another on the side thereof towards my right hand, at the distance of about two feet; but somewhat lower than the first, to the end that it might strike the optic nerve of my right eye, whilst I kept my left eye shut. Then I placed myself over against the first paper, and drew back by little and little, keeping my right eye fixed and very steady upon the same; and being about 10 foot distant, the second paper totally disappeared.

That this cannot be imputed to the oblique position of the second paper is evident in that I can see other objects further extant on the side of it so that one would believe the second paper were by a flight taken away, if one did not soon find it again by the least stirring of one's eye.

This experiment I made often, varying it by different distances, and removing or approaching the papers to one another proportionally. I made it also with my left eye, by keeping my right eye shut, after I had fastened the second paper on the left side of my point of vision; so that from the site of the parts of the eye it cannot be doubted but that this deficiency of vision is upon the optic nerve.

This discovery I communicated to many of my friends who found the same thing though not always just at the same distances; which diversity I ascribed to the different situation of the optic nerve. You have made it yourself in His Majesty's library where I showed it to those of your illustrous assembly; and you, as well as I, found the like variety, there being some, who at the distances mentioned lost the sight of a paper, 8 inches large, and others who ceased not to see it but when it was somewhat less; which appears not how it can be caused but by the differing magnitudes of the optic nerve in different eyes.

This experiment hath given me cause to doubt whether vision was indeed performed in the retina (as is the common opinion) or rather in that other membrane, which at the bottom of the eye is seen through the retina and is called the choroid. For if vision were made in the retina, it seems that then it should be made wherever the retina is; and since the same covers the whole nerve, as well as the rest of the bottom of the eye, there appears no reason to me, why there should be no vision in the place of the optic nerve where it is: on the contrary, if it be in the choroid that vision is made, it seems evident that the reason why there is none on the optic nerve is because that membrane (the choroid) parts from the edges of the said nerve and covers not the middle thereof as it does the rest of the bottom of the eye.

Upon this I desire you would give me your thoughts with freedom since I am none of those that love to obtrude conjectures for demonstrations.

Discussion by Monsieur Pecquet

Everyone wonders that no person before you hath been aware of this privation of sight which everyone now finds after you have given notice of it. But as to the sequel you draw from this discovery, I see it not cogent to abandon the plea of the retina being the principal organ of vision. For (not to insist here on other considerations) it will be sufficient now to take notice that at the place of the optic nerve there is something that may very well cause this loss of the object. There are the vessels of the retina, the trunks whereof are big enough to give a hindrance to vision. These vessels, which are no other but the ramifications of the veins and arteries, are derived from the heart, and having no communication with the brain, they cannot carry thither the species of the objects. If therefore the visual rays issuing from an object fall on these vessels at the place of their trunk or main body, 'tis certain that the impression made thereby will produce no vision and that the picture of that object will be deficient. It is not so in respect to the small ramifications that issue from those trunks and shoot into the retina; for if they be met with at the place of the bottom of the eye where vision is made distinct, they will not render the image of the object deficient because they are so small as not to be sensible.

Comment: The discovery of the blind spot was not a matter of chance. Mariotte had observed in animals the nasal entrance of the optic nerve and then set about determining the sensitivity of that area. When he found this insensitive to light he concluded that the vascular choroid was the percipient coat because of its absence at the disk, and in this opinion Mery concurred. The error was definitely rectified by Helmholtz, who showed that nerve fibers themselves are incapable of sensation.

Thomas Young in 1800 gave the first exact measurements of the visual field and of the blind spot. Von Graefe, the father of clinical campimetry, noted in 1856 the enlargement of the blind spot in disease. The extent of the blind spot is such that "at a distance of fifty feet a human figure would disappear completely" (Bjerrum). One-eyed drivers are not handicapped thereby because of the physiologic fixation nystagmus.

Because of the latent period of response the extent of the blind spot is less when tested centripetally than in a centrifugal direction. Both measurements should be made and the mean taken. Exploration should be perpendicular to its borders. Continuing from the nasal to the temporal border is an error which causes the blind spot to be displaced temporally. Diminution of the test object or of luminance enlarges the blind spot and reveals adjacent scotomata more readily. A black test object on a white field gives a blind spot 6 per cent larger than the reverse contrast. The blind spot in uncorrected aphakia is one-third larger than normal. In alleged monocular blindness the demonstration of the blind spot with the "blind" eye covered, but not with both eyes open, is presumptive evidence of malingering.

Reference

Dubois-Poulsen, A.: *Le Champ Visuel.* Chap. X. Paris, Masson et Cie, 1952.

Biographical Note

Edme Mariotte (1620–1684) lived most of his life at Dijon where he became prior of St. Martin-sous-Beaune. He was an original member of the Academy of Sciences founded in Paris in 1666, and his report concerning the discovery of the blind spot was presented in an exchange of letters between two fellow members. His subsequent letter gave the diameter of the largest disk of paper that could disappear completely from sight, and Mariotte insisted "that the whole area of the point of entrance of the optic nerve is blind." Mariotte easily explained the imperceptibility of the blind spot in binocular vision but in monocular vision he was puzzled to observe that, instead of the expected dark spot, the color of the background covered the unseen area. Helmholtz mentions that Mariotte demonstrated his experiment before Charles II of England. Unfortunately this statement, which is historically untrue, was originally based on a misreading of an abbreviated Latin footnote in Haller's *Textbook of Physiology*.

The great variety of physical subjects to which Mariotte contributed including the nature of color, the notes of the trumpet, the motion of fluids, the freezing of water and the recoil of guns. He proved that it was the reflection of light that caused an eye to be luminous. He anticipated Auenbrugger in recognizing the clinical value of percussion. His "Essais de Physique" contains a statement of Boyle's Law which he discovered independently a few years after Boyle, but which is still called Mariotte's Law in France. He was the first to demonstrate that the rate of falling in a vacuum is the same for a coin and a feather. Condorcet said, "It is Mariotte, who first in France introduced into physics a spirit of observation and of doubt."

References

Brons, J.: The blind spot of Mariotte. Acta Ophth., 1939, *17 (Suppl.)*: 1–348.
Mettler, C. C.: *History of Medicine*. Philadelphia, Blakiston Co., 1947.

On the Mechanism of the Eye

THOMAS YOUNG, M.D., F.R.S.

London

ROYAL SOCIETY OF LONDON, PHILOSOPHICAL TRANS., 1801, *16:* 23–88

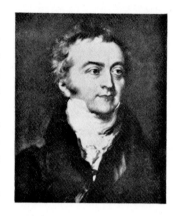

Dr. Porterfield has employed an experiment, first made by Scheiner, to the determination of the focal distance of the eye; and has described under the name of an optometer, a very excellent instrument, founded on the principle of the phenomenon. But the apparatus is capable of improvement; and I shall beg leave to describe an optometer, simple in its construction, and equally convenient and accurate in its application.

Let an obstacle be interposed between a radiant point and any refracting surface or lens and let this obstacle be perforated at two points only. Let the refracted rays be intercepted by a plane, so as to form an image on it. Then it is evident, that when this plane passes through the focus of refracted rays, the image formed on it will be a single point. But, if the plane be advanced forwards, or removed backwards, the small pencils passing through the perforations, will no longer meet in a single point, but will fall on two distinct spots of the plane and, in either case, form a double image of the object.

The same happens when we look at any object through two pin holes, within the limits of the pupil. If the object be at the point of perfect vision, the image on the retina will be single; but, in every other case, the image being double, we shall appear to see a double object: and, if we look at a line pointed nearly to the eye, it will appear as two lines, crossing each other in the point of perfect vision. For this purpose, the holes may be converted into slits, which render the images nearly as distinct, at the same time that they admit more light.

Being convinced of the advantage of making every observation with as little assistance as possible, I have endeavoured to confine most of my experiments to my own eyes; and I shall, in general, ground my calculations on the supposition of an eye nearly similar to my own. I shall therefore first endeavour to ascertain all its dimensions, and all its faculties.

My eye, in a state of relaxation, collects to a focus on the retina, those rays which diverge vertically from an object at the distance of ten inches from the cornea, and the rays which diverge horizontally from an object at seven inches distance. For, if I hold the plane of the optometer vertically, the images of the line appear to cross at ten inches; if horizontally, at seven. The difference is expressed by a focal length of 23 inches. I have never experienced any inconvenience from this imperfection, nor did I ever discover it till I made these experiments; and I believe I can examine minute objects with as much accuracy as most of those whose eyes are differently formed. On mentioning it to Mr. Cary, he informed me, that he had frequently taken notice of a similar circumstance; that many persons were obliged to hold a concave glass obliquely, in order to see with distinctness, counterbalancing, by the inclination of the glass, the too great refractive power of the eye in the direction of that inclination, and finding but little assistance from spectacles of the same focal length. The difference is not in the cornea, for it exists when the effect of the cornea is removed by a method to be described hereafter.

When I look at a minute lucid point, such as the image of a candle in a small concave speculum, it appears as a radiated star, as a cross, or as an unequal line, and never as a perfect point, unless I apply a concave lens inclined at a proper angle, to correct the unequal refraction of my eye. If I bring the point very near, it spreads into a surface nearly circular, and almost equably illuminated, except some faint lines, nearly in a radiating direction. When the point is further removed, the image becomes evidently oval, the vertical diameter being longest, and the lines a little more distinct than before. Removing the point a little further, the image becomes a short vertical line; the rays that diverged horizontally being perfectly collected, while the vertical rays are still separate. Some of these figures bear a considerable analogy to the images derived from the refraction of oblique rays, and still more strongly resemble a combination of two of them in opposite directions.

The visual axis being fixed in any direction, I can at the same time see a luminous object placed laterally at a considerable distance from it; but in various directions the angle is very different. Upwards it extends to 50 degrees, inwards to 60, downwards to 70, and outwards to 90 degrees. The internal limits of the field of view nearly correspond with the external limits formed by the different parts of the face, when the eye is directed forwards and somewhat downwards, which is its most natural position; and both are well calculated for enabling us to perceive the most readily, such objects as are the most likely to concern us. It is well known, that the retina advances further forwards toward the internal angle of the eye, than towards the external angle; but upwards and downwards its extent is nearly equal, and is indeed every way greater than the limits of the field of view, even if allowance is made for the refraction of the cornea only. The whole extent of perfect vision is little more than 10 degrees; or, more strictly speaking, the imperfection begins within a degree or two of the visual axis, and at the distance of 5 or 6 degrees becomes nearly stationary, until, at a still greater distance, vision is wholly extinguished. The imperfection is partly owing to the unavoidable aberration of oblique rays, but principally to the insensibility of the retina. The motion of the eye has a range of about 55 degrees in every direction; so that the field of perfect vision, in succession, is by this motion extended to 110 degrees.

To find the place of the entrance of the optic nerve, I fix two candles at ten inches distance, retire sixteen feet, and direct my eye to a point four feet to the right or left of the middle of the space between them: they are then lost in a confused spot of light; but any inclination of the eye brings one or the other of them into the field of view. From the experiment here related, the distance of the centre of the optic nerve from the visual axis is found to be 16 hundredths of an inch; and the diameter of the most insensible part of the retina, one-thirtieth of an inch. It appears, that the visual axis is five-hundredths, or one-twentieth of an inch, further from the optic nerve than the point opposite the pupil. It is possible that this distance may be different in different eyes.

Considering how little inconvenience is experienced from so material an inequality in the refraction of the lens as I have described, we have no reason to expect a very accurate provision for correcting the aberration of the lateral rays. But, as far as can be ascertained by the optometer, the aberration arising from figure is completely corrected; since four or more images of the same line appear to meet exactly in the same point, which they would not do if the lateral rays were materially more refracted than the rays near the axis. The weaker refractive power of the external parts, must greatly tend to correct the aberration arising from the too great curvature towards the margin of the disc. But, neither this gradation, nor any other provision, has the effect of rendering the eye perfectly achromatic. Dr. Jurin had remarked this long ago, from observing the colour bordering the image of an object seen indistinctly. The observation is confirmed, by placing a small concave speculum in different parts of a prismatic spectrum, and ascertaining the utmost distances at which the eye can collect the rays of different colours to a focus. By these means I find, that the red rays, from a point at 12 inches distance, are as much refracted as white or yellow light at 11. The difference is equal to the refraction of a lens 132 inches in focus.

But the aberration of the red rays in a lens of crown glass, of equal mean refractive power with the eye, would be equivalent to the effect of a lens 44 inches in focus. If, therefore, we can depend upon this calculation, the dispersive power of the eye collectively, is one-third of the dispersive power of crown glass, at an equal angle of deviation. Had the dispersive power of the whole eye been equal to that a flint glass, the distances of perfect vision would have varied from 12 inches to 7 for different rays, in the same state of the mean refractive powers.

The faculty of accommodating the eye to various distances, appears to exist in very different degrees in different individuals. In my eye the power is equivalent to a lens of 4 inches focus. A middle aged lady showed a power of accommodation only equal to the effect of a lens of 12 inches focus. In general, I have reason to think, that the faculty diminishes in some degree, as persons advance in life. I shall take the range of my own eye, as being probably about the medium, and inquire what changes will be necessary to produce it; whether we suppose the radius of the cornea to be diminished, or the distance of the lens from the retina to be increased, or these two causes to act conjointly, or the figure of the lens itself to undergo an alteration.

Supposing the crystalline lens to change its form; if it became a sphere, its diameter would be 28 hundredths, and, its anterior surface retaining its situation, the eye would have perfect vision at the distance of an inch and a half. This is more than double the actual change. Disregarding the elongation of the axis, and supposing the curvature of each surface to be changed proportionally, the radius of the anterior must become about 24, and that of the posterior 17 hundredths.

I shall now proceed to inquire, which of these changes takes place in nature; and I shall begin with a relation of experiments made in order to ascertain the curvature of the cornea in all circumstances.

I had an excellent achromatic microscope, made by Mr. Ramsden for my friend Mr. John Ellis, of five inches focal length, magnifying about 20 times. To this I adapted a cancelled micrometer, in the focus of the eye not employed in looking through the microscope: it was a large card, divided by horizontal and vertical lines into fortieths of an inch. I placed two candles so as to exhibit images in a vertical position in the eye of Mr. König, who had the goodness to assist me; and, having brought them into the field of the microscope, where they occupied 35 of the small divisions, I desired him to fix his eye on objects at different distances in the same direction: but I could not perceive the least variation in the distance of the images.

But a much more accurate and decisive experiment remains. I take out of a small botanical microscope, a double convex lens, of eight-tenths radius and focal distance, fixed in a socket one-fifth of an inch in depth; securing its edges with wax, I drop into it a little water, nearly cold, till it is three-fourths full, and then apply it to my eye, so that the cornea enters half way into the socket, and is every where in contact with the water. My eye immediately becomes presbyopic, and the refractive power of the lens, which is reduced by the water to a focal length of about 16 tenths, is not sufficient to supply the place of the cornea, rendered inefficacious by the intervention of the water; but the addition of another lens, of five inches and a half focus, restores my eye to its natural state, and somewhat more. I then apply the optometer, and I find the same inequality in the horizontal and vertical refractions as without the water; and I have, in both directions, a power of accommodation equivalent to a focal length of four inches, as before.

Having satisfied myself that the cornea is not concerned in the accommodation of the eye, my next object was to inquire if any alteration in the length of its axis could be discovered; and, considering that such a change must amount to one-seventh of the diameter of the eye, I flattered myself with the expectation of submitting it to measurement.

I therefore placed two candles so that when the eye was turned inwards, and directed towards its own image in a glass, the light reflected from one of the candles by the sclerotica appeared upon its external margin, so as to define it distinctly by a bright line; and the image of the other candle was seen in the centre of the cornea. I then applied the scale, in the manner already described, but without indicating any diminution of the distance, when the focal length of the eye was changed.

Another test, and a much more delicate one, was the application of the ring of a key at the external angle, when the eye was turned as much inwards as possible, and confined at the same time by a strong oval iron ring, pressed against it at the internal angle. The key was forced in as far as the sensibility of the integuments would admit, and was wedged, by a moderate pressure, between the eye and the bone. In this situation, the phantom caused by the pressure extended within the field of perfect vision, and was very accurately defined; nor did it, as I formerly imagined, by any means prevent a distinct perception of the objects actually seen in that direction; and a straight line coming within the field of this oval phantom, appeared somewhat inflected towards its centre; a distortion easily understood by considering the effect of the pressure on the form of the retina. Supposing now, the distance between the key and the iron ring to have been, as it really was, invariable, the elongation of the eye must have been either totally or very nearly prevented; and, instead of an increase of the length of the eye's axis, the oval spot caused by the pressure would have spread over a space at least ten times as large as the most sensible part of the retina. But no such circumstance took place: the power of accommodation was as extensive as ever; and there was no perceptible change, either in the size or in the figure of the oval spot.

I placed two candles so as exactly to answer to the extent of the termination of the optic nerve, and, marking accurately the point to which my eye was directed, I made the utmost change in its focal length; expecting that, if there were any elongation of the axis, the external candle would appear to recede outwards upon the visible space. But this did not happen; the apparent place of the obscure part was precisely the same as before.

From the experiments related, it appears to be highly improbable that any material change in the length of the axis actually takes place; and it is almost impossible to conceive by what power such a change could be effected.

It now remains to inquire into the pretensions of the crystalline lens to the power of altering the focal length of the eye. The grand objection to the efficacy of a change of figure in the lens, was derived from the experiments in which those who have been deprived of it have appeared to possess the faculty of accommodation.

I must here acknowledge my great obligation to Mr. Ware, for the readiness and liberality with which he introduced me to such of his numerous patients as he thought most likely to furnish a satisfactory determination. It is unnecessary to enumerate every particular experiment; but the universal result is, contrary to the expectation with which I entered on the inquiry, that in an eye deprived of the crystalline lens, the actual focal distance is totally unchangeable. This will appear from a selection of the most decisive observations:

Mr. R. can read at four inches and at six only, with the same glass. He saw the double lines meeting at three inches, and always at the same point. Miss H., a young lady of about twenty, had a very narrow pupil, and I had not an opportunity of trying the small optometer: but, when she once saw an object double through the slits, no exertion could make it appear single at the same distance. Hanson, a carpenter, aged 63, had a cataract extracted a few years since from one eye: the pupil was clear and large, and he could read most conveniently at 11 inches. With the same glass, the lines of the optometer appeared always to meet at 11 inches. But a still more unexceptionable eye was that of Mrs. Maberly. She is about 30, and had the crystalline of both eyes extracted a few years since, but sees best with the right. With the assistance of a lens of about four inches focus, she can read and work with ease. With the small optometer the intersection was invariably at the same point.

It is obvious that vision may be made distinct to any given extent, by means of an aperture sufficiently small, provided at the same time, that a sufficient quantity of light be left, while the refractive powers of the eye remain unchanged. And it is remarkable, that in those experiments, when the comparison with the perfect eye was made, the aperture of the imperfect eye only was very considerably reduced. Benjamin Clerk, with an aperture of $\frac{3}{40}$ of an inch, could read with the same glass at $1\frac{7}{8}$ inch, and at 7 inches. With an equal aperture, I can read at $1\frac{1}{2}$ inches and at 30 inches: and I can retain the state of perfect relaxation, and read with the same aperture at $2\frac{1}{4}$ inches; and this is as great a difference as was observed in Benjamin Clerk's eye. It is also a fact of no small importance, that Sir Henry Englefield was much astonished, as well as the other observers, at the accuracy with which the man's eye was adjusted to the same distance, in the repeated trials that were made with it. This circumstance alone makes it highly probable, that its perfect vision was confined within very narrow limits.

Hitherto I have endeavoured to show the inconveniences attending other suppositions, and to remove the objections to the opinion of an internal change of the figure of the lens. I shall now state two experiments, which, in the first place, come very near to a mathematical demonstration of the existence of such a change, and, in the second, explain in great measure its origin, and the manner in which it is effected.

I have already described the appearance of the imperfect image of a minute point at different distances from the eye, in a state of relaxation. The same appearances are equally observable, when the effect of the cornea is removed by immersion in water; and the only imaginable way of accounting for the diversity, is to suppose the central parts of the lens to acquire a greater degree of curvature than the marginal parts.

The truth of this explanation is fully confirmed by the optometer. When I look through four narrow slits, without exertion, the lines always appear to meet in one point: but, when I make the intersection approach me, the two outer lines meet considerably beyond the inner ones, and the two lines of the same side cross each other at a still greater distance.

Now, whether we call the lens a muscle or not, it seems demonstrable, that such a change of figure takes place as can be produced by no external cause; and we may at least illustrate it by a comparison with the usual action of muscular fibres. If we compare the central parts of each surface to the belly of the muscle there is no difficulty in conceiving their thickness to be immediately increased, and to produce an immediate elongation of the axis, and an increase of the central curvature.

In man and in the most common quadrupeds, the structure of the lens is nearly similar. The number of radiations is of little consequence; but I find that in the human crystalline lens there are ten on each side. The quantity of the nerves which proceeds to the iris, appears to be considerably smaller than that which arrives at the place of division: hence there can be little doubt that the division is calculated to supply the lens with some minute branches; and it is not improbable, from the appearance of the parts, that some fibres may pass to the cornea. The vessels coming from the choroid appear principally to supply a substance, hitherto unobserved, which fills up the marginal part of the capsule of the crystalline, in the form of a thin zone, and makes a slight elevation, visible even through the capsule. It consists of coarser fibres than the lens, but in a direction nearly similar; they are often intermixed with small globules.

But, since the whole mass of the lens, as far as it is moveable, is probably endued with a power of changing its figure, there is no need of any strngth of union, or place of attachment, for the fibres, since the motion meets with little or no resistance. The capsule is highly elastic; and, since it is laterally fixed to the ciliary zone, it must cooperate in restoring the lens to its flattest form.

The appearance of the processes is wholly irreconcilable with muscularity; and their being considered as muscles attached to the capsule, is therefore doubly inadmissible. What their use may be, cannot easily be determined: if it were necessary to have any peculiar organs for secretion, we might call them glands, for the percolation of the aqueous humour.

With respect to the eyes of insects, I have not yet had an opportunity of examining them; but there is no difficulty in supposing that the means of producing the changes of the refractive powers of the eye, may be, in different classes of animals, as diversified as their habits, and the general conformation of their organs.

Editorial comment: Young's inaugural thesis at the Royal Society, "On the Mechanism of the Eye," which was published when he was 28, is a recognized major contribution to ophthalmology. But his experiments indicating that a change in the curvature of the crystalline lens was the basic mechanism of accomodation failed to convince his contemporaries. The ciliary muscle was yet to be described; and "Physiologists, not being acquainted with any muscular elements in the eye, could scarcely imagine by what mechanism the crystalline lens could change its form, and they were little inclined to believe with Young in the contractibility of the fibers of the lens" (Donders). Young discovered his own ocular astigmatism—1.7 D inverse astigmatism attributable to the crystalline lens—through the use of his optometer based on Scheiner's experiment, and thus laid the cornerstone of our present knowledge of the subject. Young, who was somewhat nearsighted, noted no visual impairment from his astigmia. He considered it due to an obliquity of the crystalline lens as he had been informed by his optician that some nearsighted persons secured improved acuity with their lenses set somewhat obliquely. Young also introduced

44

quantitative perimetry, fixing the inner edge of the blind spot at 12° 56′ from the fixation point. It remained for von Graefe in 1856 to study the visual fields for diagnostic purposes, and for Förster of Breslau in 1868 to design the first instrumental perimeter.

Biographical Note

Thomas Young (1773–1829) was the offspring of Quaker parents and displayed from childhood extraordinary precocity. At 14 he had mastered French, Italian, Spanish, Latin, Greek, Hebrew, Persian and Arabian, and became adept soon in horsemanship, music and art. After studying medicine at London, Cambridge, Edinburgh and Göttingen he established himself as a physician in London. Fortunately for science, he was financially independent, thanks to a legacy from his grand-uncle, and his meager practice left ample leisure always for his investigative interests. In spite of his intellectual brilliance—or rather because of it—Young was never popular either as lecturer or physician. The audience was cold to his creative thinking and the ill sought elsewhere for more positive reassurance.

One year after his work "On the Mechanism of the Eye" Young wrote "On the Theory of Light and Colors" in which he demonstrated the phenomena of light interference and thus established definitively the wave theory of light. He suggested the physical dependence of color on wave length, held that heat consisted of vibrations longer than those of light, and proposed a theory of color perception by which color-blindness could be explained. Young was acclaimed by Tscherning as "the father of physiologic optics"; and in Duke-Elder's appraisal "Young was perhaps the most extraordinarily versatile genius that ever lived." His motto was: "What one has done, another can do." In physics his name is commemorated in "Young's modulus," and in medicine in "Young's rule" for calculating the proportionate dose for children (age divided by the age plus 12). When the Rosetta stone was discovered in 1799 Young realized that the Greek inscription afforded a clue to the demotic and hieroglyphic texts. By 1814 he had translated the demotic and a few years later made progress towards understanding the hieroglyphics. At the time of his death, at the age of 56, he was working on an ancient Egyptian dictionary.

Reference

Turner, D. M.: Thomas Young on the Eye and Vision, in E. A. Underwood, *Science, Medicine and History*, Vol. 2, 243–255. Oxford University Press, New York, 1953.

On Some Remarkable, and Hitherto Unobserved, Phenomena of Binocular Vision

CHARLES WHEATSTONE, F.R.S.

London

PHILOSOPHICAL TRANSACTIONS, ROYAL SOCIETY OF LONDON, 1838, *128:* 371–394

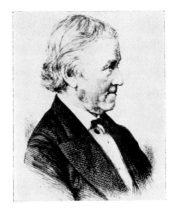

When an object is viewed at so great a distance that the optic axes of both eyes are sensibly parallel when directed towards it, the perspective projections of it, seen by each eye separately, are similar, and the appearance to the two eyes is precisely the same as when the object is seen by one eye only. There is, in such case, no difference between the visual appearance of an object in relief and its perspective projection on a plane surface; and hence pictorial representations of distant objects, when those circumstances which would prevent or disturb and the illusion are carefully excluded, may be rendered such perfect resemblances of the objects they are intended to represent as to be mistaken for them; the Diorama is an instance of this. But this similarity no longer exists when the object is placed so near the eyes that to view it the optic axes must converge; under these conditions a different perspective projection of it is seen by each eye, and these perspectives are more dissimilar as the convergence of the optic axes becomes greater. This fact may be easily verified by placing any figure of three dimensions, an outline cube for instance, at a moderate distance before the eyes, and while the head is kept perfectly steady, viewing it with each eye successively while the other is closed.

It will now be obvious why it is impossible for the artist to give a faithful representation of any near solid object, that is, to produce a painting which shall not be distinguished in the mind from the object itself. When the painting and the object are seen with both eyes, in the case of the painting two *similar* pictures are projected on the retinae, in the case of the solid object the pictures are *dissimilar*; there is therefore an essential difference between the impressions on the

45

organs of sensation in the two cases, and consequently between the perceptions formed in the mind; the painting therefore cannot be confounded with the solid object.

It being thus established that the mind perceives an object of three dimensions by means of the two dissimilar pictures projected by it on the two retinae, the following question occurs: What would be the visual effect of simultaneously presenting to each eye, instead of the object itself, its projection on a plane surface as it appears to that eye? To pursue this inquiry it is necessary that means should be contrived to make the two pictures, which must necessarily occupy different places, fall on similar parts of both retinae. Under the ordinary circumstances of vision the object is seen at the concourse of the optic axes, and its images consequently are projected on similar parts of the two retinae; but it is also evident that two exactly similar objects may be made to fall on similar parts of the two retinae, if they are placed one in the direction of each optic axis, at equal distances before or beyond their intersection.

Instead of placing two exactly similar objects to be viewed by the eyes, the two perspective projections of the same solid object be so disposed, the mind will still perceive the object to be single, but instead of a representation on a plane surface, as each drawing appears to be when separately viewed by that eye which is directed towards it, the observer will perceive a figure of three dimensions, the exact counterpart of the object from which the drawings were made.

In the instrument I am about to describe, the two pictures (or rather their reflected images) are placed in it at the true concourse of the optic axes, the focal adaptation of the eye preserves its usual adjustment, the appearance of lateral images is entirely avoided, and a large field of view for each eye is obtained. The frequent reference I shall have occasion to make to this instrument, will render it convenient to give it a specific name, I therefore propose that it be called a Stereoscope, to indicate its property of representing solid figures.

For the purposes of illustration I have employed only outline figures, for had either shading or colouring been introduced it might be supposed that the effect was wholly or in part due to these circumstances, whereas by leaving them out of consideration no room is left to doubt that the entire effect of relief is owing to the simultaneous perception of the two monocular projections, one on each retina. But if it be required to obtain the most faithful resemblances of real objects, shadowing and colouring may properly be employed to heighten the effects. Careful attention would enable an artist to draw and paint the two component pictures, so as to present to the mind of the observer, in the resultant perception, perfect identity with the object represented.

Flowers, crystals, busts, vases, instruments of various kinds, &c., might thus be represented so as not to be distinguished by sight from the real objects themselves.

The same solid object is represented to the mind by different pairs of monocular pictures, according as they are placed at a different distance before the eyes, and the perception of these differences (though we seem to be unconscious of them) may assist in suggesting to the mind the distance of the object. The more inclined to each other the referent planes are, with the greater accuracy are the various points of the projections referred to their proper places; and it appears to be a useful provision that the real forms of those objects which are nearest to us are thus more determinately apprehended than those which are more distant.

A very singular effect is produced when the drawing originally intended to be seen by the right eye is placed at the left hand side of the stereoscope, and that designed to be seen by the left eye is placed on its right hand side. A figure of three dimensions, as bold in relief as before, is perceived, but it has a different form from that which is seen when the drawings are in their proper places. There is a certain relation between the proper figure and this, which I shall call its *converse* figure. Those points which are nearest the observer in the proper figure are the most remote from him in the converse figure, and *vice versa*, so that the figure is, as it were, inverted; but it is not an exact inversion, for the near parts of the converse figure appear smaller, and the remote parts larger than the same parts before the inversion.

The same image is depicted on the retina by an object of three dimensions as by its projection on a plane surface, provided the point of sight remain in both cases the same. There should be, therefore, no difference in the binocular appearance of two drawings, one presented to each eye, and of two real objects so presented to the two eyes that their projections on the retina shall be the same as those arising from the drawings.

The preceding experiments render it evident that there is an essential difference in the appearance of objects when seen with two eyes, and when only one eye is employed, and that the most vivid belief of the solidity of an object of three dimensions arises from two different perspective projections of it being simultaneously presented to the mind. How happens it then, it may be asked, that persons who see with only one eye form correct notions of solid objects, and never mistake them for pictures? and how happens it also, that a person having the perfect use of both eyes, perceives no difference in objects around him when he shuts one of them? To explain these apparent difficulties, it must be kept in mind, that although the simultaneous vision of two dissimilar pictures suggests the relief of objects in the most vivid manner, yet there are other signs which suggest the same ideas to the mind, which though more ambiguous than the former, become less liable to lead the judgment astray in proportion to the extent of our previous experience. The vividness of relief arising from the projection of two dissimilar pictures, one on each retina, becomes less and less as the object is seen at a greater distance before the eyes, and entirely ceases when it is so distant that the optic axes are parallel while regarding it. We see with both eyes all objects beyond this distance precisely as we see near objects with a single eye; for the pictures on the two retinae are then exactly similar, and the mind appreciates no difference whether two identical pictures fall on corresponding parts of the two retinae, or whether one eye is impressed with only one of these pictures. A person deprived of the sight of one eye sees therefore all external objects, near and remote, as a person with both eyes sees remote objects only, but that vivid effect arising from the binocular vision of near objects is not perceived by the former; to supply this deficiency he has recourse unconsciously to other means of acquiring more accurate information. The motion of the head is the principal means he employs. That the required knowledge may be thus obtained will be evident from the following considerations. The mind associates with the idea of a solid object every different projection of it which experience has hitherto afforded; a single projection may be ambiguous, from its being also one of the projections of a picture, or of a different solid object; but when different projections of the same object are successively presented, they cannot all belong the another object, and the form to which they belong is completely characterized. While the object remains fixed, at every movement of the head it is viewed from a different point of sight, and the picture on the retina consequently continually changes.

Every one must be aware how greatly the perspective effect of a picture is enhanced by looking at it with only one eye, especially when a tube is employed to exclude the vision of adjacent objects, whose presence might disturb the illusion. Seen under such circumstances from the proper point of sight, the picture projects the same lines, shades and colours on the retina, as the more distant scene which it represents would do were it substituted for it. The appearance which would make us certain that it is a picture is excluded from the sight, and the imagination has room to be active.

If we suppose a cameo and an intaglio of the same object, the elevations of the one corresponding exactly to the depressions of the other, it is easy to show that the projection of either on the retina is sensibly the same. When the cameo or the intaglio is seen with both eyes, it is impossible to mistake an elevation for a depression, for reasons which have been already amply explained; but when either is seen with one eye only, the most certain guide of our judgement, viz. the presentation of a different picture to each eye, is wanting; the imagination therefore supplies the deficiency, and we conceive the object to be raised or depressed according to the dictates of this faculty. No doubt in such cases our judgement is in a great degree influenced by accessory circumstances, and the intaglio or the relief may sometimes present itself according to our previous knowledge of the direction in which the shadows ought to appear; but the real cause of the phenomenon is to be found in the indetermination of the judgment arising from our more perfect means of judging being absent.

We will now inquire what effect results from presenting similar images, differing only in magnitude, to analogous parts of the two retinae. For this purpose two squares or circles, differing obviously but not extravagantly in size, may be drawn on two separate pieces of paper, and placed in the stereoscope so that the reflected image of each shall be equally distant from the eye by which it is regarded. It will then be seen that, notwithstanding this difference, they coalesce and occasion a single resultant perception.

If the pictures be too unequal in magnitude, the binocular coincidence does not take place. It appears that if the inequality of the pictures be greater than the difference which exists between the two projections of the same object when seen in the most oblique position of the eyes (i.e. both turned to the extreme right or to the extreme left), ordinarily employed, they do not coalesce.

It now remains to examine *why* two dissimilar pictures projected on the two retinae give rise to the perception of an object in relief. I shall in this place merely consider the most obvious explanations which might be offered, and show their insufficiency to explain the whole of the phenomena.

It may be supposed, that we see but one point of a field of view distinctly at the same instant, the one namely to which the optic axes are directed, while all other points are seen so indistinctly, that the mind does not recognize them to be either single or double, and that the figure is appreciated by successively directing the point of convergence of the optic axes successively to a sufficient number of its points to enable us to judge accurately of its form.

That there is a degree of indistinctness in those parts of the field of view to which the eyes are not immediately directed, and which increases with the distance from that point, cannot be doubted, and it is also true that the objects thus obscurely seen are frequently doubled. In ordinary vision, it may be said, this indistinctness and duplicity is not attended to, because the eyes shifting continually from point to point, every part of the object is successively rendered distinct; and the perception of the object is not the consequence of a single glance, during which only a small part of it is seen distinctly; but is formed from a comparison of all the pictures successively seen while the eyes were changing from one point of the object to another.

All this is in some degree true; but were it entirely so, no appearance of relief should present itself when the eyes remain intently fixed on one point of a binocular image in the stereoscope. But on performing the experiment carefully, it will be found, provided the pictures do not extend too far beyond the centres of distinct vision, that the image is still seen single and in relief when this condition is fulfilled. Were the theory of corresponding points true, the appearance should be that of the superposition of the two drawings, to which, however, it has not the slightest similitude.

When an object, or a part of an object, thus appears in relief while the optic axes are directed to a single binocular point, it is easy to see that each point of the figure that appears single is seen at the intersection of the two lines of visible direction in which it is seen by each eye separately, whether these lines of visible direction terminate at corresponding points of the two retinae or not.

But if we were to infer the converse of this, viz. that every point of an object in relief is seen by a single glance at the intersection of the lines of visible direction in which it is seen by each eye singly, we should be in error. On this supposition, objects before or beyond the intersection of the optic axes should never appear double, and we have abundant evidence that they do. The determination of the points which shall appear single seems to depend in no small degree on previous knowledge of the form we are regarding. No doubt, some law or rule of vision may be discovered which shall include all the circumstances under which single vision by means of non-corresponding points occurs and is limited. I have made numerous experiments for the purpose of attaining this end, and have ascertained some of the conditions on which single and double vision depend, the consideration of which however must at present be deferred.

Comment: In his second paper on the Physiology of Vision (1852) Wheatstone remarks: "At the date of the publication of my experiments on binocular vision the brilliant photographic discoveries of Talbot, Niepce and Daguerre had not been announced to the world. To illustrate the phenomena of the stereoscope I could, therefore, at that time, only employ drawings made by the hands of an artist; but it is evidently impossible for the most accurate and accomplished artist to delineate by the sole aid of his eye the two subjects necessary to form the stereoscopic relief of objects as they exist in nature with their delicate differences of outline, light and shade. What the hand of the artist was unable to accomplish the chemical action of light, directed by the camera, has enabled us to effect. It was at the beginning of 1839 that the photographic art became known, and soon after, at my request Mr. Talbot obligingly prepared for me stereoscopic Talbotypes of statues, buildings and living persons." In 1849 Sir David Brewster designed the lenticular stereoscope, which Oliver Wendell Holmes later modified by giving it a handle and an adjustable picture carrier. The steroscope became popular after the Great Exhibition at London in 1851 where the French displayed a fine set of binocular daguerreotypes. During the next five years, 500,000 stereoscopes were sold. Although the accuracy of the stereoscopic sense is comparable with vernier acuity, its range is comparatively limited. With the naked eye stereoscopic vision does not extend beyond 2000 ft. The radius of stereoscopic vision is about 7000 times the interpupillary base-line. In the telestereoscope, invented by Helmholtz in 1857, the effective base-line was extended by the use of right-angled prisms with a proportionate increase in stereoscopic vision. Prism binocular field glasses and stereoscopic range finders are constructed on this principle.

Linksz, a profound student of stereopsis, has explored with penetrating insight the implications of Wheatstone's pioneering contribution. The following condensed excerpts of his evaluation is essentially in his own words: "Neither Leonardo da Vinci nor Berkeley noticed the fact that the distribution pattern of retinal images in the two eyes is different. This great discovery was Wheatstone's. He was the first to state clearly that, due to their horizontally different position, the two eyes receive horizontally different views of objects. He concluded correctly that it is the inequality of the two retinal images of an object which furnishes the means of stereopsis and he made the logical step of proving his theory by procuring for each eye a flat projection of the object as it is seen by that eye. For this end Wheatstone designed an instrument which he called a stereoscope, now usually called a haploscope. The orthoptic instruments now in use are only glorified editions of his simple contrivance. If the two uniocular images are unequal in certain respects, they are equal in almost every other respect. It is this equality, not the inequalities, that make binocular vision possible."

Reference

Linksz, A.: *Vision*. New York, Grune & Stratton, 1952.

Biographical Note

Sir Charles Wheatstone (1802–1875) was born in Gloucester, England, the son of a music-seller. At the age of 21 he established his own business in London as a maker of musical instruments; and began investigating extensively the principles involved in the various forms of musical instruments. His interest then extended to vision, light and electricity. In 1834 he was appointed Professor of Experimental Philosophy in King's College, London and was elected fellow of the Royal Society in 1836. In 1838 he presented his mirror stereoscope. The word "stereoscope" was also his invention. He is popularly known for his introduction of the Wheatstone bridge for the measurement of electric resistance (1843). Another invention was the kaleidophone which gives a visible presentation of sound; but his greatest achievement was the perfection of the electric telegraph. Numerous distinctions were conferred on him by governments, universities and learned societies. In 1868 he received both the honor of knighthood from Queen Victoria and the Copley medal of the Royal Society for his researches in acoustics, optics, electricity and magnetism. His hobby was cryptography in which he was an acknowledged expert. Though an unrivaled conversationalist, Wheatstone suffered excessively from stage-fright on facing an audience. He was fortunate, however, in having the greatest lecturer of the age, Faraday, present his papers to the Royal Institution.

Reference

Jeans, W. T.: Lives of the Electricians. London, Whittaker & Co., 1887.

Description of an Opthalmoscope for Examining the Retina in the Living Eye

HERMANN VON HELMHOLTZ, M.D.

Königsberg, Germany

ORIGINAL MONOGRAPH, "BESCHREIBUNG EINES AUGEN-SPIEGELS ZUR UNTERSUCHUNG DER NETZHAUT IM LEBENDEN AUGE," BERLIN, A. FORSTNER, 1851*

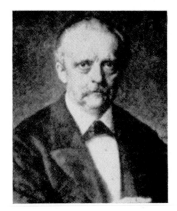

This publication contains the description of an optical instrument with which it is possible accurately to observe and examine the retina. To be of value, such an instrument must overcome two important problems. First of all, as we observe the normal eye its interior appears to be completely dark. The reason for this is that under ordinary circumstances the refractive media of the eye prevent us from observing illuminated portions of the retina through the pupil. Only by looking through the refractive media can we visualize the background of the eye. It is necessary to have a special procedure for producing the illumination, as well as an optical instrument which will allow the observer's eye to focus sharply on the retinal structures.

Illumination

This black reflex is not a property of the choroidal pigment. Even though the pigment layer could completely absorb the incident light, as do some other black substances, there are tissues present which could reflect a considerable portion of the incident light and thus become visible. This is especially true of the retina. It is even truer of the blood vessels of this tissue, since their branches carry sufficient blood to give them a definite reddish hue. Also, in the fundus of the eye there is a shining white area, the position of entry of the optic nerve, upon which there is no pigment; therefore, it reflects all light which falls upon it.

That it is the refraction of light in the ocular media and not the color

* Based on the Translation by Robert W. Hollenhorst, M.D., A. M. A. Arch. Ophth., 1951, *46:* 565–583.

of the background which causes the black reflex of the pupil is readily demonstrated by means of simple experiment. For this purpose, one can use a small camera obscura with a thoroughly blackened interior, really an artificial eye, and at the site where the image is projected one can place an opaque white panel, such as a piece of thick white drawing paper. If an attempt is made to peer through the lens from any angle whatsoever the interior of the instrument appears to be completely dark. If the convex lens is then removed, or if the distance between it and the sheet of paper is changed materially, the observer can readily visualize the white surface of the paper.

How can refraction of light produce this phenomenon? When light from a luminous point is allowed to fall on a suitably accommodated eye, a small part of it is reflected from the neural elements and blood vessels and a part from the layer of rod shaped cells. As was shown by E. Brücke, the light which returns from the latter structures passes again through the pupil, without being dispersed to other portions of the interior of the eye. The returning rays traverse exactly the same path, but in the opposite direction, as that used in converging upon the retina through the refracting surface of the eye. The angle of incidence of the departing ray is identical with the angle of refraction of the entering ray at the limiting surfaces of the medium. If we designate a as a luminous point outside the eye and b as its image at a point on the retina, we find that the ocular media focus the emergent rays from b once again into an image at a. The image of the illuminated point on the retina thus coincides with the original luminous point. Hence, all the incident light which is reflected must return to its origin and can never take another direction. Therefore, it is impossible to visualize the illuminated portions of the retina without special equipment. Furthermore, we cannot bring our eyes into the pathway of the returning light without completely interrupting the incident rays.

Up to this point we have assumed that absolutely sharp images are formed in the eye that is being observed. When this is not the case, the foregoing propositions are not universally applicable, and the reflected light may largely return to the luminous object. However, a portion of the reflected light may pass by, so that an observer who is situated very near to the line of direction of the incident light may be able to perceive a portion of the reflected light. This fact forms the basis for the methods of Cumming (Tr. Med.-Chir. Soc., London, 29: 1845–1846, 283) and Brücke (Arch. f. Anat., 1847, 225) for observing the illumination of human eyes. From what has been said, it is evident that the less exactly the rays emanating from a luminous point are focused on a point on the retina, the more intense the illumination will be. However, in these investigations it is possible for the observer to perceive only a small fraction of the returning light. In fact, he sees only those irregularly refracted rays which are of no use in the production of a definite image. For our purpose another method must be employed to make it possible to peer into the eye in exactly the same course as that of the incident light, and not merely approximately in this direction. The means whereby this could be done was discovered accidently by von Erlach and investigated by Brücke. Von Erlach, who wore spectacles, noted that the eyes of a friend would be illuminated if the latter looked directly at the image of a light reflected in the lenses of the spectacles. Unmounted lenses also could be used as illuminating mirrors, and the observer like-wise could see through these into a subject's eyes. We employ exactly the same procedure, but advantageously replace the spectacle lenses with carefully ground plane lenses.

In a darkened chamber containing only a single light source, we can set a small plane glass plate in such a position that the subject can see the reflected image of the light, although he need not look directly at this reflection. Light is thus directed into the subject's eye from the anterior surface of a lens, and the observer can simultaneously examine the eye through this same lens without being aware of the light reflected from the anterior surface. It is evident that in this way it is possible to direct the line of vision into the subject's eye in exactly the same direc-tion as that of the course of the light. Under such conditions, the observer's eye will receive light from the depths of the other eye, and the pupil will be illuminated.

With my method, the entire light is used, with the exception of the portion which is lost by passage through the reflecting glass. Moreover, the strength of illumination varies according to which portion of the retina receives the image of the flame. If it falls on the optic disk, most of the light is reflected, and the pupil is illuminated with a bright yellowish white light. The retina proper, however, reflects much less light, principally red light. In general, the image of the flame is stronger the nearer it is to the optic disk, and weaker the farther away it is from this disk. On the contrary, the yellow macula, the site of direct vision, which is used when the observed eye gazes directly at the reflected image of the flame, returns much less light than do the neighboring structures.

In order to fulfill the condition that the observer gaze into the eye exactly in the direction of the incident light, the glass plate can be adjusted by the observer. This method requires that the subject's face be shaded and the reflecting plate be made so small that it is just large enough to see through. The reflected light then will appear upon the shaded face of the subject as a small bright spot of about the shape of the reflecting glass. The observer must aim this bright spot in such a way that its center falls on the subject's eye, while he himself peers through the lens. In this way the lens may be aligned very easily, and the subject's eye can be turned to all sides without much difficulty, to permit the image of the flame to fall upon various parts of the retina.

The same simple method can be utilized advantageously to illuminate any dark cavity with a narrow opening, such as the auditory meatus or the nose. To visualize the tympanic membrane, the subject must be placed with his back against a window, preferably in sunlight; the auricle must be drawn slightly backward, and the reflected light must be directed into the auditory meatus while the observer looks in through the lens. Thus it is possible easily and conveniently to illuminate the drum head to any degree desired for purposes of examination.

If it is desired to examine closely closely the structure of the retina one must attempt to get as bright a light as possible. This objective can be reached in two ways, either by properly adjusting the angle made by the incident light or by increasing the number of the reflecting plates. If several reflecting surfaces are arranged parallel and one behind the other, and the illuminated surface is large enough that the reflected images which are produced by the various mirror surfaces superimpose themselves upon the observed eye, the various images are combined into one of greater brightness. By calculating the amount of light reflected back and forth between the various surfaces, it is possible to determine the total amount of light reflected in any system of parallel surfaces. The returning light re-enters the mirror system and divides into a part which is again reflected and a part which penetrates the system. Only the latter portion enters the eye of the observer. A value deviating slightly from the foregoing maximum is obtained if the light is reflected from one glass plate at an angle of about 70 degrees, from three plates at an angle of about 60 degrees, and from four plates at an angle of 55 degrees. These positions, therefore, are approximately the most efficient.

It is important to consider that a small portion of the light which strikes the eye of the subject is reflected from the cornea and appears to the observer as a pale light spot in the field of vision. This spot is situated in the center of the pupil as the subject directs his eye straight at the mirror and if he looks directly at the reflected image of the flame. It is of distinct advantage to the observer if the intensity of the corneal reflex can be considerably diminished. This reflex appears to be much less prominent when four plates at an angle of 56 of degrees are used than when either three plates at a 60 degree angle are employed, or one plate at a 70 degree angle, although the retinal image previously described retains practically the same intensity of illumination. Even with variation in the number and position of the plates, the apparent brightness of the corneal reflex is not proportional to the brightness of the retinal image because the light which enters the eye of the subject is partly or entirely polarized by reflection and becomes depolarized by diffuse reflection from the retina. This is a phenomenon which does not occur in the case of the specular corneal reflection. Therefore, from every point of view, the necessary intensity of light is more readily obtained by increasing the number of plates (since they reflect the light below the polarization angle of 56 degrees) than by increasing the angle of incidence because the corneal reflex can be entirely avoided by greatly multiplying the number of plates.

Formation of a Clear Image of the Retina

The problem of widening the field of vision makes it imperative that the observed and the observing eye be brought as close together as possible. It is possible, with less magnification, to permit the greater part of the visual field to be maximally illuminated; on the contrary, if greater magnification is used, this may not even take place in the center. Even though a higher magnification would be very advantageous, it is not possible to make use of it, since the illumination decreases so greatly. Moreover, the living eye cannot be held sufficiently quiet for good fixation of various parts of the image, as would be necessary if higher magnification were used. The visual field is next to be considered. That part of the retina which can be seen becomes smaller the farther the observer is from the subject's eye, and becomes greater when the observer is nearer.

Description of the Ophthalmoscope

In order to begin observations, as described above, it is convenient to combine the mirror and a concave lens in a suitable frame. I have chosen the name Augenspiegel for this combination because of its analogy to similar instruments of this name. Good blackening of the nonreflecting surfaces is essential. First of all, the inner surface of the ocular piece must be blackened and the observer must press his eye as closely as possible into the ocular piece in order to exclude all extraneous light which might come from the flame onto these surfaces. Second, the bare metal parts which are directed toward the observed eye must be blackened so that they will not produce disturbing corneal reflexes. To use the instrument, the observer places the subject in a darkened room near the corner of a table upon which a well burning double draft lamp is set at the same level as that of the eyes lateral to the face. It is advantageous to place on the table, at a suitable visual distance, a dimly lighted object upon which the eyes of the subject can fixate at definite points; an example would be a blackboard divided into quadrants, each of which is designated by a number. Then, if the

58

eye is permitted to fixate the various quadrants one after the other, the image of the flame will fall on different portions of the retina, which then may be investigated by the observer in any order desired. The observer is seated in front of the subject. Without first looking through the ophthalmoscope, he directs it in approximately the right direction, whereupon a brightly illuminated spot is cast on the face by the reflecting surface. Then the mirror is turned in such fashion that the middle of this illuminated spot falls on the eye, and if the axis of the instrument is correctly aligned, he looks through. If the retina is not seen clearly, but the pupil appears illuminated, a different concave lens must be employed. An observer who has trained himself to alter voluntarily the accommodation of his eyes can easily determine whether he sees more clearly with far-sighted or with near-sighted accommodation and whether he therefore needs more or less strongly curved lenses. As with all optical instruments possessing a focusing device, it is necessary in the use of this one to accommodate the eyes for infinity and then to adjust the instrument to the eye.

Visualization of the Retina and the Image of the Flame

If one is desirous of examining the retina thoroughly, it is necessary, as mentioned previously, to erect a numbered blackboard to use as a fixation point for the eye of the subject. If he continues to follow the course of the vessels in the direction of the larger branches, he approaches finally the place of entrance of the optic nerve. This structure is distinguished from the rest of the background of the eye by its whiteness, because it is not covered by pigment or a fine vascular network; instead, the white cross section of the nerve lies quite free, at most penetrated by a few fine vessels. Usually, the arteries and viens of the retina arise from the medial portion. Occasionally, one can see a portion of the vessels still buried in the substance of the nerve and can appreciate that this substance must be very strongly transparent in the living state. It is possible to distinguish the two types of vessels, one from the other, by the brighter color of the blood and the double contour of the walls of the arteries and their first branches. I have not been able to observe pulsations with certainty. The first main branches of the vessels border the optic nerve on the inner side and later branch out, above and below, over the expanse of the retina. The appearance of the sharply demarcated red vessels upon the bright white background is of surprising elegance.

In other parts the background of the eye looks red; here are seen larger and smaller blood red branching vessels, which may be clearly distinguished from the background. The background itself appears not to be entirely homogeneous, but indistinctly reddish. This seems to arise from the fact that the narrow capillary network is too delicate, is illuminated too faintly, and is too transparent to be clearly distinguished from the underlying light gray tissues of the retina. That the background in the vicinity of the optic nerve appears to be brighter may well be due to the fact that here the retina is thicker, as a consequence of the superimposed layers of the nerve fibers; it is always thinner toward the periphery. The site of direct vision (the yellow spot) is especially well distinguished from its immediate surroundings. In order to bring this spot into view, the subject's eye must gaze directly at the reflected image of the flame. In such a view the retina appears to be much darker; also, no traces of any capillary vessels are visible upon it. In observing this site, however, one is very much disturbed by the corneal images, which are situated exactly in the center of the field of vision, whereas when more lateral portions of the retina are examined these reflexes are situated somewhat more to the side.

After one learns to recognize the characteristics of the retina in the normal eye, I have no doubt that it will be possible to diagnose all the pathologic conditions of the retina by visual observation, as is done in examination of other transparent parts, such as the cornea. Engorgement of the vessels or varicosities of the vessels can easily be perceived. Exudates in the substance of the retina, or between the retina and the pigment layer, can be recognized by their light appearance against the dark background, similar to what can be seen in corresponding lesions in the cornea. If they are situated partly in front of the retina, the blood vessels will be hidden as by a veil. In this respect, I recall that, according to Brücke, the living retina is almost as transparent as the other ocular media. Fibrinous exudates, which are much less transparent than the ocular media, must therefore considerably increase the reflex if they are situated in the fundus of the eye. I also believe that opacities of the vitreous body will be recognized much more readily and exactly. It is easily possible to estimate the extent of the opacity by means of the degree of blurring of the retinal vessels. If scintillating particles have become detached from such an opacity, these also may be perceived readily. In short, I believe I do not exaggerate when I anticipate that all those changes in the vitreous body and the retina previously noted in cadavers will be recognized in the living eye. This fact appears to offer the greatest impetus to development of the pathologic study of these structures.

Moreover, it is possible, when it is necessary to do so, easily to determine objectively the presence and the degree of myopia or hyperopia of the observed eye. The observer should first examine a normal eye. He should allow this eye to fixate objects at various distances and should note which concave lenses are needed at the various stages of accommodation of the eye. Then, in investigating another eye, he can determine, by the strength of the concave lens needed to give a clear view of the retina, the state of accommodation of the subject's eye. The observer is thus entirely independent of the statements of the subject, since he himself can see, as though with the other's eye, the refractive media of this eye. In this way, for example, I was able to examine a completely amaurotic eye and determine that this eye was highly myopic as well.

These investigations led me to an important physiologic deduction. The isolated cross section of the optic nerve evidently is so transparent that light falling upon it can penetrate deep into the substance of the fibers, inasmuch as at times the tortuous loops of the central artery and the central vein can be seen shimmering through the substance of the nerve. If the image of the flame is cast upon the site of entry of the optic nerve, all the nerve fibers, or at least a very large portion of them, are exposed to more or less intense light, and yet apparently no light is perceived. We must, therefore, conclude that the fibers of the optic nerve are insensitive to objective light, although every other kind of stimulation is perceived as subjective light. It is not difficult to make the assumption that all stimuli which are able to act on the visual nerve system produce sensations of light, but that the vibrations of the ether are able to act only on the retina. This similar situation may be noted in the reaction of the nerves of touch to warmth and cold. In this case as well there is a different response in the peripheral ramifications than there is in the trunk. Furthermore, it is possible to conclude that in the retina it is the cellular elements which are sensitive to light, and not the nerves which radiate over the inner surface. We are able to postulate further that the continuations of the visual nerve fibers in the retina are insensitive to light.

Comment: No instrument has developed ophthalmology as much as the ophthalmoscope. It stimulated likewise the progress of other fields of medicine by inspiring other endoscopic instruments. The ophthalmoscope was first publicly presented by Helmholtz before the Physical Society in Berlin on December 16, 1850. In acquainting his father with the discovery, Helmholtz wrote: "Formerly a number of ocular diseases were designated 'black cataracts,' as the changes in the living eye were not understood." Von Graefe, who realized the immense practical importance of the invention, in a letter to Helmholtz said: "Forgive one not known to you an inquiry about a subject of the greatest personal interest. Professor Brücke told me of your success in constructing an instrument which permits the examination of the living retina. I am anxious to try this much longed for diagnostic instrument and beg you to send to Berlin one or two constructed according to your specifications." The Helmholtz ophthalmoscope was rapidly modified. In 1852, Reute improved the illumination by using a concave mirror with a central perforation and also evolved the indirect method of ophthalmoscopy. In the same year, Rekoss, Helmholtz's instrument maker, added movable disks bearing a battery of lenses which facilitated the inspection of the fundus and permitted a rough determination of the refraction. The first practical ophthalmoscope, designed for the measurement of refraction, however, was that of Loring in 1869. With its use the general employment of an objective method for the determination of refractive errors was initiated. In 1873 Cuignet observed that at a distance of 1 meter the apparent movement of the illuminated area depended on the refraction of the eye and utilized this phenomenon as an objective test. In 1878 Mengin christened the procedure "retinoscopy" and Landolt explained the optical principles involved. By 1870 the fundus pictures revealed by the ophthalmoscope were incorporated in atlases by Sichel, Eduard von Jaeger and Richard Liebreich. An atlas of the comparative ophthalmology of mammals by Lindsay Johnson appeared in 1897 and of the fundus oculi of birds by Casey Wood in 1917. The modern period of ophthalmoscopy has been marked by refinements of the electric ophthalmoscope, first introduced by Dennett in 1885.

Reference

Sachs, M.: Nearly 100 years of the ophthalmoscope. Arch. Ophth., *40:* 268–272, 1948.

Biographical Notes

Hermann von Helmholtz (1821–1894) was born at Potsdam, Germany. His father was a teacher of classical languages; his mother was Caroline Penn, a descendant of William Penn, founder of Pennsylvania. He received his medical degree in 1842, from the Royal Friedrich-Wilhelm Institute where he made firm friends with Brücke, du Bois-Reymond and Ludwig. In 1849 he became professor of physiology at Koenigsberg and while preparing his lectures conceived the idea of the ophthalmoscope. After occupying similar chairs at Bonn and Heidelberg, he was appointed director of the Physical Institute at Berlin. In 1893, at the request of Hermann Knapp, von Helmholtz attended the World's Fair at Chicago. On his return home he suffered a serious fall aboard ship and died the following year.

Helmholtz ranks as one of the greatest scientists of all time. Like Thomas Young, he preferred research to medical practice; and like Young, his important contributions to vision and optics were but facets of a manifold interest. His works on acoustics, nerve conduction, electro- and thermo-dynamics, and the conservation of energy (written independently by Joule and Robert Meyer) were equally fundamental. His writings inspired Hertz to search for Maxwell's electromagnetic waves, an investigation that led Marconi to the invention of wireless telegraphy. In 1890, in an address commemorating the 600th anniversary of the medical school at Montpellier, he said: "No one can work scientifically without aiding his country and, at the same time the entire civilized world." The last edition of his *Physiologic Optics,* edited by Gullstrand, von Knies and Nagel, was translated into English by the American Optical Society in 1924.

Reference

Koenigsberger, L.: *Hermann von Helmholtz.* English translation by F. A. Welby. Oxford, Clarendon Press, 1907.

Examination of the Visual Field in Amblyopic Disease

ALBRECHT VON GRAEFE, M.D.

Berlin, Germany

ARCHIVES FÜR OPHTHALMOLOGIE, *2:* 258–298, 1856*

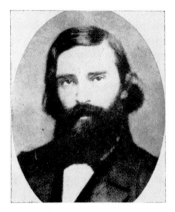

In determining central visual acuity, we are yet not at all informed concerning the patient's faculty of vision. The second and equally important part is the examination of the field of vision, or in other words the determination of the dimension and modality of eccentric vision. If this part of the examination were neglected, extensive visual disturbances of prognostic significance might be overlooked. A number of pathologic conditions are manifest for a time only by the changes in eccentric vision and it is only the last stage which induces progressive dimness of central vision. Even the patient's complaints may often remain to us unintelligible. Some patients who can read the finest print yet experience the greatest difficulty in walking abroad alone. In examining their eyes we find an almost complete intact central vision with a highly restricted eccentric vision. As an illustration I may demonstrate a subject who figures in the streets of Berlin as the blind musician, and who actually has to be led about, although he can distinguish letters (No. 4) of Jaeger's letter test. The opening of his visual space is about 10 degrees horizontal by 10 degrees vertical, in comparison to the normal of 174 degrees horizontal by 160 degrees vertical. To realize the situation of such a subject, we need but roll a sheet of paper into a tube which permits surveying at a 1½-foot distance an area of the above mentioned size in order to convince ourselves of the difficulty of orientation under such conditions. Though normally very eccentric impressions may be very indistinct yet they remind us of the presence of larger objects and induce us to confirm their presence by looking in their direction. If eccentric vision is interrupted, then every impression not exactly

* From the translation by Ralph I. Lloyd, M.D., Eye, Ear, Nose & Throat Monthly, *14:* 117–122, 164–167, & 192–196, 1935.

received in the axis of vision is missed and it becomes impossible to avoid obstacles in walking. Patients having a restricted field of vision frequently distinguish far objects better than near, and small better than large ones. This apparent mystery finds its quite natural explanation in the fact that large objects exceed the field of vision, but the image will fit into the small visual field only if the visual angle is sufficiently decreased. These conditions may be well illustrated by the above mentioned tube test.

No special method is required to determine the limits of the field of vision. For instance, we may mark any ocular object drawn on a board, if only we take care to have the axis of vision fixed immovably. We may then gradually displace any other ocular object from the direction of the axis of vision towards the limits of the field of vision by simultaneously performing slight lateral motions which will drive home the impressions. Finally, we mark the position in which this object becomes invisible. In order to guard against after-images and unreliable statements, we cause this object repeatedly to disappear and reappear in this position. At the most outward position from which reliable data is obtainable, we then mark definitely as the limiting position. The eccentric object should be large, well lighted, but not shiny or strongly reflective. I am not in favor of choosing a candle flame because the large diffusion of light makes it difficult for many test subjects to distinguish absolutely between the qualitative perception of the ocular object and the quantitative illumination which may be conducted by the sclera. Trial tests have convinced me that results fluctuate very widely when using candle light. It is also difficult to avoid disturbing reflexes due to the motions of the candle flame when the candle is already beyond the limits of the field of vision. Finally we must guard against after-images that will appear in the candle test even with highly peripheral impression.

In a highly restricted case the patient should be placed at a distance of several feet from a board with a fixed ocular object at the center. The surface of the board should be divided into many squares by two systems of vertical cross lines, and the squares should be numbered. While the patient fixes the central object we move a piece of chalk successively through the different squares towards the periphery of the board and note the number of the square in which the piece of chalk disappears. If this test is repeated in many directions it will give the exact shape of the field of vision, which may be marked on the board at the time or later. In order to infer from it the opening of the field of vision, it is but necessary to mark the distance of the eye from the board. For practical purposes I recommend adopting a standard for this distance. Most fields of vision observed in amblyopia were measured at the distance of 1½ feet.

We frequently observe patients whose field of vision is still extended and who yet manifest a remarkable clouding of eccentric impressions in certain directions. Usually this fact is brought to our attention because the patient is unable to find his way in spite of good visual acuity. It was first brought home to me while observing a patient whose unilateral blindness was due to glaucoma and whose other eye was in the unfortunate preliminary stage of periodical obscurations. Examination by the above described method during intervals when the patient could still read the finest print proved his field of vision to be of normal extent. But when I placed before him a sheet of paper and asked him to fix the central black spot, from which lines radiated in eight directions, every line bearing black spots at regular small distances, the pathologic condition of his eccentric vision was established by the fact that in certain directions he received distinct impression of numerous eccentric points, while in outward and upward directions he did not. When I re-examined this patient at the onset of clouding—indicated by the onset of temporal pain—the restriction in eccentric vision had considerably increased and closely approached the center.

Our third consideration concerns the interruptions in the field of vision. Certain spots in the field of vision conduct none or very imperfect impressions in spite of no decrease in the extent of the field of vision nor in the clearness of eccentric impressions in certain retinal radials. The retinal portions involved may be wholly deprived of function, whereupon the phenomenon appears about like the normal blindspot, that is, the patients do not perceive some dark shape, but at the spot in question they have absolutely no visual impression. I have proved to my satisfaction that with smaller defects of this type and an otherwise normally functioning retina, a filling-in by superposition, a psychic process, occurs as in Mariotte's spot. Usually the retinal function is not completely paralyzed, but the retina retains a certain degree of sensibility to subjective and even to objective stimulation. Thus these interruptions will appear sometimes as light, sometimes as dark spots, conducting either no impression at all or enveloping the images seen in a cloud or a solar fog. These interruptions have extremely variable shapes, due to the basic causes of the disease. Often they appear as small round spots, which the patient may completely overlook because of their very eccentric position. They might even possibly be overlooked at examination, had not the ophthalmoscope indicated to us the study of a definite section of the field of vision.

In this respect there is one important disease which I must discuss in detail. We observe in the equatorial areas dark masses of pigment attached to the inner aspect of the choroid, radiating in starlike formation and often appearing like bone corpuscles. The intervals between these are free and almost bare of pigmentation; the large vessels actually appear so bare as to give the impression of a destroyed or atrophied choriocapillaris. This change, which is originally restricted to the equatorial sections, gradually progresses toward the posterior pole of the eye and simultaneously distinct symptoms of optic nerve atrophy present themselves. The optic papilla turns white and highly reflective, while the central vessels, and particularly the arteries, undergo progressive shrinking. Since this process starts in the equatorial sections, it results in progressive contraction of the visual field. I must again emphasize that in spite of marked changes in the optic nerve and in the central vessels, which constitute an essential part of the findings, the central vision may be preserved for a long time. No other disease presents in the majority of the cases such a disparity between visual acuteness and dimension of the visual field. As a rule the contraction is a regular concentric one, so the point of fixation remains exactly in the center of the visual field; yet sometimes this is not so. Judging by its course and the basic changes present, we cannot very well consider it an inflammatory process; the frequently occurring hereditary diathesis would also indicate other trophic changes.

The restrictions of the visual field in paralysis of the optic nerve due to central causes are likewise very interesting. In some cerebrospinal diseases we sometimes observe concentric contractions, which, however, never proceed as regularly as in the choroid disease just discussed. Usually the shape of the visual field becomes irregular and the point of fixation is as a rule eccentric. Often the shape of the visual field is absolutely identical in both eyes. Contractions in central diseases differ, moreover, from those in choriod disease just described, in that the central sight simultaneously depreciates considerably. Evidently this concentric contraction or restriction of the visual field corresponds to the gradual atrophy of the retina; the peripheral portions which are less highly innervated fading out first; here, too, the border of the visual field is not clearly defined, so that there is a certain transitional area within which retinal activity is depreciated to a minimum of quantitative perception. Ophthalmoscopic examination fails in such cases to detect any structural differences to mark off the border between the sensitive and the insensible portions. Usually only the general symptoms of atrophy of the optic nerve are apparent.

Particularly instructive for the physiology of the optic nerve are the hemianoptic restrictions in cerebral diseases. It happens not infrequently that in both eyes one-half of the visual field is wanting. There are numerous cases wherein the right eye has lost the right half of the visual field and in the left eye also the right; or vice versa, in both eyes the left half is wanting; while it is rather rare that the right half in the right eye and the left half in the left eye is wanting. The first kind of hemianopia is in itself far more disturbing to the patient; in the other, however, both visual field losses are compensated. How can we explain these extraordinary restrictions which occur with such great regularity? Retinal anesthesia beyond a vertical dividing line is observed as distinctly as in anesthesia starting at the meridian line after severing of the trigeminal nerve. Typical cases, moreover, experience no visual sensation whatever in the anesthetic portions. This can only be due to the distribution of the nerve elements. When we examine these cases more accurately and when we carefully consider all the other symptoms of the disease, we find that they apparently confirm the recent established theory of a semidecussation of the optic nerve. We learn that the symptom complex for the first (homonymous) type of hemianopia indicates a unilateral cerebral disease. For instance, if bilaterally the left half of the visual field is wanting, we observe frequent phenomena of left sided hemiplegia. If we assume this hemiplegia due to right sided cerebral disease causing paralysis and atrophy of the right optic stem, then we would satisfactorily explain this hemianopia by the statement that the right bundle of the paralyzed stem supplies the temporal section of the right retina, and the crossed bundle supplies the nasal side of the left retina. I am well aware that I am not stating anything new with this theory and its practical application; but as the matter is still so little known I feel impelled to communicate my observations concerning it, which I shall amplify in the future by corresponding autopsy findings. Let me now but briefly state that the simultaneous occurrence of the hemianopia described with its associated hemiplegia is not a rare finding, and I particularly urge the attention of hospital clinicians to it. The second (crossed) kind of hemianopia, in which both inner retinal halves are anesthetic, usually presents symptoms indicating a tumor or some pressure at the base of the cranium. If such a pressure is effective at the median line, then the crossed bundles (fasciculi cruciati—those close to the median line anterior as well as posterior to the chiasma) and thus the inner retinal halves will be especially involved. This kind of hemianopia never stops so sharply in the median line as does the other kind.

In diseases of the retina, retinitis apoplectica, degeneration of Bright's disease, and exudative processes, inequality of eccentric sight is still more frequent than actual restriction of the visual field and almost always associated with it. I have already mentioned that in retinal detachment indistinctness of eccentric vision occurs within an area adjoining the detached portions; also that exceptionally the detachment induces incomplete losses only and merely reduction of eccentric impressions to quantitative sensation. Granular exudations in the optic nerve are usually associated with the anomaly in question but as a rule, there is simultaneous intracranial disease which may possibly take a prominent part; at least as far as the ophthalmoscopically observed changes are concerned; with complete obscuring of the papilla, the visual field often shows not the least fluctuation.

It is really remarkable how many choroidal changes may be observed which are widely distributed throughout the eye-ground but with no portion of the visual field completely wanting. The interruption in posterior sclerotic choroiditis is particularly instructive. In this disease the conditions vary extraordinarily according to the stage and degree of the affection. In the beginning conduction is but slightly diminished in that part of the retina (largely) deprived of choroid. This may be on account of the excessive dazzling of this portion of the retina. It is then impossible to demonstrate by any means enlargement of the blind spot. Because of possible additional changes in the bared retina we may later on observe an enlargement of the blind spot which does not, however, correspond to the dimension of the white spot in the eye-ground, but is smaller. Extensive improvements in visual acuteness are rather frequently attained, even in prolonged and stationary affections; while changes in the visual field are but moderately attained and not at all in the majority of cases.

The prognosis in amaurotic affections with extremely depreciated central visual acuteness but perfect retinal conduction elsewhere is far better than in amaurotic affections with comparatively higher visual acuteness but severe anomalies of the visual field.

Comment: Von Graefe's pioneer contributions to clinical perimetry were based on a simple apparatus comparable to the Peter hand campimeter. In his article on the glaucomas in 1869, he described in amazing detail the visual field in glaucoma simplex including the fingerlike defects about the blind spot and the nasal step. After the advent of Foerster's arc perimeter, von Graefe's method of campimetry fell into desuetude until revived by Bjerrum in 1889. Bjerrum added the conception of isopters and quantitative perimetry. The modern projection perimeters are ideally adapted to quantitative perimetry permitting a rapid diminution in the size and contrast of the test object and of the general illumination. In some cases even more delicate methods are required to reveal a reduction in sensitivity. The simplest of these is the exposure of two targets simultaneously on opposite sides of the fixation point and at equal distances from it. The inability to see then the target in the affected field is explained by gradients of excitability (Bender, 1952) or of visual attention (Allen, 1948). This phenomenon is observed in disturbances of the brain, but not of the optic nerve. Flicker fields are superior to standard perimetry in detecting regions of minimal depression including the central area in retrobular neuritis. Haitz utilized the Holmes stereoscope to maintain steady fixation. To extend the usable field of the stereoscope, Lloyd developed the stereo-campimeter.

68

When the media are cloudy, the field for color may be more reliable than that for white as color perimetry is less influenced by blurred images. Colored test objects are likewise useful in the central field as the presence of a 3 mm. red object is easier to determine than that of a 1 mm. white object. In 1953, Harrington introduced test objects of sulfide inks rendered fluorescent by ultraviolet light. As these colors are of greater purity and saturation than those previously available, this innovation should give color perimetry a new impetus. The tachistoscopic device of Harrington and Flocks (1955) provides a satisfactory screening test that can be performed in a few seconds. This simplified test could well be included in the visual examination of motor vehicle drivers.

Reference

Lebensohn, J. E.: Evolution of clinical perimetry. Am. J. Ophth., *42:* 316–318, Aug. 1956.

Test-Types for the Determination of the Acuteness of Vision

HERMAN SNELLEN, M.D.

Utrecht, Holand

Monograph in English, French, Italian, German and Dutch
Utrecht, van de Weyer, 1862

The formula for the acuteness of vision (v) is expressed by the utmost distance at which the types are recognized (d), divided by the distance at which they are seen at our standard angle of five minutes (D).

1. The smallest angle, at which objects of known size and known form can be distinguished, determines the degree of the acuteness of vision.

The size of the image found on the retina depends on this angle. The increase, however, is not in direct proportion: a double sized image does not enlarge the distinctive power in a double ratio inasmuch as the percipient elements are not equally distributed over every part of the retina, but decrease in number from the center of the yellow spot to the periphery.

2. To determine the smallest visual angle we measure the utmost distance at which objects of definite size can be recognized.

The angle, if small, can be considered as in inverse proportion to the distance at which the object is seen.

3. A visual angle and corresponding distance being taken as a unit of measure, the proportion between such distance and that at which the object is actually seen expresses the acuteness of vision.

4. We take as unit of comparison the recognition of letters seen at an angle of five minutes.

We have adopted as proper objects square letters, the limbs of which have a diameter equal to one-fifth of the letters' height. Such letters are clearly distinguished by a normal eye at an angle of five minutes. As the limbs and subdivisions of the letter just measure one-fifth of their height, they present themselves at an angle of one minute; for instance, our letter *C* shows an opening, as compared with the *O*, of one-minute visual angle. In testing accuracy of vision, we accept perfect recognition and not uncertain perception of the letters.

5. The numbers placed above each type express in feet the distance, at which the letters are seen at our standard angle of five minutes.

6. The dimensions of our letters, as well as those of the interstices by which they are separated, have been accurately measured.

7. The utmost distance at which the types are recognized (d), divided by the distance at which they appear at an angle of five minutes (D), gives the formula for the acuteness of vision (v). $v = d/D$.

If d and D be found equal, and No. XX be thus recognized at a distance of 20 feet, then v is $20/20$; in other words, there is normal acuteness of vision. But d may sometimes be greater than D, and No. XX be visible at a greater distance than 20 feet; in such cases the acuteness of vision is greater than the normal average.

8. The normal acuteness of vision decreases with age. This is caused partly by decreased transparency of the media of the eye, which lessens the perfection of the retinal image; partly, by decreased perceptive and conductive power of the nervous structures.

9. The value of v should be found equal in testing with different types, each at its corresponding distance. If such is not the case, and v appears to diminish considerably within or beyond a certain distance, it may be inferred that the refraction is in fault, or that the eye is not adjusted for such distance.

In case of diminished acuteness of vision, v must still—within the limits of adjustment—be equal for different numbers of type each at its own distance: if therefore, *e.g.* at 20 feet, v is proved to be $20/200$, then at 10 feet v cannot differ considerably from $10/100$. In case any other value for v were stated, it would imply carelessness or simulation.

10. If acuteness of vision is found considerably greater for near than for distant objects, myopia must be assumed to exist. The farthest point of clear sight expresses approximately the degree of myopia.

11. If the distinction of distant objects increases with positive glasses, hypermetropia is proved to be present, and the strongest glass with which it still improves, or at least remains unaltered, determines the degree of manifest hypermetropia.

12. Should the horizontal and vertical strokes not be discerned with equal clearness, the focus of the eye is not the same for the horizontal and vertical meridians. The cylindrical glass which equalizes such difference shows the degree of astigmatism.

Difference in sharpness of horizontal and vertical lines produces an apparent alteration in the form of the letters. This distortion constitutes a rather important indication of the existence of astigmatism.

13. Positive lenses magnify, negative lenses diminish the size of the retinal image.

14. The size of the pupil is not without its influence upon the value of v. If the light be insufficient, v increases in proportion to the dilatation of the pupil; contraction of the pupil on the contrary improves the amount of v where the retinal image is confused from imperfect adjustment of the eye or from irregular refraction of the media.

15. The amount of v is dependent on the entensity of light. The most favorable amount of light is variable and depends especially upon the degree of light to which the eye has been exposed immediately before.

Independently of the strength of light, v is influenced moreover by the contrast between the white and black of the letters. The contrast as well as the illumination of the letters is therefore required to be of constant value during our tests.

16. Colored letters or white letters with colored illumination supply the means of ascertaining the acuteness of vision for each color. If the refractive media of the eye have a certain color, that color is seen better than its complimentary color.

17. The recognition of our isolated letters is a better test of v than reading a line of words in the corresponding types. In reading tests, however, fluency is chiefly to be desired.

18. Square figures, constructed in the proportion of one to five, may be considered equal to our test-types for people who cannot read.

19. Round dots of a certain diameter cannot be placed on an equal footing with parallel lines of the same diameter. The dots require a larger visual angle.

Comment: Snellen initiated his scientific study of visual acuity at the suggestion of von Graefe. In spite of numerous proposed modifications, his optotypes are still the generally accepted standard. Snellen recognized that visual acuteness must be measured in the same way as tactile sensibility, that is by the minimum distance at which two simultaneous impressions produce two independent sensations, the "minimum separabile." Snellen described two ways of measuring visual acuity. Using one size of type, he ascertained the maximum distance at which it was visible; or he placed the person examined at a fixed distance and displayed different sizes of type. The latter method is admirably adapted to the needs of the refractionist, but the former is preferable for mere visual rating as it permits the use of an unlearnable letter chart, such as that designed by Grow (1910) or Lebensohn (1943). These charts contain about ten rows of 20/20 letters. If the eye tested cannot read the indicated line at 20 feet, the person examined slowly approaches the chart, thus providing a gradual increase in the size of the visual angle. The furthest distance at which an accurate reading is secured assesses the visual acuity with this distance as numerator, and /20 as denominator.

Snellen amplified his views on visual acuity in the *Graefe-Saemisch Handbuch* (1874) and in Norris and Oliver's *System of Diseases of the Eye* (1900). He objected to the decimal notation, stating: "Reduction to a decimal does not indicate at what distance and with what letters the test has been made; and in such arithmetical series, the intervals are too great for the larger visual angles." In 1868 Snellen published a test card for illiterates, using the incomplete square (the Snellen prong), each side of which subtended the angle of five minutes with one side omitted. In 1873 he added a middle bar to the incomplete square, making the figure now known as the Snellen E. The 1868 edition of his monograph also presented a near-vision test based on his distant types, each letter being a square subtending an angle of five minutes at the designated reading distance. These charts were not as easily read as ordinary type and were soon abandoned for standardized lower-case texts. In these near charts, a number above each section signified the distance in the metric system at which the letters subtended the five-minute visual angle. Louise Sloan pointed out that in such metric charts if the reading distance is 40 cm. (16 inches), the near vision is readily convertible to its distance equivalent by dividing both terms of the fraction by two, *e.g.* 0.40/0.50 equals 20/25.

The diversity in letter discrimination, inherent in all forms of the Snellen chart, helped the refractionist to detect slight modifications in visual acuity. Scientific accuracy, however, demanded a test that was invariable, unlearnable and repeatable. To meet these requirements the Landolt ring was introduced in 1888, and has been favored for precise studies since. As astigmatism may cause the gap to be seen in one position but not in another, Ferree and Rand in 1934 proposed a test circle with gaps at right angles. Walter Fink suggested in 1945 that testing would be facilitated if the circles were varied with two, three, and four gaps as the person examined need then but register the number of gaps. This method seems ideal for illiterate adults who often resent as too puerile the manipulations required for the usual illiterate test.

The visual angle in minutes and the fractional notation of visual acuity are reciprocals of each other. If the visual acuity is noted as 20/40, 6/12, or 0.5, the visual angle is hence 2. The fractional notation is often misconceived by the laity as a measurement of visual efficiency. This misunderstanding could be avoided by designating visual acuity by the visual angle. The term "snellen" uncapitalized would be appropriate for this measurement. The acuity by visual angles has been added to the chart devised by Louise Sloan in 1959. Besides its many excellent features, this chart is among the best for the examination of patients with relatively low absolute acuity. In the ordinary chart, the progression of the visual angles downward is 10 snellen, 5 snellen, 3.3 snellen, but Sloan's chart doubles the intervals in this area with 10 snellen (20/200), 8 snellen (20/160), 6.25 snellen (20/125), 5 snellen (20/100), 4 snellen (20/80) and 3 snellen (20/60).

References

Lebensohn, J. E.: Visual rating. U. S. Navy Med. Bull., *41:* 744–749, (May) 1943.
Lebensohn, J. E.: Snellen on visual acuity. Am. J. Ophth. *53:* 152–155, (Jan.) 1962.

Biographical Note

Herman Snellen (1834–1908) was the son of a physician and received his medical degree at Utrecht in 1857. From then on he became increasingly associated with Donders as his pupil, intern, office assistant and co-worker both at the Netherlands Eye Hospital and the University of Utrecht. In Snellen's thesis for the doctorate he reviewed his experiments that demonstrated that keratitis neuroparalytica was due simply to mechanical injuries, such as dust, which the insensitive eye did not feel, and not to trophic disturbance. In 1862, Snellen was appointed docent; and Donders, who was then called to fill the chair of physiology, relegated practically all his former duties to him. Snellen's scientific work reached its high point in the study of visual acuity with which his name will be ever linked. His abiding interest in subjective examinations had previously led to an ingenious test for feigned unilateral amblyopia in which the tested person, wearing red and green glasses, viewed letters in red and green. His many contributions to ophthalmic surgery included the Snellen sutures for entropion and ectropion, an improved form of artificial eye, and the aluminum shield for the postoperative care of cataract patients. He promoted school hygiene by improving the construction and gradation of seats. In the Bowman Lecture of 1896 he discussed his researches on retinal perception. He received many honors, including fellowship in the Royal College of Surgeons of Ireland (1892), membership in the Ophthalmological Society of the United Kingdom (1896) and presidency of the ninth International Congress of Ophthalmology at Utrecht (1899). Snellen followed Donders in the chair of ophthalmology (1877–1899) and was succeeded by his son and assistant, Herman Snellen, Jr. In 1894 he supervised the construction of a palatial eye hospital, named after Donders, which replaced that built for Donders in 1858. Snellen, who had married a woman of English origin, spoke fluently Dutch, English, French and German.

Reference

Straub, D. M.: Obituary. Am. J. Ophth., 25: 91–93, 1908.

An Addition to the General Examination of the Field of Vision

J. P. BJERRUM, M.D.

Copenhagen, Denmark

SKAND. O. MAG., *2:* 141, 1889*

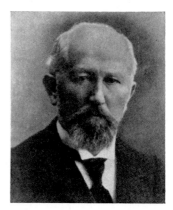

The ordinary examination of the field of vision with white and colored objects in daylight is one of our most important clinical examinations and its theoretical and practical value cannot be overestimated. The diameter of the objects generally used in field examinations varies from 1 to 2 cm.; equal to a visual angle of 2° to 4° if the perimeter radius is 300 cm. These visual angles must be considered large and the examinations therefore coarse. The ideal examination of retinal functions will ascertain not only the function of large groups of retinal elements but the function of a single element. One retinal element is equal to a visual angle of one minute or about that. When we, therefore, in measuring the field of vision use an object with a visual angle of 2°, the retinal image will cover several thousand of these elements so we will be very far from a fine point examination of the retina.

In order that I may work with small visual angles, I move the patient away from the test surface 2 meters as a rule. For test surface, I use a large broad roller shade that reaches from the ceiling to the floor and which is placed opposite two windows getting good light from both. The shade must be dull black without visible markings, otherwise the observation of small objects would be disturbed.

On the usual perimeter, the blind spot is about 1 inch in diameter but at two meters distance, this becomes 7 inches. As test objects, I use small round white ivory discs with diameters of 20 mm.; 10 mm.; 9 mm.; and so on to 1 mm. The usual procedure of the examination is as follows: First is the general perimeter examination with a test

* From the translation by M. K. Povlsen Ph.G., Eye, Ear, Nose & Throat Month, *13:* 221, July, 1934

74

object of 10 mm. and a perimeter radius of 300 mm. Next the table with the chin support is placed 2 meters from the screen and the field is examined with a test object of 3 mm. The visual angle is indicated on the record as the diameter of the test object over the distance of the eye from the screen. In the first instance the visual angle is 10/300 and the last is 3/2000. When I then speak of 10/300 or 3/2000, it means white test objects of 10 and 3 mm. respectively, at a distance of 300 mm. and 2000 mm., respectively. If the visual angle in degrees or minutes is desired, these figures may be multiplied by $180°/pi$. Thus the visual angle in the first case is $2°$; and the last becomes about 5 minutes.

In an examination with a 10/300 test object, the normal border is externally $90°$, internally $60°$, below $70°$ and above $55°$. It is well known that one cannot figure too closely because of individual differences but these will not exceed $5°$ one way or the other. If the patient has one normal eye, this may be used as a standard. If the visual angle is 5 minutes (3/2000) the normal minimum border is outward $35°$; inward $30°$; down $28°$ and up $25°$.

You should not put too much weight upon small concentric narrowings of the visual field. It is the irregular encroachment from one side; the sector defects and the scotoma which have the most significance. The individual fluctuations show themselves only as somewhat concentric variations and not as indents or scotomas. Variations of ordinary daylight in which the visual field is measured, play no important role for a normal eye in an ordinary perimetric examination with 1/30 test object. If the visual angle is smaller, that influence is greater but it must not be understood that the visual field of a normal individual is in any principal degree different with a 3/2000 test object whether it is a lighter or a darker day. In consequence of that there is only very little variation. But it can happen with a patient that a defect shows easier in duller light than in a stronger but that is only because there is actually diseased perception. Individual variations in the diameter of the pupils have the same consequence as variation in the light as they change the amount of light upon the retina. If a patient has very small immobile pupils and the light also happens to be poor, there may be indents in the field outline for small objects and it will be proper to re-examine in good light. But never will these conditions in themselves cause irregularities like sector shaped or scotomatous defects nor will they be caused by individual physiological peculiarities.

Refractive errors may bring about a narrowing of the visual field for small objects and the more so the smaller they are. Therefore must you correct myopia and possible hypermetropia with proper glasses when using small test objects. The statements of a single individual vary very little in defining the outline of the field for small white objects and they are, according to my experience, less variable than the answers for colored test objects. It is not easy to decide when a color is seen as such. Normally the size of the field declines with the visual angle of the test object used. If this angle is $1/2°$, the field is about the normal size; but if the visual angle of the test object is smaller than $1/2°$, the borders become narrower, the smaller the test object is. For $6/2000$ ($10'$) a normal minimum is: out $50°$; in $40°$; down $37°$; up $35°$. For $3/2000$, ($5'$): out $35°$; in $30°$; down $28°$; up $25°$. For $1/3000$ ($1'$) the field is much smaller, not even $10°$ from the fixing point. Something like this, one finds in examining the Mariotte blind spot; for $20/2000$ it has its customary size; but if one takes an object of 2 or 3 mm. diameter, one finds that it gets larger; all around it is a zone in which the object, at a distance of 2 meters, is not seen, but an object of 20 mm. is seen all over the zone. The width of this zone is about $1°$. The retinal anatomy must therefore be incomplete.

Sometimes I found in choroiditis disseminata, scotomas in the shape of rings and fractions of rings, bow-shaped scotomas; with the inside concave edge near the fixation point and the outside convex edge 10 to $20°$ away. These scotomas are easily overlooked in the usual perimeter examination with objects of $2°$ or thereabouts, either because the function in the scotoma area is only diminished, not extinguished; or because the scotoma is so small. In retinitis pigmentosa and chorio-retinitis luetica diffusa, one finds ring scotomas. These do not lay as near the fixation point as those just described; they are $20°$ between the fixing point and the inner border. Oftener with these diseases a concentric narrowing of the field occurs which can be considered as a form of zonular defect. I have examined several cases of typical pigmentary retinitis with small objects and could always prove a noticeable even strong concentric narrowing of the field borders in ordinary daylight even if the limits for large objects were normal. A similar strong contraction of the field for small white objects only have I now and then met in some diseases with such objective symptoms as keratitis punctata, iritis with synechia, opacities in the vitreous.

In the circumpapillary zone of choroidal atrophy which accompanies myopia of high degree, you may with small test objects find that the blind spot is very much enlarged, caused by a diminution of the function in the atrophied area. A very large scotoma approaching the fixing area is not a good sign even though it be merely a relative defect. As a matter of fact, you sometimes find (equal to choroidal changes or hemorrhages) a scotoma in the macular area in cases wherein the blind spot in spite of circumpapillary choroidal atrophy does not show enlargement. In amblyopia centralis a scotoma can always be demonstrated in which a sufficiently small object is absolutely invisible.

Finally I have examined many cases of glaucoma simplex. Certain peculiarities of the visual field in that disease formed by the glaucomatous process are characteristic symptoms. Only in exceptional cases is it possible to show these peculiarities by ordinary perimetry. That I have found them is due to the method of examination. Consider the visual field of a patient with glaucoma simplex—vision 5/12. For a 10/300 test object there is a scotoma defect inward. The 4/2000 test object is only seen in a small central island from near the fixation point to a point 12° to 13° outside of that, or the blind spot as near as one can tell. What I want to call attention to in this field is the following: the sector shaped, partly absolute, partly relative defect, reaching inward with a trailer, under the fixing point right up to the blind spot and the defect in the upper half of the field also reaching the blind spot. The better functioning part of the field is connected with the blind spot, an edge on each side. The visual field is narrowed internally (as always in glaucoma), and this in a very high degree while it is not narrowed externally. The visual field of another patient with glaucoma simplex shows the same type as the previous, except that the peripheral area wherein the small object is seen is much larger, forming a half circle. For 10/300 the visual field has a fairly satisfactory extension. 5/2000 is only seen in a moderately small central island and in a half ring figure. The two functioning areas are divided by the Mariotte spot and the strips that extend up and down from it. Position and size of the Mariotte spot in normal eyes is subject to small variations.

In the next case the visual field of the right eye for 10/300 is seen all over within a fairly good-sized area and much better than in the other eye. For 5/2000 on the contrary, the whole lower part of the visual field is missing but it is seen in a good expansion from 26° to 35° in the upper half. The defect for 5/2000 makes a tangent with the blind spot. In another case the vision of the left eye is 5/60, the border for 10/300 is good and there is no scotoma for this size of test object. 5/2000 is seen only in a half ring shaped portion but not in the macular area. The vision of the right eye is 5/36. The patient's diary indicates that the visual field began to retrograde with a central scotoma as just noted on the field for the other eye.

In the following case the limits for 10/300 are considerably indented down and in, nearly to the fixing point, but elsewhere are almost normal. 3/2000 is not at all seen in the central areas of the field but it pops up at the outside edge of the blind spot and is thereafter seen all the way to 45°. The area is a little more than one-fourth of a ring and corresponds to the general shape of the field obtained for 10/300. In the next patient vision is reduced to 3/72 by glaucoma simplex. The object is not seen at all in the whole inner part of the visual field and not in the central area.

When one considers the glaucoma effects upon the nerve threads, operating at the disc edge or in the walls of the glaucomatous excavation, one gets a simple explanation of the condition of the visual fields that I have so far spoken of. If all of the fibers are completely destroyed at some one point where the fibers stream out from the papilla, we get a complete defect in the visual field, which reaches right up to the papilla edge, a sector spreading toward the periphery because these fibers spread out into a fan. If contrarywise, those from a certain spot in the papilla are only partially destroyed, we get an amblyopic condition of the corresponding area to be found only by smaller test objects. There is nothing remarkable that a disease, which operates upon the nerve fibers in the papilla, should not always produce an effect upon the whole area supplied by the fibers passing over the edge at that point. If the cause does not work upon the entire thickness of the nerve fiber layer, one will not get a defect which reaches to the periphery. In the visual fields mentioned in this article, I have been able to follow the functional defect in the visual field right up to the blind spot; but it has often happened that this was impossible. If we look at the fields aready pictured, we will find a reversed picture of the nerve fibers streaming from the papilla. In the first, the nerve fibers which go up and out (corresponding to the down and in of the field record), and those that go downward (corresponding to the upward portion of the record) are affected while those that go straight out to the macular area and those that go inward and also up and in, are almost untouched.

In some of the cases mentioned herein, the glaucomatous narrowing of the field continues over the macular area to the blind spot. On the contrary, some cases have a normal outer border while the central areas are amblyopic. It seems to show that the nerve fibres laying closest to the corpus vitreum are most affected but that sometimes the deeper fibres are more affected. It seems to have been proven that the nerve fibers ending farthest from the papilla, are the superficial ones. The fibers running straight supply the macular region and a central scotoma is then analogous to a peripheral defect as far as the operating causes are concerned. The outward going fibers are affected as well as those going slightly askew; up and out, and down and out; and which after an arc-like course supply that part of the retina from the papilla out to the periphery. Bunge published two cases of glaucoma with central scotoma, in 1884, and in each the scotoma formed an arc over the fixing point which in the one case reached the blind spot, in the other not. Furthermore, he emphasized the constancy with which the glaucoma simplex defects (indents) are internally located; also, that the part of the field functioning longest is outside of and near the blind spot. He uses this last condition as an argument that it is the intraocular pressure that affects the nerve fibers during the process of excavation formation. First, the superficial fibers are affected (those going outward to the periphery); both upward and downward, also to the macula. Last affected are the deep fibers which run inward. Although the field forms usually found uphold this theory of pressure damage, one must not attribute too large a significance to it. With some right, I think one can conclude that the cause for visual debility in glaucoma simplex most often works from the papilla edge or in the wall of the excavation. One must remember that in addition to the nerve fibers, the vessels radiate from the disc to all sides. A disease process could very easily produce phenomena in respect to the visual field geography by operating upon the arteries at the disc edge, very similar to those set forth.

Central and paracentral scotomas are not at all rare in glaucoma and examples have been shown here. These do not as a rule resemble in shape or position the scotomas of amblyopia centralis (toxic amblyopia) or of optic atrophy. The glaucoma defects are most often paracentral, running upward and downward from the blind spot and never spreading outward from the blind spot, but inward, to reach the periphery. The central scotomas of glaucoma are thus in their geographic relation different from the scotomas of genuine atrophy of the optic nerve. If a glaucoma defect once in a while resembles these, it is only for a time in its process of development.

Comment: To Bjerrum is due the conception of quantitative perimetry based on the isopters of white targets of different sizes at a distance of 1 to 2 meters. When his classic article appeared in 1889, von Graefe's method of campimetry, pioneered in 1856, had fallen into disuse, displaced in popularity by Foerster's arc perimeter introduced in 1869. Lloyd comments: "The mad rush from the perimeter to the campimeter which followed the publication of his article was much like the earlier stampede from the campimeter to the perimeter." As compared to the qualitative perimetry of von Graefe, the quantitative perimetry of Bjerrum is a signal advance as it gives a precise picture of a deficit in the visual field and presents an accurate evaluation of its progress. A defect with a sloping edge encourages the neursurgeon to hope for some recovery. In glaucoma, a defect with a steep slope suggests neural involvement, while a gradual slope would indicate a circulatory disturbance. In brain lesions even a slight reduction in sensitivity can be revealed by exposing two targets of the same size simultaneously on opposite sides of the fixation point. The inability to see the target in the affected field is dependent on a reduced gradient of excitability or of visual attention. When the media are cloudy the field for color may be more reliable than that for white as color perimetry is less influenced by blurred images. Colored test objects also are useful in the central field as the presence or absence of a 3 to 5 mm. red object is easier to determine than that of a 1 mm. white object. The tachistoscopic method of Harrington and Flocks, ushered in in 1955, expedites routine central field examinations. It is the simplest technique for screening purposes and can be performed in a few minutes.

Campimetry by projected light is ideally adapted to quantitative perimetry since it permits a rapid shift in the size, contrast and illumination of the test object. Projected targets never become faded or smudged and, like magnetic campimeters, avoid the obtrusive wand. Projective campimetry can be photographically recorded by placing a Land Polaroid self-developing camera with a wide angle lens above the patient's head and facing the screen. As quickly as the patient responds to the presence of the target, the camera is snapped and all responses are recorded rapidly on the same film.

References

Lebensohn, J. E.: Evolution of clinical perimetry. Am. J. Ophth., *42:* 316–318 (Aug.), 1956.
Michaels, D. D.: Projection campimetry and photographic recording. Am. J. Ophth., *55:* 107–115 (Jan.), 1963.

Biographical Note

Jannik Petersen Bjerrum (1851–1920), the son of a dyer and farmer, was born in Skjarbak, Denmark. He received his medical degree in 1876 in Copenhagen where he continued his study and training in ophthalmology. In 1882 he secured his doctorate with a notable thesis on the form and light sense in various eye diseases, which revealed his dominant interest in functional investigation. In 1884 he first showed that the visual acuity in strabismic amblyopia, in contrast to that in organic amblyopia, is either unaffected or improved by reduced illumination—a finding that was recently confirmed by Burian (Arch. Ophth., *62:* 396, 1959). In 1886 he began studying the field defects in glaucoma by quantitative perimetry and discovered the significant Bjerrum scotoma. In 1896 he succeeded Grut in the chair of ophthalmology at the University of Copenhagen and became Associate Editor of the Nordisk Ophthalmogisk Tidsskrift. In 1900 Bjerrum was elected the first president of the newly founded Copenhagen Ophthalmological Society. While professor of ophthalmology, he authored compact textbooks on *The Ophthalmoscope* and *The Investigation of Visual Capacity*.

Reference

Lundsgaard, K. K. K.: Obituary. Klin. Monatsbl. Augenh., *65:* 371, 1920.

Atlas of the Slitlamp-Microscopy of the Living Eye

ALFRED VOGT, M.D.

Basle, Switzerland

BERLIN, JULIUS SPRINGER, 1921*

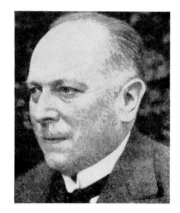

Preface

For the illustrations I am very much indebted to the artist, Mr. J. Iseli, who made the greater number of them. In executing the illustrations special care was taken to produce reproductions true to nature. Sketches and schematic presentations were avoided as much as possible.

Introduction

The slitlamp, in combination with the corneal microscope, permits us to observe the living endothelium on the posterior surface of the cornea. Every individual endothelial cell on Descemet's membrane, as well as each pathologically deposited lymphocyte, is revealed. The nerve fibers of the cornea can be traced to their finest ramifications. In Descemet's and Bowman's membranes we have observed pathological folds, manifested by characteristic reflexes. We can see the blood corpuscles as they roll along in newly formed corneal vessels as well as those within the vessels that form the vascular loops at the limbus. Edema of the corneal epithelium or endothelium is revealed by a deposit like fine dew.

A multitude of previously unknown manifestations in cataract formation have been disclosed. We learned to recognize the subcapsular striae of vacuole formation in advanced cataract, the folding or wrinkling of the capsule when shrinking begins, the types of nuclear sclerosis, peripheral concentric clouding, the various forms of wreath and rosette shaped cataract, the genesis of spokes and cystic spaces and the characteristic picture of lamellar separation in posterior cortical cataract. The slitlamp distinguishes also the acquired from the various forms of

* Excerpts adapted from translation by Dr. Vonder Heydt.

81

congenital cataract; it likewise gives a definite differentiation between cataracta complicata and cataracta senilis.

Our knowledge of the normal youthful and the normal ageing lens is enriched beyond expectation. We can see the lens epithelium and the anterior and posterior graining (shagreen) in normal and changed conditions. The laminations of the lens of which we had only a vague conception previously can now be studied with the bundle of light as to form, arrangement, number and degree of luminosity. We discover the surface of the senile nucleus in relief. The embryonal segmentations are made visible both in youth and in extreme age.

The slitlamp discloses the normal vitreous body and such pathological changes as absorption of supporting structure, senile and pathological opacification, and deposits of crystals, blood, lymphocytes and pigment.

In addition, we are given an "optical section" of the living eye and the location of areas in cornea, lens and vitreous can be as exactly fixed as in anatomical preparations.

Technic

Within the last two years I have introduced a modification of the Gullstrand apparatus. Instead of focusing the light on the slit opening I let the image fall on the illuminating lens. By this means the bundle of light is of greater luminosity and more homogeneous. This modification (Köhler's method) has been applied to the nitrogen lamp by Henker. The luminosity of the nitrogen lamp is greater, and its light whiter than that of the Nernst rod. For this reason the less expensive and more easily handled nitrogen lamp is to be preferred.

During the examination the patient uses his other eye for fixation, for which we use a light of very low candle power. The magnification most commonly used is 24 times. The binocular microscope is well adapted for investigating the dimensions of ocular structures. We use a measuring ocular and find it of great value, especially in the lower powers of magnification (10 to 37 times). It would be of great service if the slitlamp had a device by means of which we could measure the depth of the anterior chamber, the thickness of the cornea and that of the lens.

Methods of Examination

The slitlamp allows four methods of examination: (1) Focal illumination (direct lateral), (2) Transillumination by light reflected from iris or lens, (3) Specular illumination of reflecting surfaces, (4) Indirect lateral illumination at the margins of illuminated areas. Focal illumination is the most important. Transillumination is used principally for the study of surfaces apparently covered by a dewlike deposit and for transilluminating the iris. Thanks to specular illumination we are able to observe the living endothelium of the cornea. The last method, indirect lateral illumination, is often of value in observing certain lens conditions, especially the vacuole formation in the subcapsular area.

Examination in Focal Illumination

The opalescence of cornea, lens and vitreous body increases with age. The anterior chamber is relatively "optically empty, therefore dark." The presence of exudates and cells is betrayed by the luminous shaft becoming visible. In some cases after operations for cataract or glaucoma, the anterior chamber is so shallow that we are in doubt as to whether it may exist. In this only the slitlamp can give reliable information. In a similar manner we can determine in peripherally situated anterior synechiae exactly the extent of adhesions.

Depth can be determined in two ways: (1) roughly, by simple binocular stereoscopic observation, (2) precisely, by the linear optical section. For the purpose of determining depth the slit must be reduced to about 0.5 mm. The axes of observation and illumination must be at least at 60 to 80 degrees.

When examining in diffuse light, the patient looks straight ahead; the angle between the axis of observation and the direction of the light is 40 degrees. Changes in the media appear in their natural color. Precipitates appear gray to whitish-gray, and if brown the luster is in proportion to the amount of pigment they may contain. Opacities of the lens, if very thin and flat, appear blue or bluish-green. In transillumination, however, they are brown to brownish-yellow. Opacities of the lens of greater density appear white; in transillumination, black. Red blood cells are a luminous light yellow.

Pigment particles of less than one micron are visible by reflection. In direct focal illumination they appear as luminous spots, comparable to the dust made luminous by rays of sunlight in a dark room. In parenchymatous keratitis, blood vessels may be invisible in diffuse focal light, while with transillumination they as well as the blood corpuscles in them can be seen. On the contrary, homogeneous media present more favorable conditions for observation by direct light, as in viewing the striations of keratoconus, corneal nerve fibers or ruptures in Descemet's membrane.

In the normal lens, focal illumination will show the laminations of the lens, the embryonal sutures and remnants of the anterior and posterior vascular membrane. We see also the supporting structure of the vitreous body and remnants of embryonic vessels.

Observation by Transillumination

In transillumination the light is directed onto more or less opaque tissues (iris' cataract) from which it is reflected. It is chiefly utilized in examining the cornea. In edema of the epithelium or endothelium, the cells become visible when their refractive index is changed by absorption of fluid. A uniformly delicate dewlike change results. In characteristic cases of bedewing of the posterior corneal surface we can differentiate two types of droplets: (1) uniform fine droplets; (2) round, oblong or club-shaped, less transparent droplets which are irregularly scattered, that signify precipitates on the posterior corneal surface.

In the iris the transillumination technique can reveal atrophy of the pupillary border and the retinal pigment layer. In age, the retinal pigment usually disappears, leaving a membranous translucent sheath. Ecchymosis of the iris after contusio bulbi is visible only by transillumination. The blood-stained area shows red when the light is reflected just to its border. Atrophic areas, perforations and iridodialysis appear luminous.

In the lens, as in the cornea, transillumination often reveals deposited crystals of cholesterin, invisible in focal illumination, because it is veiled by opacities.

Examination of Reflecting Zones in General

On the surfaces of the limiting optical media, we see, in addition to diffused light, definite reflected images. The easiest to focus are the clearly outlined images of the anterior corneal and posterior lens zones, because of their luminosity. We must bring the reflected zone into an exact focus in order to see the detail on it clearly defined. For instance, on the anterior corneal surface we must see the corpuscular elements of the tears, and on the anterior or posterior lens surface the graining (shagreen). To explore surfaces that are convex anteriorly, such as the anterior and posterior surfaces of the cornea, and the anterior surface of the lens, the patient must be directed to look in a direction opposite to that we wish to examine.

The opacities and irregularities of a reflecting surface, which appear black on a luminous background, are like defects in the mercury film of a mirror. Consequently, we can observe changes in the reflecting zone so minute as to be invisible in diffuse light

Examination with Indirect Lateral Illumination

By the method of indirect lateral illumination with the slitlamp we focus the microscope onto the margin of the luminous zone. In this manner the vacuole formations in the areas of the anterior and posterior lens surfaces (subcapsular vacuolar layers) are more distinctly seen than by any other method. If we examine deposits or individual cells under indirect lateral illumination they assume a plastic form giving the impression of prominences—or depressions, by an inversion of relief. Thus, projections arising from the posterior corneal surface may act as small concave mirrors and produce this effect.

Comment: Before the advent of the slit-lamp, the microscopic study of the living eye proved futile. Henker launched the modern type slit-lamp apparatus in 1916 when he joined the Czapski microscope, devised in 1897, to the Gullstrand illuminating unit, first exhibited in 1911, and provided adjustments for the ready manipulation of the two elements. Vogt recognized the vast potential of this arrangement and greatly amplified its possibilities by changing the optical arrangement, introducing the adjustable slit and varying the methods of illumination. In 1920 Vogt directed the first international slitlamp course. His atlas of slitlamp microscopy, published the following year, and the 3-volume second edition (1930–1940) rank among the great creative books of ophthalmology. Vogt and his disciples added a technical slitlamp vocabulary to the lexicon of ophthalmology. The term, biomicroscopy, as a succinct equivalent for "slitlamp microscopy of the living eye," was suggested by Mawas in 1925.

Leonhard Koeppe and Hans Goldmann are chiefly responsible for the further advances in this field. In 1918, Koeppe extended slit-lamp microscopy to the fundus. Though his technique was cumbersome, he demonstrated the essential requirements for success: (1) nullification of the refractive power of the eye by the Koeppe contact lens, (2) reduction of the observation-illumination angle to 5 degrees. Goldmann's reduction prism neatly solved the second requirement and promoted remarkable progress. As a feasible alternative to the Koeppe lens, Hruby popularized in 1941 a precorneal planoconcave lens of 55 D., and in 1953 El Bayadi demonstrated indirect ophthalmoscopy with the slit-lamp using a precorneal planoconvex lens of 60 D. Koeppe also extended the slit-lamp technique to gonioscopy but the perfected method is Goldmann's achievement. Furthermore, in 1955, Goldmann announced the slit-lamp application of applanation tonometry—a method of registering ocular tension that was not influenced by variations in ocular rigidity and corneal curvature. A desideratum sought by Vogt, an accurate measurement of the thickness of the cornea and the depth of the anterior chamber, is now possible with Lobeck's split-field depth micrometer, that uses the coincidence method.

By endowing the slit-lamp and microscope with a common axis of rotation, Comberg, in 1933, enabled both to be turned together and thus maintain the slit image constantly in the field of view. The Goldmann slit-lamp of 1937 embodied in addition a fixation lamp, a steering lever and the reduction prism. At the 1958 International Congress of Ophthalmology, the slit-lamps displayed by the various manufacturers had a new look as well as advantages that made all previous models outdated. The objectives in the turret automatically focused on changing magnification; the illuminating system, contained in a freely movable vertical shaft, permitted the illumination-observation angle to be varied from 90 degrees to zero; and the slit-image could be rotated to any angle.

The slit-lamp added a new perspective to the study of the living eye. Minute colorless foreign bodies of glass or plastic, which were undetectable by other means, could be definitely located. In 1942, Karl Ascher, then at the University of Cincinnati, noted aqueous veins intercalated between Schlemm's canal and the episcleral and conjunctival veins—a discovery that definitely proved the aqueous to be in continuous circulation. Biomicroscopy has made diagnoses not otherwise possible. Burki in 1940 established the appearance of cystine deposits in the cornea and conjunctiva as an early and pathognomonic sign of cystinosis. The slit-lamp frequently reveals the first signs of many diseases such as Fuch's dystrophy, cyclitic glaucoma, sympathetic ophthalmia and cataracta complicata. The slit-lamp facilitates the certain diagnosis of posterior detachment of the vitreous, retinoschisis and central serous retinopathy and positively differentiates a macular cyst from a macular hole. Indeed, the numerous advances in biomicroscopy are a tribute to the tempo of progress in the past half-century.

Reference

Lebensohn, J. E.: On the golden anniversary of slit-lamp microscopy. Am. J. Ophth., *52:* 5–10, 1961.

Biographical Note

Alfred Vogt (1879–1943) was born near Aarau, Switzerland, the son of a school-teacher farmer. After receiving his medical degree at the University of Basle, he continued his studies there at the Ophthalmic Institute directed by Mellinger, and wrote his dissertation, "On the danger of aniline dyes to the eyes." He then returned to his home town, Aarau, where he combined the private practice of ophthalmology with independent research. While there he demonstrated the susceptibility of the crystalline lens to prolonged infrared radiation and introduced ophthalmoscopy by red-free light. In 1918, Vogt made the unprecedented transition from private practice to the academic appointment of Professor of Ophthalmology at the University of Basle, and in 1923 he accepted the invitation to head the Ophthalmic Institute at the University of Zurich. His range of interests covered all ophthalmology. He introduced cyclodiathermy for the treatment of complicated cases of glaucoma, popularized Gonin's technique in the operation for retinal detachment and studied intensely the hereditary factors in ocular pathology. But his primary interest was always the slit-lamp, and he completed the 3-volume second edition of his atlas of slit-lamp microscopy only 3 years before his death. Vogt was honored with the Donders medal, the Gullstrand medal and in 1939 on his 60th birthday with a Festchrift containing 90 papers from all over the world. His demise was due to a chronic kidney ailment complicated by severe vascular disease from which he had suffered for 20 years. His only son died tragically in an avalanche accident in the Swiss Alps. But, in spite of mental anguish and physical distress, a supreme devotion to his mission enabled him to complete his task.

Reference

Stocker, F. W.: Obituary. Arch. Ophth., *31:* 172–174, 1944.

Part Four
Physiologic Optics

Magnifying-Glasses

FRIAR ROGER BACON
Oxford, England
EXCERPT FROM OPUS MAJUS, 1267*

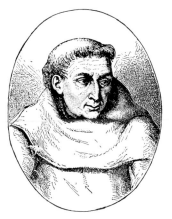

If anyone examines letters or other minute objects through the medium of crystal or glass or other transparent substance, if it be shaped like the lesser segment of a sphere, with the convex side towards the eye, and the eye being in the air, he will see the letters far better, and they will seem larger to him. For according to our canon concerning a spherical medium beneath which the object is placed, the centre being beyond the object, the convexity being towards the eye, all causes agree to increase the size, for the angle in which it is seen is greater, the image is greater, and the position of the image is nearer, because the object is between the eye and the centre. For this reason such an instrument is useful to old persons and to those with weak eyes, for they can see any letter, however small, if magnified enough. But if a larger segment of a sphere be employed, then, according to our canon the size of the angle is increased, and also the size of the image, but propinquity is lost because the position of the image is beyond the object, the reason being that the centre of the sphere is between the eye and the object seen. Therefore such an instrument is not of so much use as the smaller portion of a sphere.

---

* From the Translation by J. H. Bridge, M.D., The Opus Majus of Roger Bacon, Oxford, 1897.

Objects are greater when the vision is refracted; for it easily appears by the above-mentioned canons that very large objects may seem to be very small and conversely, and those at a great distance away may seem very near and conversely. For we can so form glasses and so arrange them with regard to our sight and to objects that the rays are refracted and deflected to any place we wish, so that we see the object near at hand or far away beneath whatever angle we desire. And so we can read the smallest letters or count grains of sand or dust from an incredible distance owing to the magnitude of the angle beneath which we see them, and again the largest objects close at hand might be scarely visible owing to the smallness of the angle beneath which we view them; for it is on the size of the angle on which this kind of vision depends, and it is independent of distance save *per accidens*. So a boy can appear a giant, a man seem a mountain, and in any size of angle whatever, for we can see a man under as large an angle as though he were a mountain and make him appear as near as we desire. So a small army might seem very large, and though far away appear near, and conversely: so, too we could make sun, moon, and stars apparently descend here below, and similarly appear above the heads of our enemies, and many other similar marvels could be brought to pass, that the ignorant mortal mind could not endure the truth.

As to double refraction, what is causally manifest with regard to it we can verify in many ways by the results of experiment. For if anyone holds a crystal ball or a round urinal flask filled with water in the strong rays of the sun, standing by a window in face of the rays, he will find a point in the air between himself and the flask at which point, if any easily combustible substance is placed, it will catch fire and burn, which would be impossible unless we suppose a double refraction. For a ray of the sun coming from a point in the sun through the centre of the flask is not refracted, because it falls perpendicularly on flask, water, and air passing through the centre of each. . . . But all the other rays given forth at the same point in the sun from which this perpendicular ray comes are necessarily refracted in the body of the flask, because they fall at oblique angles, and since the flask is denser than air, the refraction passes between the straight path and the perpendicular drawn from the point of refraction to the centre of the flask. And when it passes out again into the air, then, since it comes upon a less dense body, the straight path passes between the refraction and the perpendicular drawn from the point of refraction, so that the refracted ray may fall upon the first perpendicular which comes without refraction from the sun. Now since an infinite number of rays are given off from the same point of the sun, and one only falls perpendicularly on the flask, all the others are refracted and meet at one point on the perpendicular ray which is given off along with them from the sun, and this point is the point of combustion. On it are collected an infinite number of rays, and the concentration of light causes combustion. But this concentration would not take place except by double refraction, as shown in the diagram.

Comment: The beginnings of spectacles is veiled in medieval mystery. They first appeared toward the end of the 13th century in both Europe and China, but the differences between the earliest spectacles of West and East suggest a possible independent development. In ancient Greece and Rome lenses were used only as "burning glasses." The Opus Majus of Roger Bacon contains the first mention of the employment of lenses as a means of assisting sight. The Friar's knowledge may have been inspired by the writings of Alhazen or derived from eastern missionaries; in turn, the transfer of Bacon's ideas to Italy by a member of his order would account for the introduction of spectacles there, first by Salvino d' Armati and subsequently by Alessandro di Spina.

At first the use of glasses was opposed by both priest and physician. The clergy regarded the device as an impertinent effort to defeat the divine purpose of inflicting disabilities on the aged; and the physicians, fearing that the eyes were thereby eventually weakened, regarded the prescribing of glasses as beneath their dignity. By the 15th century spectacles had attained social approbation and it became customary to picture with spectacles characters of dignity and importance. In 1480 Ghirlandajo painted Saint Jerome at a desk from which dangled a pair of nose-glasses. This detail inspired the legend that the learned saint was the inventor of spectacles and so Saint Jerome became the patron of the spectacle makers' guild.

Lenses were orginally used for the relief of presbyopia and "for old sight in young people." A myopic correction is first pictured in the portrait of Pope Leo X, painted by Raphael in 1517, which now hangs in the Palazzo Pitti of Florence. In 1628 Daca de Valdes of Seville published the first discussion of refraction in a quarto of 100 pages in which cataract lenses are mentioned.

Reference

Lebensohn, J. E.: The history of spectacles. Bull. Soc. Med. Hist. of Chicago, *4:* 229, 1930.

Biographical Note

Roger Bacon (1214–1294) was born in England of a noble family. He studied at Oxford and then at Paris for the degree of Doctor of Theology, mastering at the same time physics, mathematics, Latin, Greek, Hebrew and Arabic. At the age of 36 he returned to London, joined the Franciscan monks, and became an instructor at Oxford. His scientific experiments were looked upon with suspicion. After a few years his lectures were interdicted and he spent the next 10 years in a Paris prison in solitary confinement, until the accession of Pope Clement IV. The world owes a great debt to this dignitary, a man of liberal culture, who requested from Bacon to whom he was friendly some treatises on science. In 18 months Bacon completed three immense volumes, the Opus Majus, the Opus Minus, and the Opus

Tertium—works which inspired a new era in the world of physical science. With the advent of the next pope 3 years later Bacon was thrown again into prison and all his books were condemned. This second confinement lasted 14 years, just 2 years before his death at the age of 80. For centuries this martyr of science was regarded as a wizard. "The Famous Historie of Fryer Bacon" related how by the wave of a magic wand he summoned excellent music such as had never been heard before; and by another wave of the wand brought tables covered with the richest fruit, and so on.

Reference

Holden, S.: Friar Roger Bacon. Pop. Sci. M., *60:* 253–262, 1902.

Diffraction of Light

FRANCESCO MARIA GRIMALDI, S.J.

Physicomathesis de Lumine, Coloribus et Iride, 1665

A Source Book in Physics, McGraw-Hill, N.Y., 1935*

Proposition I

Light is propagated or diffused not only directly, by refraction, and by reflection, but also in still a fourth way, by diffraction.

FIRST EXPERIMENT

A very small hole is made in a window shutter and through it the sunlight from a very clear sky is admitted into a room which is otherwise closed so as to be dark. The diffusion of this light will be in a cone or what is nearly a cone, and becomes visible if the air is filled with dust or if some smoke is set up in it. In this cone there is placed an opaque body at a great distance from the hole, and so that at least one end of the opaque body is illuminated. Then the before mentioned cone is received on a white board or on a sheet of white paper laid on the floor, and there is seen its illuminated base with the shadow cast by the opaque body which has been placed in the cone.

What should be especially noticed is that the shadow appears considerably larger in fact than it ought to be, if the whole thing is supposed to act by straight lines.

In addition, at its sides there is some color, always bluish at the side which is nearer the shadow and reddish on the further side. These bright bands apparently depend on the size of the hole because they are not seen if it is very large.

It may further be observed of the before mentioned bands of colored light, that the first is wider than the second, and the second is wider than the third (it has never yet happened that more than three have been seen). These decrease in the intensity of the light and of the colors in the same order in which they recede from the shadow. Yet the individual bands are wider and further apart, the further the white board on which they are received is from the opaque body casting the shadows, and further also by how much the more this is set obliquely to the solar radiation. This reason itself demands, because they are made by the

* Extract based on translation by W. F. Magie.

rays which are part of the luminous cone and which become more and more separated from one another the further they proceed.

There may be someone perhaps who, because of his failure to consider this observation, is unwilling to recognize that the before mentioned bands are bands of light, as we have said they are, but will contend that they should rather be called bands of shadow, because he has not paid enough attention to those obscure colors which we have said appear at the sides of these light bands.

SECOND EXPERIMENT

An opening is made, perhaps a finger breadth wide, in the window shutter of a well darkened room, and in this opening is placed a thin opaque plate and through a very narrow opening in this plate sunlight is admitted and forms a cone of light. At a great distance from the plate another plate is placed so as to cut this cone at right angles. In it there is also a small hole through which some of the before mentioned cone of light, which is interrupted by the plate, is admitted. This plate is so placed that the base of the cone considerably exceeds the size of the hole, so that the hole is all lighted or filled with light. Then the light which enters through the hole will again form a cone or almost a cone. When this is cut orthogonally or is terminated by a smooth white surface it will show on this surface an illuminated base, notably greater than the rays would make which are transmitted in straight lines through the two holes.

For the experiment to succeed there should be bright sunlight because, as has been said, the holes should be very small, especially the first one, and also the white surface on which the base is received should be at a great distance from the hole, otherwise the base is received should be at a great distance from the hole, otherwise the base observed is either not at all or only a little larger than the base deduced by calculation.

Further it should not be omitted that the illuminated base appears in the middle suffused with pure light, and at either extremity its light is colored, partly reddish, partly also strongly bluish.

Comment: "The discovery of diffraction and its successful mathematical analysis became most important arguments in favor of the wave theory of light. Light can be diffracted, meaning 'broken away' from its rectilinear path" (Linksz). Diffraction is a fundamental property of light, though not apparent when the wave front is relatively unrestricted. The image of a point is always a diffraction disk, which in contrast to other aberrations decreases in diameter as the size of the aperture increases. Hence, for the best visual acuity the pupil must be neither too small nor too large. For pupillary diameters between 3 and 5 mm. the resolving power of the eye is fairly constant.

The mathematics of the diffraction pattern was investigated by R. Airy in 1834. The central disk receives 84 per cent of the energy transmitted and the successive rings receive 7, 3, 1.5 and 1 per cent respectively. The diffraction patterns of the different waves of white light are superposed and the resultant image is characterized by variously colored rings. Because the threshold of the light-adapted eye is so high the rings of the diffraction pattern do not register and their overlapping is ignored. The situation is otherwise in dark adaptation and the increased sensitivity then present is consequently detrimental to the perception of fine detail.

Under proper circumstances certain structures of the eye can act as a diffraction grating and induce a diffraction spectrum seen as halos. When a normal eye observes a small bright source in dark surroundings a physiological halo is perceived produced by the radial structure of the crystalline lens. In such halos the angular diameter of the outer red ring is about 7°. The large halos produced by mucus on the corneal surface,—with a diameter up to 14°—is due to the distance of this source from the retina. Edema of the deeper layers of the corneal epithelium, as occur in acute glaucoma and photophthalmia, gives rise to vivid halos. The size of a glaucomatous halo varies from 7° to 12°, presumably because the edematous globules formed vary in size as the attack progresses, small droplets producing larger halos.

If parallel lines are etched closely on glass the rulings absorb the rays while the very narrow strips of unscratched glass allow the light to pass through. With white light this grating produces a diffraction spectrum in which the colors are uniformly distributed according to the difference in wave length, while in a prismatic spectrum the longer waves are crowded and the shorter waves are spread out.

No microscope can resolve details that are closer together than one-third of a wavelength of light because of the overlapping of diffraction disks from adjacent elements. With ordinary light this limit of resolution is realized with a magnifying power of 800, with which an eye having an acuity of 20/20 can just distinguish an interval of 0.19 micron. In microphotography using ultra-violet light of 275 millimicrons wave length the resolving power is nearly double.

References

Linksz, A.: Vision. New York, Grune & Stratton, 1952.
Emsley, H. H. and Fincham, E. F.: Diffraction halos in normal and glaucomatous eyes. Trans. Opt. Soc. *23:* 4, 1921–22.

Biographical Note

Francesco Maria Grimaldi (1613–1662) was born and died in Bologna, Italy. In 1632 he became a Jesuit and for 25 years taught literature and mathematics. His chief interest, however, was in natural science. He made a chart of the moon and we owe to him much of the lunar nomenclature. With Newton and Huygens he inaugurated the first great era in the study of light. He first described and named the phenomenon of diffraction in a 16-page brochure that was published posthumously in 1665 three years after Grimaldi's death. Robert Hooke, in 1672, independently communicated similar observations to the Royal Society of London. More than a century elapsed before it was realized that the strongest possible argument for the wave theory of light lay in this discovery.

Bifocal Spectacles

BENJAMIN FRANKLIN
Philadelphia, Pennsylvania

To George Whatley   Passy, 21 August, 1784.

Your eyes must continue very good, since
you can write so small a hand without spectacles. I cannot distinguish a letter, even of
large print, but am happy in the invention
of double spectacles, which serving for distant objects as well as near ones, make my
eyes as useful to me as ever they were. If all
the other defects and infirmities were as
easily and cheaply remedied, it would be
worth while for friends to live a great deal
longer, but I look upon death to be as necessary to our constitution as sleep. We shall
rise refreshed in the morning.

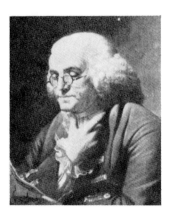

B. Franklin

To Benjamin Franklin   London, 15 November, 1784.

I have spoken to Dolland about your invention of double spectacles,
and, by all I can gather, they can only serve for particular eyes, not in
general.

George Whatley

To George Whatley   Passy, 23 May, 1785.

By Mr. Dolland's saying that my double spectacles can only serve
particular eyes, I doubt he has not been rightly informed of their construction. I imagine it will be found pretty generally true, that the same
convexity of glass, through which a man sees clearest and best at the
distance proper for reading, is not the best for greater distances. I therefore had formerly two pairs of spectacles, which I shifted occasionally,
as in travelling I sometimes read, and often wanted to regard the pros-
pects. Finding this change troublesome, and not always sufficiently
ready, I had the glasses cut and half of each kind associated in the same

94

circle. By this means, as I wear my spectacles constantly. I have only to move my eyes up or down, as I want to see distinctly far or near, the proper glasses being always ready. This I find more particularly convenient since my being in France, the glasses that serve me best at table to see what I eat not being the best to see the faces of those on the other side of the table who speak to me; and when one's ears are not well accustomed to the sounds of a language, a sight of the movements in the features of him that speaks helps to explain; so that I understand French better by the help of my spectacles.

B. Franklin

Comment: In the Franklin bifocal the lenses for distance and for near were cut across, the two parts being held together simply by the frame. An improvement, the "perfection bifocal," changed the design by fitting the reading correction into a semicircular cut-out of the distance glass. One hundred years after Franklin's invention, in 1884, came the cement bifocal in which the presbyopic addition was cemented to the spherical surface of the distance lens by Canada balsam, a substance having almost the same refractive index as crown glass. This bifocal was inexpensive and allowed the near correction to be changed readily, but the wafer was conspicuous, its edge collected dust, and the cement tended to separate. The cosmetic fused and one-piece bifocals followed; the Kryptok in 1908, the Ultex in 1910. After the expiration of their patents, "flat-top" segments with a short optical radius (distance from optical center of segment to its upper edge) were introduced (Panoptik, Fulvue, Univis-D, Ultex-K). These segments permit myopes of moderate degree to wear bifocals with less discomfort, and their minimal "jump" is helpful to workers who move about much and read only occasionally such as waitresses, saleswomen and taxi drivers. On the other hand, reduction of displacement in the reading field is desirable for professional and sedentary occupations and this can be accomplished in hyperopia by the appropriate selection of segments of longer optical radii; and in high myopia by adding to the flat-top segments "slab-offs" (prism base up in the bifocal area). Occupational bifocals with a large near-vision field and a distance window is preferred by dentists and book-keepers. Three types are available: the inexpensive Rederite, which can be recommended only when the distance correction totals less than one diopter; extra large Ultex segments (AA); and "minus adds" in which the near correction is flint glass and the distance window is a fused crown-glass segment. Bifocals in anisometropia pose a special problem because of the prismatic differential in looking down. Not infrequently the presence of a natural anisophoria simplifies the solution. Otherwise optical compensation can be effected by dissimilar segments, slab-off, or prism in the segment. In anisometropic myopia when binocular vision is not necessary and the correctable acuity of each eye is good, instead of bifocals, the less myopic eye may be fitted for distance and the more myopic eye for near.

Reference

Lebensohn, J. E.: Practical problems pertaining to presbyopia. Am. J. Ophth., *32:* 22, 1949.

Biographical Note

Benjamin Franklin (1706–1790) was born in Boston, and after only four years of formal schooling became a printer's apprentice at age 12. Starting in Philadelphia as an independent printer he rapidly prospered and at age 23 purchased *The Pennsylvania Gazette* from which the recent *Saturday Evening Post* claimed lineal descent. Three years later he launched *Poor Richard's Almanack* which has since been translated into 15 languages. Its aphorisms are still quoted such as: "No man e'er was glorious who was not laborious"; "What signifies knowing the names, if you know not the nature of things." The community-minded Franklin inaugurated in the colonies the first lending library, the first police force and the first fire department. He also helped in founding the Pennsylvania Hospital, the University of Pennsylvania and the American Philosophical Society. The general recognition of Franklin's political and executive gifts made him ambassador of the colonies to Great Britain and later to France and also a member of the Continental Congress and the Constitutional Convention. Before leaving for France at age 70 he gave the Continental Congress a personal loan of about 4000 pounds. His various diplomatic missions required a prolonged sojourn abroad, totalling 16 years in London and 9 years in Paris. He consequently became the most cosmopolitan spirit of his age and knew more men of eminence in science, letters and politics than any other man of his time.

Franklin retired from business at age 42 to devote himself to science. For six years he did so exclusively and his scientific interests continued to occupy the intervals of his subsequent varied activities. Franklin was concerned with every sort of natural phenomenon including many phases of medical science. His detailed studies in electricity, culminating in the famous experiment identifying lightning and electricity, established firmly his place as a scientist. Honorary degrees were bestowed upon him by universities at home and abroad, M.A. from Harvard, Yale, and William and Mary, LL.D. from Edinburgh, D.C.L. from Oxford; and he became an honorary member of the Medical Society of London and the Royal Medical Society of Paris. The French translator of his scientific works, Barbeu Dubourg, did much to facilitate Franklin's reception in France. Science was the one activity which Franklin pursued from some compelling inner impulse. He was a true child of the Enlightenment. His last public act was to sign a memorial to Congress for the abolition of slavery.

Reference

Pepper, W.: *The Medical Side of Benjamin Franklin*, 122 pp. W. J. Campbell, Philadelphia, 1911.

On the Manufacture of Glass for Optical Purposes

MICHAEL FARADAY, F.R.S

PHIL. TRANS. ROY. SOC. LONDON, 1830, 120: 1–57

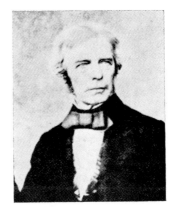

Perfect as is the manufacture of glass for all ordinary purposes, and extensive the scale upon which its production is carried on, yet there is scarcely any artificial substance in which it is so difficult to unite what is required to satisfy the wants of science. Its general transparency, hardness, unchangeable nature and various refractive and dispersive powers render glass a most important agent, but when the philosopher desires to apply it in the construction of perfect instruments, it is found liable to certain imperfections. These are so important and so difficult to avoid, that science is frequently stopped in her progress by them.

It must be well known to the scientific world, that these difficulties have induced some persons to labor hard and earnestly for years together, in hopes of surmounting them. Guinand was one of these: and died engaged in it in the year 1823. Fraunhofer labored hard until science was deprived of him also by death. But the public are not in possession of any instruction, relative to the method of making a homogeneous glass fit for optical purposes, beyond what was possessed before their time.

A room and furnaces were built at the Royal Institution in September 1827. At first, the inquiry was pursued principally as related to flint and crown glass; but in September 1828 it was directed exclusively to the preparation and perfection of peculiar heavy and fusible glasses, from which time to the present continual progress has been made.

Process of Manufacture

The general properties which render glass so valuable as an optical agent, are easily obtained: but there is one condition essential in all delicate cases of its application, which is not so readily fulfilled; this is, a perfectly homogeneous composition and structure. Many a disk, which upon the most careful examination has appeared perfectly free from striae and quite uniform, has been found incapable of giving a good image on account of the existence of irregularities in the mass which still produce a confused effect.

Besides these, there are other faults in glass. Occasionally appearances are observed in it, which seem to indicate crystallization, or an irregular tension of its parts: these, there is every reason to believe, may be avoided by careful annealing. Bubbles are not usually considered as of much consequence, but objectionable when the glass is looked at, rather than when looked through. In practice, it is said that no other real evil than loss of light is dependent on them.

Of all these faults, that of the irregularity constituting streaks, striae and waves, is the most difficult to avoid, and the most injurious in its effect. It is not an improvement that is required, but absolute perfection, a homogeneity equal to that of pure water. Crown glass consists of silica, lime, sometimes a little alkali, and small quantities of other matters: these substances are not very different in their refractive powers, and when fused do not produce very strong streaks. Again: the specific gravity of the different materials used is not very different so that the mixing agencies which affect the contents of the pot are more energetically exerted, and the whole mass approaches nearer to uniformity in a given time.

With flint glass many circumstances are altogether different. Oxide of lead enters into its composition to the amount of one-third of its weight, or more, and by its presence gives that proportion of refractive and dispersive power, which makes the glass valuable in conjunction with crown: and it makes the glass heavy also, because of its own great specific gravity. A third property, namely its high fluxing or dissolvent power, it also confers upon the glass. Now these three properties are unfortunately very conducive to the formation of striae.

The difficulties introduced into the manufacture of flint glass fit for optical uses compelled the subcommittee to consider seriously the possibility of making other glasses than those ordinarily in use, which, at the same time that they had the high dispersive power enabling them to replace flint glass, might have also such fusibility as would allow of their being perfectly stirred and mixed.

The borate of lead, and the borate of lead with silica, were the substances which, after some trials, were found to offer such reasonable hope of success as to justify a persevering series of experiments. The glass with which I have principally worked is a silicated borate of lead, consisting of single proportionals of silica, boracic acid and oxide of lead.

It appears that this very heavy glass has the power of developing the color of mineral substances far beyond what flint glass possesses; just as flint glass surpasses in the same property crown glass. The utmost care is necessary to preserve all the materials from metallic contamination.

The heat should not be raised too high or the operation hastened, and then the ebullition will proceed very gradually and favorably, the rough materials being by degrees converted into glass. Before the first charge is entirely melted a second is put in, and when that is fused down, sometimes a third. When all is fused, the temperature is allowed to rise; the glass is then well agitated and mixed by a platina stirrer.

Experiments were made on the means of cleansing the entering air; consisting merely of a plug of clean dry sponge into the end of the tube, which, at the same time that it allowed sufficient air to pass, seemed, from the appearance of the tube afterwards, to have excluded every impurity.

There are two conditions of the finished glass, each of great importance. The most essential is the absence of all striae and irregularities of composition; the other, the absence of even the most minute bubbles. The first is obtained by agitation and perfect mixture of the whole; the latter, principally by a state of repose. Hence a mixed process has been adopted.

The heat which has to be borne during the operation of stirring is very considerable, especially upon the hands; but at such a moment no retreat from the work, because of mere personal inconvenience can be allowed. But the circumstance renders the use of a cover for the stirring hand very advantageous.

For entering upon the considerations relative to the bubbles, it will be evident that these are at first very numerous. It occurred to me that its formation might be hastened and the final separation advanced by mixing some extraneous and insoluble substance with the glass, to act as a nucleus.

The substance I resorted to for this purpose was platina in the spongy state. It was found to assist powerfully in the evolution and separation of bubbles, and afterwards to sink so completely to the bottom, that not a particle remained suspended in the mass.

We can at pleasure obtain a glass perfectly free from striae, unexceptional in hardness, and with less color than crown glass.

A great variety of glasses have been formed by the use of different proportions of ingredients. The specific gravity rises very high; often 6.4, double that of some specimens of flint glass. As the proportion of oxide of lead diminishes, so also does the specific gravity lessen, and it is in some of the specimens as low as 4.2.

The refractive and dispersive powers of the glasses increase with their specific gravity, as was to be expected. The refractive index for maximum yellow, ascertained by Mr. Herschel, for the borate of lead glass was 2.0652; and for the silicated borate of lead, 1.8735.

One important circumstance connected with the application of these glasses is their color. The usual color is more or less yellow, and is perhaps almost altogether dependent upon the presence of a little iron.

There is one very important action of the glass upon light which may perhaps interfere more with its application, i.e., its reflective power. This is very strong in all the heavy glasses, far stronger than in flint, and exceedingly surpassing the similar power of crown glass.

In hardness, these glasses differ from each other as much as in any other quality. The borate of lead is very soft; the biborate of lead is harder, and the triborate equal to flint glass in hardness. The silicated borate of lead is softer than flint glass.

The superficial changes of glass which interfere with its optical uses are of two kinds. The one is shown by a tarnish upon its surface, which when strong is iridescent. It is quickly produced by the intentional presence of sulfureted hydrogen, which acting upon the oxide of lead present, reduces it, and forms a sulfuret of lead. In plate glass the change is of another kind, and is shown by the appearance of minute crystallizations, which spread obstructing the light.

A very curious and important influence of alkali in facilitating the tarnish of glasses containing oxide of lead, was discovered during the course of these investigations. Ordinary flint glass consists of 33.28 oxide of lead, 51.93 silica, and 13.77 potassa. Provided the alkali be away, the quantity of oxide of lead may be enormously increased; and a glass containing 64 per cent of oxide of lead, in combination with 36 per cent of silica, has not tarnished by an exposure for 18 months on the same shelves with flint glasses that have tarnished.

Hence the reason why the absence of alkali has been earnestly insisted upon in the preparation of the ingredients for the heavy optical glasses.

If a small quantity of flint glass be very finely pulverized in an agate mortar, then placed upon a piece of turmeric paper, and moistened with a drop of pure water, strong indication of free alkali will be obtained. The same effect is produced by using plate glass. Glass may be considered rather as a solution of different substances one in another, than as a strong chemical compound; and it owes its power of resisting agents generally to its perfectly compact state, and the existence of an insoluble and unchangeable film of highly silicated matter upon its surface.

An extraordinary difference exists between the electrical relations of this glass and other glasses, due principally to the same absence of alkali.

Ordinary glasses freely conduct electricity under common circumstances. Thus if a gold-leaf electrometer be diverged, and then touched with them, the electricity is instantly discharged. If a similar experiment be made with these heavy glasses, they have no sensible power of discharging the electricity, but insulate as perfectly as sealing wax or gum lac. Hence the glass may probably be found hereafter to answer many useful electrical purposes. But the great point at present is the proof which such electrical properties give of the absence of that film of moisture which is so constant upon other glasses.

The corrosion or crystallization which takes place principally upon plate glass, is doubtless also due to the alkali present.

Comment: The varieties of fine optical glass now available were achieved only after more than a century of labor and costly research. Without them neither the quality microscopes nor the high grade ophthalmic lenses of today would be possible. Though Faraday toiled four years on this project (1825 to 1829), the new glasses that he produced were but a laboratory success as their commercial manufacture was apparently not feasible. However, his pioneer work had a directive influence on all subsequent investigations. Signal results of practical importance were finally attained through the happy collaboration of the optical physicist, Ernst Abbe and the glass manufacturer, Otto Schott. Their experiments, which extended from 1880 to 1885, demonstrated that the incorporation of sundry new elements into the glass melt led to many desirable variations in refractive index and dispersive power. Whereas refractive index and dispersive power are simultaneously increased by lead, both properties are decreased by boron and fluorine, while barium oxide increases the refractive index much more than the dispersive power. The tendency of glass to crystallize can be minimized by the addition of zinc oxide, alumina or magnesia.

The optical glass for ophthalmic lenses is first rolled into plate glass form. This method, an American innovation, has proved superior for spectacle lenses. Since 1934 American research laboratories (Eastman Kodak Company, Corning Glass Works and Haywood Scientific Glass Corporation) have studied further the optical properties of glass in relation to chemical composition, experimenting with rare elements such as thorium, lanthanum and titanium. Lanthanum effectively contributes to higher refractivity without increasing the dispersion. These projects have resulted in 17 additional types of valuable optical glass. As these rare-element borate glasses are very corrosive to standard pot refractories, platinum lined pots must be used—a technic that recalls Faraday's work. The new high-index glass (1.70/55) is a significant improvement over prewar dense barium crown (1.61/57).

References

Kingslake, R. and De Paolis, P. F.: Sci. Monthly, *68:* 420, 1949.
Lebensohn, J. E.: Arch. Ophth., *16:* 284, 1936.
Obrig, T. E.: *Modern Ophthalmic Lenses and Optical Glass.* New York, Chilton Company, 1935.

102

Michael Faraday (1791–1867) was born near London and had but meager schooling. When 22 years old he left his employment as bookbinder, at which he had worked since the age of 10, to become the assistant of Sir Humphry Davy at the Royal Institution. After an experiment on the liquefaction of chlorine, 13 glass fragments were removed from his eye. He continued intensive research in chemistry, optics and especially electricity for over 40 years. He proved the identity of electricity from different sources, discovered induced electricity, developed electroplating and demonstrated the interrelation of magnetic and electric forces. The idea of the interconvertibility of the forces of nature dominated him. Ampere had caused electricity to produce magnetism. Faraday, believing that the converse should be true, in 1837 caused magnets to elicit a current of electricity,—from which experiment the giant turbo generators of today have evolved. This same intuition led Faraday to the discovery of magneto-optical relations. He found that if a bar of his heavy glass was freely suspended by a silk thread between the poles of a powerful electro-magnet, the bar would point across the magnetic lines of force, a property that he christened diamagnetism. With his heavy glass he demonstrated also that a magnet could rotate the plane of polarized light, the effect depending on the strength of the electro-magnet and the direction of the current. Clerk Maxwell credited Faraday with the first conception of the electromagnetic theory of light.

Faraday had an abiding interest in optics. For nearly 30 years he was the official scientific advisor on lighthouses. In 1831 he discussed the illusions of movement and showed how pictures of successive phases of motion could give the impression of continuous movement and, on the other hand, that an object in motion might be seen stationary or with its motion reversed when watched through the cogs of a revolving wheel, observations that inspired the much later inventions of the cinema and stroboscope.

Faraday rarely made mistakes notwithstanding the immense amount of his published researches. Helmholtz said: "It is the highest degree astonishing to see what a large number of general theorems, the methodical deduction of which requires the highest powers of mathematical analysis, he found by a kind of intuition, with the security of instinct, without the help of a single mathematical formula." Faraday contributed to the scientific vocabulary anode, cathode, diamagnetic, dielectric and electrolysis and in turn his memory is honored by the term farad, used to denote the unit of electrical capacity. He had an exceptional gift of popularizing science. Charles Dickens, then editor of Household Words, asked for an account of his lectures on the breakfast table and of those addressed to children.

References

Kendall, J.: *Michael Faraday, Man of Simplicity*. New York, Roy Publishers, 1955.
Randall, W. L.: *Michael Faraday*. Boston, Small, Maynard & Company, 1924.

Astigmatism

FRANS CORNELIS DONDERS, M.D.

Utrecht, Holland

EXCERPTED FROM *On the Anomalies of Accommodation and Refraction of the Eye,* CH. VIII, PP. 449–556, LONDON, 1864

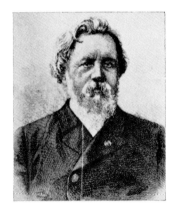

Sometimes it happens that in the several meridians of the same eye the refraction is very different. This aberration, dependent on an asymmetry of the eye, may be designated astigmatism. By the word astigmatism, used without more precise definition, regular astigmatism will be understood.

The theory of refraction by asymmetrical surfaces was developed by Sturm in 1845. He showed that when a homocentric bundle of light falls on a convex asymmetrical surface, after the refraction it no longer continues homocentric, but that the refracted fasciculus of rays forms a certain skew surface which is bounded by lines intersecting in space at right angles in different planes. Sturm assumed that the focal interval, which is the result of asymmetry, should make any accommodation of the eye for different distances superfluous. This opinion no longer needs refutation.

We do not call regular astigmatism abnormal until it attains to such a degree that the accuracy of vision perceptibly suffers from it. For equal lengths of the focal interval, this is the case sooner, in proportion as the pupil is larger.

1. The disturbance manifests itself first, when stripes of different directions lying in the same plane have to be distinguished.

2. There exists a certain indifference for spectacle-glasses of nearly equal power. It is impossible to make a definite choice. This phenomenon led me long ago to suspect that the diminished acuteness of vision, often peculiar to hypermetropia, might be dependent on abnormal astigmatism.

3. The diffusion-image of a point of light alters. This is already the case in the ordinary degree of regular astigmatism but at high degrees

103

thereof it is particularly striking. In such we soon find a spherical glass, with which a point of light at a distance exhibits itself as a stripe of light, and at the same time a modifying spherical glass which, placed over the first, makes the stripe of light assume a precisely opposite direction. In the required strength of this modifying glass we possess a means of determining the degree of astigmatism.

4. The alternating distinctness of such stripes is very striking, while on a line, which cuts the two opposite stripes at an angle of 45°, it has scarcely any influence.

5. Lines of equal length in the two opposite directions do not appear equally long: a square exhibits itself as an oblong.

6. If the direction of the principal meridians is known, a narrow slit is rotated before the eye, first in the direction of one principal meridian, then in that of the other. In these two meridians, the strongest convex lens, or the weakest concave one by which the best distant visual acuity can be gotten, is to be employed. The degree of astigmatism is obtained by the difference of refraction in the two meridians. If emmetropia or hypermetropia be present in one of the meridians, it is well, so as to obtain a very exact result, to previously paralyze the accommodation by means of atropine.

7. Determination of astigmatism by the optometer often produces variable results, because of the difference of accommodative power of both meridians in two successive examinations.

All the above phenomena we may observe in ourselves. The only thing necessary for this purpose is to make the eye astigmatic, and this is effected by holding a cylindrical lens before it.

In the anomaly under consideration, the subjective examination first presents itself. Absence of the normal acuteness of vision supplies the first indication. We must now determine in what direction the principal meridians are situated. For this purpose we make use of a remote point of light. Subsequently, we obtain a still better result by determining in what direction of the axis of the most neutralizing cylindrical glass the patient sees best. What is the state of refraction in each of the principal meridians? This appears from the strength of the positive or negative glass, with which in each of these meridians the greatest acuteness of vision is obtained. The determination is unattended with difficulty when a certain degree of myopia exists in both principal meridians. But if hypermetropia be found this knowledge is accurately obtained only during artificial paralysis of accommodation. The degree of astigmatism is found from the difference of refraction in the two principal meridians.

Abnormal astigmatism is to be considered as a higher degree of the same asymmetry which belongs to normal eyes: similarity of the seat and conformity of direction of the principal meridians in the two cases afford the proof thereof. As to the normal, the cause is in general to be sought in the cornea; and the direction of the principal meridians, for the whole dioptric system, as well as for the cornea in particular, is of that nature, that the meridian of maximum of curvature usually approaches to the vertical. For the abnormal degrees of asymmetry the same rules obtain. What is more, they here present still less of exception. Precisely the high degree of this asymmetry explains, why it preponderates over the influence of the lens. The investigations recently carried out with Dr. Middleburg have supplied me with proof, that with a high degree of asymmetry of the cornea asymmetry of the crystalline lens exists, acting in such a direction, that the astigmatism for the whole eye is nearly always less than that proceeding from the cornea.

In using cylindrical glasses the eye, in order to maintain the acuteness of vision, is somewhat limited in its movements. However, every spectacle-glass, as such, necessarily causes limitation, and, in fact, experience shows that in the use of cylindrical glasses this is productive of no particular inconvenience.

Airy discovered abnormal astigmatism is his own left eye. At the same time he conceived that a cylindrical glass might correct the asymmetry, which he actually found to be the case. The form of his astigmatism was the compound myopic. He correctly gave preference to a negative spherico-cylindrical glass, whereof the concave spherical surface was to correct the common myopia of the two principal meridians, the concave cylindrical the still remaining astigmatism. In truth, bi-cylindrical glasses are never necessary; they may always be advantageously replaced by spherico-cylindrical glasses.

Astigmatism is often hereditary. Not unfrequently one of the parents labors under the same defect. More frequently still, different children, born of the same parents, exhibit this anomaly, and mostly in the same form. In the majority of instances both eyes are affected. When a high degree of ametropia occurs only on one side, asymmetry of the bones bounding the orbit is a very common phenomenon. Slight cases first present themselves when the range of accommodation is perceptibly diminished, while in high degrees of astigmatism the disturbance is early remarked.

Illustrative Case Reports

Simple myopic astigmatism. A student of divinity, now 21 years of age, consulted me three years since, because of amblyopia. Finding no improvement, the patient ceased his visits. Some weeks ago he again presented himself. His power of vision was so defective that he feared he should not be able to continue his studies. I immediately suspected that astigmatism, previously overlooked by me, must exist in this case. The acuteness of vision was, for the right eye 1/4, for the left eye, 1/5. Negative lenses improved the sight but comparatively little. We therefore proceeded to the trial with the point of light. The right eye saw the point of light as a line inclining nearly 30° outwards. The left eye presented a remarkable correspondence with the right. Here too the vertical principal meridian inclined about 30° outwards. The case described is one of the thousands, in which astigmatism has been looked upon as amblyopia, and has been treated as such. If the aimless treatment was only vexatious to the patient, his joy, when he found his sight at all distances improved by suitable glasses, was indescribably great.

Compound myopic astigmatism. In the following case the patient had not been aware that she saw less acutely than other people. I therefore think it probable that Young also, whose astigmatism was of about the same degree, incorrectly ascribed perfect acuteness of vision to himself. My patient drew and painted very respectably. She was loud in her commendation of the advantage obtained from a cylindrical glass; little pictures especially were with it seen much more acutely. So far I had never yet combined a cylindrical surface with a bifocal. Such a combination cannot, however, in my opinion, produce any inconvenience.

Hypermetropic astigmatism. Most cases of abnormal astigmatism belong to the hypermetropic form. Those eyes are also most subject to the highest degrees of astigmatism. With this a great degree of asthenopia is connected. For a short while large print can still be read, but soon fatigue, and even pain, occurs. One of my patients recorded the following: "My occupation is that of a clerk. The first effort to work was the most painful. After that my work went on somewhat better, but I found it impossible to work all the forenoon; I was constantly obliged to leave off. At the end my eyes were painful, and I felt best when I walked for a considerable time in the open air, out of the sun." He got 2.25 C✕ 90 in each eye to work with and to wear. Thereupon he communicated to me: "On using the spectacles I found, even on the first day, an incredible improvement (his acuteness of vision was, in fact brought from 2/7 to 3/4. Next day I experienced no painful affection, and I found it easy to work uninterruptedly the whole morning. I saw everything infinitely sharper. In the evening I experienced not the slightest inconvenience from the light. In the open air, too, I am free from pain. Spectacles which I had tried before (ordinary spherical glasses) had been of no use to me."

Abnormal Irregular Astigmatism

Astigmatism may also be recognized as the result of corneal diseases, but in such cases it is usually associated with much irregular astigmatism. The same is the case when, through partial luxation, the crystalline lens attains an oblique position. If a portion of the lens disappears from the pupillary area, a high degree of irregular astigmatism becomes one of the results.

Until a short time ago I thought acquired astigmatism of little importance. I supposed that cylindrical glasses would not remedy the disturbance of vision. The result has, however, proved the contrary. In the case of a central speck upon the cornea, I performed iridectomy and obtained a well-formed pupil. Nevertheless, the acuteness of vision was very imperfect. I tried the combination of a convex sphere with a cylindrical glass and ordinary print could now be read. The existing astigmatism may be resolved into a regular and irregular astigmatism, and after correction of the regular, the irregular causes less disturbance. After the extraction of cataract, too, the cornea often acquires a form, which gives great value to the combination with a cylindrical glass.

Comment: Donders was the first great ophthalmologist to investigate assiduously the problems of refraction and the first to impress upon the profession the prevalence and importance of astigmatism. His initial paper on this subject, which appeared in von Graefes Archiv, 1860, 7: 176, introduced the term, "Astigmatismus," to the German language.

The primary discoveries relating to astigmatism were made by physicists and mathematicians. In 1670 Newton noted the astigmatism of oblique bundles of rays. Euler, who flourished in the generation after Newton, worked out the currently used general formula of the power of cylinders at various angles from the axis. The first scientific use of a cylindric lens was made by Fresnel in 1819 for the purpose of obtaining a luminous line. Young, while using his own optometer based on the Scheiner principle, was the first to reveal and measure the astigmatism of a human eye in 1801. In 1827 the astronomer, Airy, first utilized a cylinder for the correction, fitting a spherocylindrical lens for the compound myopic astigmatism of his left eye. In 1829 Airy reported a change in this eye; both the myopia and astigmatism had diminished. He referred to the latter as "a geometrical phenomenon to which the term astigmatism was very happily affixed by the present master of Trinity College, Rev. Dr. Whewell." Edward Jackson and Swan Burnett, however, preferred "astigmia," as this term is etymologically more correct and harmonizes with all other words relating to the optical condition of the eyes, such as myopia, asthenopia, esophoria, exotropia and so on.

The articles of Airy stimulated intellectuals in England and America to note their own astigmatism and to attempt correction. In 1828 John McAllister of Philadelphia ground a plano lens with a concave cylinder axis horizontal for Rev. Goodrich, which was the first ever made in this country.

The ophthalmometer of Helmholtz, invented in 1854, permitted an accurate determination of the radii of the principal meridians of the cornea. Calculation showed that each millimeter of difference of these radii produced 6 diopters of astigmatism. Extensive use of the Helmholtz ophthalmometer by Donders enabled him to demonstrate in 1860 the hitherto unsuspected prevalence of significant corneal astigmatism. To learn the total astigmatism, Donders used an optometer provided with a stellate figure and measured the foci of the principal meridians. In 1862 Donders published in Dutch a 136-page monograph on "Astigmatism and Cylindrical Lenses," which was forthwith translated into German by Schweigger and into French by Dor. As a consequence of this work, cylinders were henceforth added to the trial case.

After ascertaining the principal meridians by the changes in the apparent form of a remote point of light after the successive application of spherical lenses, Donders then determined the refraction in each meridian through the use of the stenopeic slit. His book is, in the words of Duke-Elder, "one of the few classics that have caused a revolution in ophthalmology." Ophthalmologists flocked to Utrecht to study under the great Donders. After John Green arrived in 1865, he was inspired to devise a more reliable test for the detection and measurement of astigmatism. The astigmatic charts in optometers had been unsatisfactory because of the disturbing influence of accommodative efforts. To eliminate this factor Green introduced large test diagrams, hung on the wall at a distance of 20 feet. Among the variety of charts he devised are radiating lines, rotating dials and duplicated, triplicated and dotted lines.

Javal and Schiøtz perfected an accurate but simplified ophthalmometer in 1884 which encouraged the examination for astigmatism, and the prescribing of cylinders soon became widespread.

A paralysis of accommodation caused by diphtheria led Edward Jackson to read Donders. This masterwork so fascinated him that he gave up general practice for ophthalmology and soon became the Donders of America. His "Skiascopy and its Practical Applications to the Study of Refraction," published in 1896, clarified the technique of retinoscopy and emphasized its importance. In 1893 he announced his cross cylinder test as a superior subjective method for determining the amount of astigmatic error, and in 1907 he described the even more valuable cross cylinder test for astigmatic axis. Mounting familiarity with the shadow test and the cross cylinder caused the ophthalmometer to follow into desuetude the optometer and the stenopeic disk as equipment for measuring astigmatism.

References

Lebensohn, J. E.: The story of astigmatism. Sight-Saving Rev., *30:* 139, 1960.
Lebensohn, J. E.: The correction of astigmatism. Eye, Ear, Nose and Throat Month. *39:* 885, 1960.

Biographical Note

Frans Cornelis Donders (1818–1889) was born at Tilburg, North Brabent, Holland, the son of a merchant who died a year later. Of the nine orphans, he was the only boy. After receiving his medical degree from the University of Leyden, he lectured on physiology at the School of Military

Medicine at Utrecht. In 1845 he became editor of two leading Dutch medical journals. In his physiologic research he specialized on the eye and contributed studies on the movements of the eye, entoptic visual phenomena, prismatic spectacles, the association of accommodation and convergence and regeneration of the cornea. In 1848 he joined the University of Utrecht, where he taught ophthalmology and general biology. In his inaugural address he spoke on evolution, reviving the theories of Lamarck, but adding, independently of Darwin, the idea of natural selection. "Organic beings adapt themselves to the circumstances in which they are placed or perish." Continuing his interest in the eye, he wrote on the causes of squint, micropsia and colored vision. When the Chair of the Ophthalmic Clinic became vacant, Donders was persuaded to devote himself to clinical ophthalmology. To qualify himself further, he studied with Bowman in London, at whose home he met Albrecht von Graefe in August, 1851. Although his ophthalmic practice flourished, his scientific investigations continued and produced notable articles on the variation of accommodation with age, the imbibition of cornea and sclera and the development of cilia. Among his disciples was J. A. Moll, the discoverer of the "glands of Moll." The Netherlands Hospital for Diseases of the Eye was built for him in 1858 through public subscription—an indication of his popularity and influence. His famous book was based on the dissertations he included in the annual reports of the hospital. After its publication in English, it was translated into German by Otto Becker, into Italian by Quaglino and into French by de Wecker. Donders published a revised summary thereof in Dutch in 1869. In 1862, Donders assumed the chairmanship of the Department of Physiology and made Snellen, his former pupil, the acting head of the hospital. After his retirement at age 70, he revisited London. While in that city he suffered a stroke, and on March 24, 1889, he passed away.

Reference

Connor, R.: Donders. Detroit M. J., *12:* 274, 1912.

Headaches from Eye Strain

S. WEIR MITCHELL, M.D.

Philadelphia, Pennsylvania

AM. J. M. SCI., 1876, *71:* 363–373

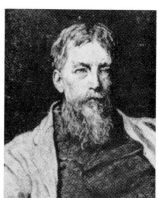

During the year 1874, I called the attention of the profession to the cerebral symptoms resulting from disorders of the refractive or accommodative apparatus of the eye. Many of the patients treated successfully by the correction of optical defects never so much as suspected that their eyes were imperfect. What I desire to make clear is—

1. That there are many headaches which are indirectly due to disorders of the refractive or accommodative apparatus of the eyes.

2. That in these instances the brain symptom is often the most prominent and sometimes the sole symptom of the eye troubles, so that while there may be no pain or sense of fatigue in the eye, the strain with which it is used may be interpreted solely by occipital or frontal headache.

3. That the long continuance of eye troubles may be the unsuspected source of insomnia, vertigo, nausea, and general failure of health.

4. That in many cases the eye trouble becomes suddenly mischievous, owing to some failure of the general health, or to increased sensitiveness of brain from mental causes.

The form of head-pain to which I refer is certainly not of the nature of migraine, and, as it soon disappears when the eyes are corrected, is lacking happily in the obstinacy of that distressing malady. The following cases illustrate the propositions I have stated. First I put the following case, because it was the one which opened my eyes on this subject.

Case 1. A prominent merchant consulted me for pain in the upper spine and occiput. It increased every winter, and left him during the summer, which was spent in shooting and fishing. He was aided by nothing I did. Some friend suggested that his eyes might be weak, and he consulted Dr. William Thomson, who gave me the following particulars: "Writing has become so distressing to this gentleman, that for a year past all letters have been written by a secretary, at his dictation. It was suspected that this would prove to be a case of compound astigmatism. On paralyzing his accommodation with atropia, this was found to be correct." On using these glasses habitually, his distressing symptoms quickly disappeared; he has long since forgotten his apprehensions of an impending apoplexy; he can see as sharply as any, and he can use his eyes continuously in any near work.

The following case will show how profoundly the whole system may be perturbed by an ocular defect.

Case 2. An accomplished and energetic single lady, aged 30, began some five years ago to have evening headaches, pain in the back of the head and neck, sense of extreme fatigue and violent flushing if she persisted in writing or reading. Unfortunately a portion of her income depended upon her ability to write. I confess that for nearly two years I looked everywhere but to her eyes for the cause of mischief. At length I asked her to consult an ophthalmologist. Dr. Thomson sent me the following note: "Vision, R.E. 20/20, L.E. 20/30. Refraction under atropine indicated the following correction: R.E. +0.75 S/+0.75 C x 90, 20/20; L.E. +0.87 S/+1.12 C x 90, 20/20. No muscular insufficiency." When I saw this lady six months later, the change in her appearance was remarkable. The headache left early, and with it went the sleeplessness. Once able to slumber, the body swiftly repaired damages, and a general gain in flesh, color, and strength were the results.

Case 3. A housewife, aged 35, suffered from neuralgic pain in the eyes and head, which was never relieved by any method of treatment. This pain would be induced by a visit to any brightly lighted place of amusement, or by an effort to read at night. No relief would follow until she slept. Dr. Thomson reported that her vision was R.E. 20/40, L.E. 20/40. Refraction under atropine indicated the following correction: R.E. +1.50 S/+0.75 C x 75, 20/20; L.E. +0.87 S/+1.50 C x 90, 20/20. She reports that there is no strain with the glasses on in reading even at night and that she has had but one or two slight headaches.

Case 4. A woman, aged 36, stated that at 16 years of age she had typhoid fever, and that since that time she has been unable to use her eyes for any near work. During the past years she can only glance over the headings in the newspapers. She cannot read ordinary print for more than half a minute without pain, which, if she persists, becomes a severe headache that continues for hours. Dr. Thomson found: Vision, R.E. 20/25, L.E. 20/100. Refraction under atropine indicated the following correction: R.E. $+0.75$ S/$+0.75$ C x 60, 20/20; L.E. $+2.00$ C x 100, 20/20. A relief from pain followed in a short time upon the constant use of the correction. Her photophobia disappeared and she was able to read for several hours daily. Who that had not seen it could believe that the correction by glasses of the eye trouble could have given a relief so speedy and so perfect that she herself described it as a miracle?

Case 5. A well nourished intelligent lady, aged 27, consulted me for certain nervous troubles, pain in the back and intense and frequent headaches. The nervous symptoms usually followed her headaches, and consisted in slight but prolonged hysterical states. Almost every day she had severe headache, usually frontal, increasing towards nightfall. Other means failing, I came to suspect there was an optical disorder. The following are Dr. Norris's notes of the ocular condition: "Visual acuity, R.E. 20/200, L.E. 20/30. Refraction: R.E. -2.25 S/-1.12 C x 90, 20/20; L. E. $+2.25$ S/$+0.75$ C x 90. I ordered R.E. -1.12 C x 90; L.E. as noted. With these glasses she has been able to write and read with comfort, and has entirely lost her headaches." The relief given in this case was almost immediate.

Case 6. A single woman, aged 22, complained that for five years past she has been obliged to abandon any useful occupation and most of her amusements, in consequence of severe neuralgic headaches, much aggravated by any attempt to use the eyes. If she persists in using her eyes, these symptoms are accompanied by nausea and vomiting. She has never had any pain in her eyes. Dr. William F. Norris found: Vision each eye, 20/100. Refraction under atropine indicated the following correction: R.E. $+1.50$ S/$+5.00$ C x 105, 20/40; L.E. $+0.75$ S/$+4.50$ C x 75, 20/30. She was directed to wear them from the time she gets up till she goes to bed. Six weeks later she stated that the headache and nausea had entirely disappeared, and that she can employ herself in reading, writing, and sewing like other people.

Case 7. A lady, 40 years of age, of nervous temperament had been annoyed with an indistinctness of vision and slight pain in the eyes, which were attributed to severe headaches to which she was subject. The headache was almost constant, but was more violent after an attempt to use the eyes in any near work. Dr. Harlan found that she needed the following correction: R.E. -1.25 C x 180, 20/30; L.E. -1.50 C x 15, 20/30. As the power of accommodation was found deficient, another pair of glasses was ordered for reading. In a few weeks she wrote that her eyes were quite at ease, and the headaches had disappeared.

Case 8. A young woman, aged 16, found that she had headaches which came only upon use of the eyes. I advised that her eyes should be corrected, but as her family physician insisted that she could not be suffering suddenly from what had always been present, she was easily persuaded to yield to her own dislike of glasses. After a year more, she came back to me with an addition to her symptoms of occasional un-steadiness of gait with sudden sense of vertigo. The headaches were no better. Of late, too, her rest was disturbed by dreams. I could only urge anew the correction of the eyes, and persuaded her to wear her glasses steadily. Soon the vertigo, headaches, and insomnia passed away. In a month she was able to sew, write, or read for hours at a time.

There is an ocular vertigo as well as an aural vertigo. Usually it comes only after the eye trouble and some other cause of general weakness have made the intra-cranial circulation unstable. Such as are in sturdy health are often able for years to overcome, without sense of strain, muscular difficulties in binocular accommodation, and to endure un-harmed astigmatism with accommodative troubles. But with increase of years their powers fail. Or else it chances that to one of these comes an attack of illness, or a time of over-work with worry, when at once the eye trouble leaps into prominence, and once felt is felt more and more by a brain which, in the language of the photographer, I might aptly describe as having become over-sensitized. The following case attests the truth of my statement.

Case 9. A lawyer, aged 51, was in good health until September 7, 1874. At this time he experienced the most intense anxiety, owing to the extreme illness of a near relative. From this time he began to have certain head troubles on reading or writing. After using the eyes an hour, the pain became fixed on the vertex, and lasted all day. I felt sure he had ocular defects, and asked him to see an ophthalmologist. Dr. William Thomson writes as follows: "This gentleman informed me that for the past five days he had not been able to read at all. He had never used glasses except for near work. The acuity of each eye was 20/30. Refraction under atropine indicated the following distant cor-rection: R.E. +0.87 S/+0.62 C x 120, 20/20; L.E. +0.87 S/+0.62 C x 120, 20/20. His old sight was likewise corrected. One month later, he reported that he could not dispense with the distant glass, and that with the others he could use his eyes all day without any pain, and considered himself entirely relieved." This case seems to me in all ways instructive. The symptoms were such as to point rather to cerebral troubles than to the eyes as the cause of distress; the comparatively slight character of the optical defects and the rapid relief from glasses are all worthy of consideration.

The accommodative effort needed in hypermetropia, especially with astigmatic trouble, is extreme, owing to the instinctive craving for

114

distinct vision—and hence the source of fatigue. The use of the eyes is so incessant that it is impossible for the victims, by any means save glasses, to put the eyes at rest. A low degree of hypermetropia may not be detected in persons under 40 without the use of atropia since the power of accommodation must be paralyzed.

Comment: The discomfort resulting from errors of refraction or from ocular muscle imbalance originates primarily from irritation of the trigeminal nerves supplying the eyeball. In a sensitive individual, the irritability is diffused and headache is experienced referred from the meningeal branch of the fifth nerve. As the connections of the trigeminal nucleus are particularly extensive, the irritability may likewise diffuse to the splanchnic nerves, and reflexly maintain functional gastric disorders. Dr. Charles G. Stockton, in his contribution to Osler's Medicine, states: "Most frequently the causes of gastric asthenia are to be found in eyestrain. The subject has been so widely discussed in America that it is somewhat threadbare; yet its signal importance remains largely disregarded. Asymmetrical astigmatism is the defect most often responsible, but it is not always in astigmatism of high degree that the trouble arises. It is most commonly found in instances of moderate degree of astigmatism with axes differing in the two eyes, and especially in anisometropia. The nervous disturbances following these visual defects are apt to appear after the age of puberty, and are especially active when the crystalline lens begins from age to lose its pliability."

Gastric disorder of asthenopic origin may manifest itself in disturbances of secretion, motion or sensation with resulting heartburn, belching, nausea, anorexia or constipation. Evidence from the laboratory has both confirmed and clarified the nature of this reflex effect. Using a stomach balloon connected with a water manometer, Lebensohn (1929) made tracings to demonstrate the effect on gastric motility of astigmatic errors and muscular imbalances artificially produced by the wearing of cylinders and prisms, respectively. Such errors were shown to exert a definite depressive effect on the motor function of the stomach. Release from inhibition occurred regularly upon the removal of the asthenopia-producing irritant.

References

Lebensohn, J. E.: Oculovisceral reflexes. Am. J. Ophth., *12:* 562–568, 1929.
Gould, George M.: *Biographic Clinics.* Rebman, London, 1903.

Biographical Note

Silas Weir Mitchell (1829–1914) was born in Philadelphia, the seventh physician in three generations of his highly cultured family. At the University of Pennsylvania, his record was poor, for he had an aversion to certain required subjects, especially mathematics. In 1850 he graduated from Jefferson Medical School and forthwith boarded a clipper ship for a year in Europe. His interest in physiology prompted him to study under Claude Bernard from whom he learned high standards of research. After Mitchell's return to Philadelphia he soon acquired a large practice but still carried on scientific investigations. In 1853 he was admitted to the Academy of Natural Sciences, in 1857 he helped launch the Pathological Society in Philadelphia, and in 1887 he initiated the founding of the American Physiological Society to which he annually donated sums for prize essays. Before the Civil War he contributed a toxicologic study of snake venoms. The War was a turning point in Mitchell's career. From his experience as head of a military hospital for nervous diseases came his most valuable monograph on *Injuries to the Nerves and Their Treatment* (1872). The book was the first complete study of ascending neuritis, traumatic neuroses, traumatic neurasthenia and psychic phenomena after amputations. Mitchell was the first to describe causalgia (1864) and erythromelalgia (1872). He confirmed Rolando's view that the cerebellum augments and reinforces movements initiated by the cerebrum. The relation of eyestrain and astigmatism to headaches and other neurotic symptoms was first suggested by him in 1874 and amply confirmed by William Thomson in 1879. The extent to which small, rather than gross, errors of refraction can create poor health was constantly emphasized by George M. Gould, Mitchell's most ardent apostle in this field, in numerous writings. Mitchell's assertion that "Many neural diseases are pictures painted on a hysterical background" anticipated Charcot and Freud. Although Mitchell became the most prominent figure in early American neurology, he occupied himself with literary as well as professional pursuits. He wrote popular treatises, fiction, drama, verse, essays and juvenile stories. In *Wear and Tear* he called attention to the indisposition of Americans to play, and to the increase in nervous disorders that inevitably followed. The historical novels, *Hugh Wynne* (1897), *Adventures of François* (1898) and *The Red City* (1908) are considered his best works. Mitchell's complete poems were published in 1914.

Mitchell was a tall, vigorous man with a distinctive face and fertile mind. He was probably the most versatile American since Benjamin Franklin. Yet he had one keen disappointment—he never obtained an official university position. Among his intimate friends were Oliver Wendell Holmes, Williams James, Walt Whitman, Andrew Carnegie, John Shaw Billings, Osler and Noguchi. To medical history Mitchell contributed studies on instrumental precision, and on Harvey.

Mitchell's early investigations included an experimental contribution to ophthalmology, concerning the production of cataracts by injection of sugar into the dorsal subcuticular sac of frogs. Mitchell never wore glasses through his life span of 85 years, as one eye remained essentially emmetropic while the other developed a convenient degree of myopia.

References

Earnest, E. P.: *Weir Mitchell, Novelist and Physician*. University of Pennsylvania Press, Philadelphia, 1950.

Snyder, C.: Silas Weir Mitchell and research in ophthalmology. Arch. Ophth., *67:* 528–530, April, 1962.

A Contact-lens

ADOLPH EUGEN FICK

Zurich, Switzerland

Arch. Ophth., 1888, *17:* 215–226*

Among the numerous diseases of the cornea, there are many which change its normal form, and accordingly vision suffers. Attempts have been made to correct the optical error due to keratoconus by hyperbolic and conical glasses; the practical improvement obtained is insignificant or nil. In defects of vision due to irregular corneal astigmatism, Donders recommended stenopaic glasses. He and his pupil, von Wijngarden, demonstrated that the improvement of vision was often astonishing, and that the narrowing of the visual field did not occasion disturbance in near vision, as, for instance, in reading and writing. For distant vision, stenopaic glasses cannot be used, since a patient with a greatly contracted field and good central vision would be much worse off than one with poor vision and a field of normal extent.

Searching for another means of correcting the different forms of irregular corneal astigmatism cannot be regarded as superfluous. The most radical means would be to replace the cornea by another surface of regular curvature. This can actually be done; I have succeeded in excluding the defective cornea by a small glass shell, and thus, without narrowing the field of vision have increased the acuteness of vision. However, I could not advise the possesor of this eye to use the remedy, which I call "a contact-lens", because the fellow eye was normal. If I publish my views before any patient is wearing the "contact-lens" it is because I am justified in stating that, as a result of my studies, I have solved the principle of the problem.

The "contact-lens" consists of a thin glass shell, bounded by concentric and parallel spherical segments. It is placed upon the eye, and the interspace between it and the eyeball is filled with a liquid having the same refractive index as the cornea. I began my observations upon animals in order to ascertain whether and how long the eyeball would suffer a contact-lens to be placed upon it without suffering injury. Large rabbits proved to be admirably adapted for these experiments. Plaster-of-Paris casts of the eyeball showed that the radius of curvature of the cornea

---

* Translated by Charles H. May, M.D., New York.

did not differ materially from that of the sclera, and that the eyeball of the rabbit is pretty nearly a perfect sphere. Then I had small glass globes blown, 21, 20 and 19 mm. in diameter, and a segment separated, the base of which was distant but a few millimeters from the equator. It was found that well-fitting glasses adhered to the globe. Hence it follows that the glass accompanies the eyeball in all its movements and that not a drop of the liquid escapes. It is impossible to distinguish an eye supplied with the glass from the naked eye, unless a careful examination be made. After six to eight hours there is quite a change in the picture, owing to milky clouding of the liquid. If the glass be removed, the epithelium of the cornea appears slightly clouded and the conjunctiva shows moderate injection.

The cause of the clouding of the cornea is found in its epithelium. If a little of the clouded epithelium be scraped off and examined after staining, the cells show fat-globules in greater or lesser quantity. The injection of the eyeball disappears with rapidity after removal of the glass. The injection is apt to be absent in those rabbits which have been utilized in a long series of experiments. Apparently, a sort of toleration is established.

That clouding of the liquid is partly due to corneal epithelium in a state of fatty degeneration, is evident from what has been stated. The problem was to find a liquid which would cause as little irritation as possible to the cornea. This could only be discovered by numerous trials. Finally a two-percent solution of grape sugar was found to answer all requirements. A well-fitting glass filled with sterilized two-percent solution of grape sugar is borne by the rabbit's eye for eight to ten hours without the production of any apparent clouding of the liquid, and with no clouding of the cornea or injection of the conjunctiva. I would also say that any possible injection of the conjunctiva will disappear within half an hour, and any corneal clouding in the course of the night.

In order to obtain properly fitting contact-lenses for the human eye, I resorted to taking plaster-casts again—naturally of the eye of the cadaver. The cast of a human eye shows plainly that the cornea is the segment of a sphere of smaller radius of curvature than the rest of the globe. The next step was to have a glass vesicle made which fitted upon the periphery of the plaster cast; then a portion of this small globe was heated and a protrusion blown out. A segment was separated and the broken edge was made smooth by melting. Such a glass was placed in the conjunctival sac of my left eye; I wore it for two hours without any other subjective symptom, except some flow of tears. The liquid between the cornea and the glass remained clear, and contained, as the microscope showed, only a few organized elements. Other persons subjected themselves to experiment; and as subsequent trials proved still more satisfactory in relation to the subjective and objective disturbances than the first had, I concluded to have the contact-lens ground. Prof. Abbe, in Jena, was kind enough to fulfil my request. The formula in the construction of a contact-lens is the following: A glass cornea, having a radius of curvature of 8.0 mm. rests upon the glass sclera; the latter has a breadth of 3 mm, and a radius of curvature of 15 mm. The weight of the contact-lens is about 0.5 gram.

Introduction is best accomplished by seizing the small glass between the index finger and thumb of the right hand, at the same time lifting the upper lid of the patient's eye with the left, and requesting him to look down; now the glass is pushed beneath the upper lid, and whilst the patient looks up and thus carries the contact-lens upward, the lower lid is drawn forward somewhat, and the contact-lens adjusted to the eyeball. In order to supply the liquid: While the patient lifts the upper lid, the upper portion of the margin of the lens is slightly drawn from the eyeball by a squint-hook, and with the unemployed hand the sugar solution, warmed, is allowed to drop upon the eyeball from a pipette with bent extremity. To remove the lens again, it is only necessary to lift the lower margin of the glass with a squint-hook, while the patient is looking up, and then to have the patient look down; during the downward movement the lens becomes detached and is caught in the patient's handkerchief. If the lens fits well, the patient does not complain, has no flow of tears, and either has no injection of the ocular conjunctiva, or very little. If symptoms of irritation show themselves, the glass must be removed. The irritation is usually produced by the margin of the glass sclera rubbing against the lid during movements of the eyeball. Despite clumsy manipulation on the part of the patients, injury to the corneal epithelium did not occur in a single case.

Possibly contact-lenses will be worn for cosmetic reasons. Those eyes which are deformed by leucomata can be changed so that they no longer attract attention, by the use of a contact-lens upon which the iris and a black pupil is painted.

Comment: In 1827, following the announcement by Airy of the correction of his own astigmatism, the English astronomer, Sir John Herschel, first suggested the possible use of a glass shell placed on the cornea to nullify irregular corneal astigmatism. The idea proved impracticable until the discovery of local anesthesia by Koller in 1884. Three years thereafter, in 1887, the concept was revived simultaneously and independently by Fick of Zurich who introduced the term "contact-lens"; by August Mueller of Kiel, a medical student with a myopia of −14 D., who sought a substitute for his strong spectacles; and by F. A. Mueller of Wiesbaden, a maker of artificial eyes, who evolved for Prof. E. T. Saemisch of Bonn a blown shell with a central transparent cornea to protect an eye with lagophthalmos.

The present public interest in contact lenses dates from 1929, when at the International Congress of Ophthalmology, Prof. Heine of Kiel reported his experience in substituting contact lenses for unsightly spectacles. After methyl metacrylate plastics were invented, Theodore Obrig and Ernest Mullen worked out the process of making contact lenses from this material in 1938. Within a year the substitution of plastic for glass had gained almost universal acceptance. Contact glasses at this time were of the scleral type, and consisted of a spherical corneal portion with a diameter of 12 mm. surrounded by a peripheral scleral rim having a diameter of 20 mm. The comfortable fitting of the scleral rim was all-important but not always successful. The fluid in this helmet-shaped device had to be changed frequently; otherwise Fick's phemonenon, now better known as Sattler's veil, developed—a mistiness of vision, usually accompanied by seeing colored halos around lights. This resulted from corneal edema due to impaired circulation of tears and oxygen to the cornea.

A significant step forward was the advent of the Tuohy corneal lens in 1948. It consisted of a round plastic disk, the inner surface of which touched the cornea at its center while the rim stood out slightly to allow the free passage of tears. The precorneal film provided enough capillary attraction to permit the lens to adhere quite strongly. The design proved too simple; the lids felt the edge of the corneal lens and blinking often dislodged it completely. Moreover, because of the corneal contact, some epithelial erosion was not infrequent. Among the modifications designed to overcome these drawbacks are the vented lens (1953), the microlens (1954) and the contour lens (1955). A lenticular form of the corneal contact lens has enabled aphakic corrections to be fitted more successfully. The Lacrilens and the similar Invisalens are nonfluid, corneoscleral types, vented to provide lacrimal irrigation.

The improvements in contact lenses have been accompanied by a marked expansion in their use and a corresponding increase in professional interest. Contact lenses should only be fitted to strongly motivated patients. Adaptive symptoms are trying but usually subside in a few days if the lenses are worn 2 or more hours daily. After fitting young persons the power of the contact lens should be checked under cycloplegia—a procedure too seldom used. The eyes must be checked every 3 to 4 months to rule out corneal trauma. Among the ocular contraindications are chronic blepharoconjunctivitis or ocular allergies, entropion or trichiasis, marked epiphora or excessive dryness of the eyes, corneal disease or neuroparalytic state, marked exophthalmos or local neoplasm.

The nonoptical uses of contact glasses are important. For concealing a disfiguring corneal scar a contact glass with a black pupil is simpler than tattooing and the results are more cosmetic and more permanent; likewise, a blind squinting eye can be thus given a normal appearance.

References

Lebensohn, J. E.: Contact glasses. Hygeia, *15:* 717, 1937.
Obrig, T. E., and Salvatori, P. L.: *Contact Lenses,* Ed. 3. Obrig Laboratories, New York, 1957.
Agatson, H., Barnert, A. H., and Feldstein, M.: Corneal lenses in ophthalmic practice. Am. J. Ophth., *49:* 277, 1960.
Welsh, R. C.: Contact lenses for aphakics. Arch. Ophth., *64:* 251, 1960.

Biographical Note

Adolf Eugen Fick (1853–1937) taught and practiced in Zurich, Switzerland. Shortly after the beginning of World War I, however, at the age of 63, he volunteered for duty with the German army as medical officer. He commanded military hospitals in France and in Russia until taken prison of war in the Crimea. Upon his release he settled in Herrshing am Ammersee, a suburb of Munich, and occupied himself with popular writing for the lay press. His ophthalmologic contributions include monographs on the microorganisms of the conjunctiva (1887) and on skiascopy (1891). In 1888 he designed an applanation tonometer, which was widely used until superseded by the impression tonometer of Schiötz in 1905. Applanation tonometry has been revived recently by Hans Goldmann, also of Switzerland, who combined Fick's method with slit-lamp observation, and has shown that with this technique the findings in the lower levels of elevated ocular tension are more reliable than with the Schiötz instrument. His manual of ophthalmol (German edition, 1894) was a well illustrated compact book of 488 pages, which emphasized the whys and wherefores. It was translated into English by Arnold B. Hale of Chicago, who considered it the most suitable of extant texts for students, in 1896. Fick contributed to the second edition of the Graefe-Saemisch Handbuch the articles on blindness and on ocular hygiene (1918).

Reference

Obituary (unsigned). Klin. Monatsbl. Augenh., *98:* 812, 1937.

A Metric System of Numbering and Measuring Prisms

CHARLES F. PRENTICE

New York, New York

ARCH. OPHTH., 1890, *19:* 64–75; 128–135

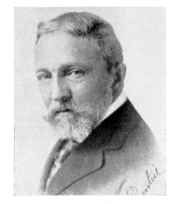

The present method of designating prisms by the angular deviation of their refracting surfaces, is open to the objection that we thereby define only an isolated feature of their construction, to the utter disregard of the varying powers of refraction, which must result from the use of refracting substances having different indices.

With a view of securing greater accuracy and uniformity in our utilization of the refractive properties of prisms, the following system of numbering, which I believe to be feasible, as well as suited to the requirements of ophthalmologists, is presented.

The prismatic refraction is in inverse proportion to the distance at which the unit deflection is produced, being fully in harmony with the refraction of a lens, which is in the inverse proportion to the distance at which the image is formed.

Provided, therefore, a standard amplitude of deflection be adopted as the unit, and which shall be measured in a plane one meter from the refracting surface of the prism, we shall be enabled to designate prisms, in dioptries, for instance, with the same significance as in lenses.

Thus prisms of two, three or four dioptries will produce the same unit deflection at one half, one third, or one quarter of a meter, respectively.

We shall also find the same prisms to produce two, three, or four times the unit deflection *in the meter-plane*, so that the problem reduces itself to the selection of a series of prisms which shall produce tangent deflections, at this distance, which are multiples of the adopted unit.

Supposing the chosen unit of deflection to be exactly equal to 0.01, or one centimeter, our series of prisms would then be:

1^Δ producing a tangent deflection $= 1$ cm. in the meter-plane.

2^Δ " " " " $= 2$ cm. " " " "

3^Δ " " " " $= 3$ cm. " " " "

A system of numbering prisms in terms of dioptries (to be designated as Prism-Dioptries, ($^\Delta$) could therefore be adopted which would satisfy all the conditions here set forth.

Such prisms could be measured by noting the deflection they produce upon the index line of a coarse centimeter scale, placed at right angles to the line of sight, at the distance of one meter.

If the scale were rendered adjustable, relatively to a vernier, it would be possible to determine fractional parts of the unit deflection.

The Prism Mobile, which consists of two prisms rotating before each other in opposite directions, will afford the most ready means of filling a demand for definite deflections, inasmuch as the rotation of the prisms, from 0° to 180°, produces all possible deflections from one millimeter upward. The instrument could easily be graduated to read to centimeters, and tenths, or millimeters of deflection. For the determination of muscular insufficiencies of comparatively low degree, and to render the instrument as light as possible, a special cell, to contain weak rotating prisms, could be devised, similar to that of Dr. Risley, to fit the trial frame.

I may venture to assert that the prism, although the simplest element in Dioptrics, is the most difficult to manufacture, when required to be *exact*; and we shall therefore be obliged, for the present at least, to use existing commercial prisms for spectacle glasses.

By actual experiment I have found prisms, represented as being of one degree (1°), to produce deflections varying between 9 and 12 millimeters, and which, if reduced to the basis of our standard of one centimeter, are to be designated as 0.9 and 1.2 dioptries, respectively.

For each pupillary distance, we find a different prism necessary to supplant the meter-angle. This is but natural, since greater demands for convergence will be necessary in wide than in narrow pupillary distances.

This leads us to the final and simple rule:

Read the patient's pupillary distance in centimeters, when half of it will indicate the prism-dioptries required to substitute one meter-angle for each eye.

One could scarcely hope for a more convenient method than to find the prism-dioptries, corresponding to one meter-angle, expressed in the patient's features.

The Relation of the Prism-Dioptry to the Lens-Dioptry of Refraction

Some of the advantages of the prism-dioptry, as the unit of measure for the refraction of simple prisms, having been shown, and whereas prisms are frequently combined with spherical lenses, it is here proposed to further consider the relations of the prism-dioptry to such combinations, as well as to the equivalents which are to be obtained by a mere decentration of the spherical lenses themselves.

Thus prepared we may proceed to a consideration of the prism-dioptry.

Supposing a lens to be 1 D., and the deflection sought to be 1 cm. = 1^Δ, at the meter plane, which corresponds to the focus of the lens, it would require a decentration of one centimeter to produce this result.

A lens of 2 D., being decentered the same amount, would produce a tangent deflection equal to *1 cm. at its focus, half a meter,* which would be equivalent to 2 cm. at the meter plane, or 2^Δ, it having been shown that the prismatic refraction is in the inverse proportion to the distance at which the unit deflection is produced.

A lens of 2 D., limited by its size to a decentration of 3 mm., will afford 0.6^Δ. A lens of one half or one third the power will require to be decentered twice or three times as much to secure the same number of prism-dioptries.

We have consequently but to remember that *the prism-dioptries in decentered lenses are in direct proportion to their refraction and decentration.*

Our present lenses will, however, not permit of a decentration of 1 cm., owing to their limited size, yet, if required, larger ones could be furnished the trade at a comparatively small increase in cost, which could be utilized specifically in corrections involving prism-dioptries.

However, in cases where the size of the lens proscribes the limits of decentration, it becomes necessary to add to it a constant prism. Since the slightest decentration of a simple lens is certain to produce a prismatic effect, it is evident that the *constant* value of any prism, which it may be desired to add to a lens, will only be retained when the optical axis of the lens strictly coincides with the visual axis.

The effect of decentration will naturally be to increase or diminish the prismatic action of the constant prism, which has been combined with the lens.

Supposing a 5 D. lens to be combined with a 2 D. prism, the former being decentered 2 mm., by shifting the visual axis toward the apex of the prism. We know that a 5 D. lens will produce 5^Δ when decentered 1 cm., and therefore will produce 0.2 of 5^Δ when decentered 2 millimeters, which is equal to 1^Δ. The constant prism of 2^Δ has therefore been increased by 1^Δ, making it 3^Δ. A decentration of the lens to an equal amount in the opposite direction will leave but 1^Δ for the entire combination.

Two millimeters have in this case affected the value of the constant prism by 50 % of its active function.

We can now realize the importance and necessity of an accurate adaptation of spectacles, with regard to the pupillary distance, when high spherical corrections are resorted to.

The prism-dioptry and the meter-angle being directly dependent upon the pupillary distance, it behooves us, in any endeavor to secure accurate results, to be exceedingly particular as to its measurement.

Dr. Maddox, in his exhaustive work on prisms, calls attention to a unique, most simple, and accurate device for determining it.

Dr. Stevens having fully shown the disturbances occasioned by hyperphoria, I may here be permitted to call attention to the danger of artificially producing it by improperly centering the lenses in the vertical meridian in a simple case of hyperopia in which no real hyperphoria exists.

We shall admit that the lenses are decentered vertically, in opposite directions, by 5 mm. above and below the horizontal plane, which will be equivalent to a decentration of one of the lenses by 1 centimeter, provided the other is properly centered.

Our hyperope being corrected by lenses of 2 D., would under these circumstances, be forced to overcome 2^Δ at the meter plane, and therefore a vertical diplopia of 12 centimeters at 6 meters.

Inversely, in making Dr. Stevens' test for hyperphoria, in emmetropia for instance, supposing a means to be devised to enable the patient to exactly indicate the distance between the images which he sees at a 6-meter distance. Admitting, by way of illustration, that he has decided them to be 6 centimeters apart, vertically, which, being equivalent to 1 cm. at 1 meter distance, will lead us at once to decide that a prism of 1^Δ, properly placed before the eye, will correct his *manifest* hyperphoria. The same patient would have to struggle with a vertical diplopia amounting to $3\frac{1}{3}$ mm. at a reading distance of $33\frac{1}{3}$ cm., being quite sufficient to cause consecutive lines of type to appear intermingled with each other.

As a third demonstration, supposing it to be desired to afford binocular vision to an emmetrope at a distance of $\frac{1}{3}$ of a meter, *without his powers of accommodation or convergence being called into requisition.* His pupillary distance being 60 mm., for instance, half of it will be 3 centimeters, which gives us 3^Δ for his meter-angle, making 9^Δ requisite to set aside his convergence to $\frac{1}{3}$ of a meter, while 3 D. of lenticular refraction are necessary to substitute accommodation for the same distance. A 3 D. lens would require to be decentered 3 cm. to afford 9^Δ, so that a pair of such lenses, placed before the eyes with their bases in, would accomplish the desired stereoscopic result. Two properly centered lenses of 3 D. combined with 9^Δ would serve the same purpose.

The above illustrations suffice to show the value of the prism-dioptry in leading to our conception of the actual work performed by prisms at different distances, and which the prevailing degree-system of numbering must continue to keep us in ignorance of.

Besides, a degree-system of numbering prisms cannot be brought to a convenient relation to any of the following points, which have been shown to exist in favor of the metric system:

1. A direct relation between the meter-angle and the prism-dioptry for variable pupillary distances.

2. A direct relation of the prism-dioptry to the lenticular dioptry, for any amount of decentration of lenses.

3. Simple measurement of the pupillary distance determining the prism expressing the meter-angle.

4. All fractional intervals of the prism-dioptry being rendered available for differing pupillary distances.

5. The prism-dioptry being capable of measurement by a simple instrument.

6. The resultant deflection produced by similarly placed superimposed prisms being equal to their sum expressed in dioptries.

7. Can be applied to existing commercial prisms, without increasing the cost or revolutionizing the present market.

A possible objection to the new system of measuring might arise in the fact that it does not define the minimum deviation, yet, as the prisms used in spectacles are of small angles, and as long as it is understood that prisms of greater angle are to be held with one side parallel with the base-line, from the eye, which is the case in measuring by the instrument, we obtain the desired uniformity.

Comment: The diopter unit was introduced by Monoyer in 1872. Previously, the power of a lens was expressed in the inch system with *one* as the numerator and the focal length in inches as the denominator. Prisms continued to be numbered by their refracting angle in degrees, though Edward Jackson had advocated a designation according to their deviation. The prism-diopter nomenclature that Prentice suggested was adopted by the Ophthalmic Section of the A.M.A. in 1891 and by American manufacturers in 1894. Since then both lenses and prisms are known by the work they perform. Prentice championed the superior value of the prism-diopter over the meter-angle as a measure of convergence and the usefulness of the prism-diopter conception in relation to the decentration of lenses. The triangle sign is appropriately symbolic of the compound word, prism-diopter, as it suggests both the principal section of a prism and the letter delta. Since the decentration of a spectacle lens should be confined to its nonaberrational area, it must not exceed 4 mm. Prentice preferred base-up in the correction of hyperphoria since the internal reflections near the base of a prism are then less noticeable because of the habitual downward use of the eyes. For the same reason a vertical prism prescribed in a bifocal segment should likewise be base-up. Thanks to the law of decentration elucidated by

126

Prentice, optical compensation for anisometropia can be done as effectively but with less expense by prescribing appropriate dissimilar segments. A theoretical objection to the prism-diopter as a unit of measurement is that 20 prism-diopters is 0.27^Δ less than 20 times one prism-diopter, but up to 20^Δ the difference is too slight to be of ophthalmic importance.

References

Prentice, C. F.: Lenses and prisms, ophthalmic. American Encyclopedia of Ophthalmology, Vol X, pp. 7233–7406. Cleveland Press, Chicago, 1917.
Lebensohn, J. E.: The management of anisometropia. Eye, Ear, Nose & Throat Month., *36:* 217–222, 1957.

Biographical Note

Charles Frederick Prentice (1854–1946) was born in Brooklyn, N. Y., and graduated in mechanical engineering from the Royal Polytechnicum, Karlsruhe, Germany, in 1875. He abandoned this vocation in 1882 to join his father's lucrative optical business where his technical training proved a great asset. He soon became recognized as an authority on ophthalmic optics through his original articles published in the leading ophthalmic journals. In 1886 he wrote a treatise on ophthalmic lenses and in 1917 contributed on this subject to eight volumes of the American Encyclopedia of Ophthalmology. He was the first to develop the formulae for converting obliquely crossed cylinders to the equivalent sphero-cylindrical combination (1888). This was later simplified to a graphical method by S. P. Thompson (Philos. Mag., 1900, *49:* 316–324). The prism-diopter system as well as the designation of lens power according to the back vertex refraction, which was advocated by him in 1915, are now in universal use. In 1897 he introduced the reading slit under the name "typoscope", a device that has proved extremely serviceable to many with incipient cataract. His friends included many distinguished ophthalmologists—Noyes, Stevens, Herman Knapp, Casey Wood and Swan Burnett. He was the first American optician to charge a professional fee for an eye examination. As he never approved of the term optometrist adopted by the New York Optometry Law enacted in 1908, he called himself a "physical eye specialist". He retired in 1921 and spent his final years between Florida and his home in Nelson, British Columbia, where he died at the age of 92.

Reference

Prentice, C. F.: *Legalized Optometry and the Memoirs of Its Founder.* Fletcher Press, Seattle, 1926.

The Crossed Cylinder

EDWARD JACKSON, M.D.

Philadelphia, Pa.

OPHTHALMIC RECORD, 2: 464–466, JUNE, 1893

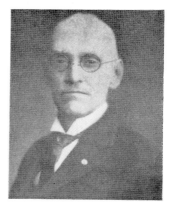

While this term applies strictly to any combination of cylindrical lenses with the axes perpendicular to one another, it is here intended to speak of such a combination of a convex cylinder and concave cylinder of equal strength, or their optical equivalent sphero-cylindrical lens, as a convex 1 D. cylinder combined with a concave 1 D. cylinder, axes perpendicular; or its equivalent, a convex 1 D. spherical combined with a concave 2 D. cylinder; or a concave 1 D. spherical combined with a convex 2 D. cylinder.

The advantage of such a lens in the use of the trial set, was referred to at the meeting of the American Ophthalmological Society in 1887. But the hint then given has not received the attention this matter deserves. It is the lens I use most constantly and would find most inconvenience from losing, of any in my trial set; and my assistants and students have come, by working with it, to place the same estimate on its value. It can, of course, be imitated by taking a convex and a concave cylinder from the trial case, placing them with their axes perpendicular and using in the manner to be presently indicated; but a combination that is used so constantly, in every case, whether hyperopic, myopic, or astigmatic, it is much better to have constantly at hand ready for use.

When we have placed before the eye a sphero-cylindrical combination of lenses, supposed to be approximately the correction, and wish to test it by varying its strength, it is perfectly easy to alter the strength of the spherical without in any way effecting the cylindrical factor of the combination. When, however, we attempt to change the strength of the cylinder by holding before it the proper convex and concave cylinders from the trial set, we at the same time alter the general convex and concave effect of the lens. And so, without the corresponding change in the spherical, we do not get simply a change of cylindrical effect, but a double alteration that may be very misleading.

This can best be illustrated by taking a special case. Suppose the combination hit upon to be a $+2D.$ spherical with a $+0.50$ D. cylinder, while the glass really required is a $+1.5$ D. spherical $\bigcirc + 1$D. cylindrical. The holding of a convex 0.5 D. cylinder in front of the first combination, would be certain to make the vision worse. And although just that additional strength is needed for the cylindrical, the natural inference from such a trial would be that it was not needed. The same difficulty about fixing the strength of the cylinder will be experienced so long as the proper strength of spherical has not been exactly obtained. And each error of the kind into which the surgeon is led entails a considerable loss of time in finding out it is an error and correcting it.

Of course, by using in every case both a convex and a concave cylinder and turning them each, first, to correspond with the axis of the cylinder already before the eye and then perpendicularly to it, such errors may be avoided. But besides the additional time this requires, the transition from the lens which improves the vision to the lens, which most remarkedly impairs it, requires a complete change of the glasses held before the eye, as well as a change of their direction, and the lost time, diminishes the force of the contrast between improvement and impairment, by which, the patient has to judge.

The use of the lens is simply, as has been indicated by the foregoing remarks, to hold in front of the approximate correction already placed before the eye and by alternately placing it so that it will first increase and then diminish the strength of the cylinder in the combination already fixed upon, to ascertain whether the cylindrical factor is of exactly the best strength.

The writer, instead of the actual crossed cylinder, has always employed the sphero-cylindrical equivalent with a concave spherical, and a convex cylindrical side. In this case, the axis of the cylinder marked on the glass corresponds with the axis of the convex cylinder that is increased by it, or is at right angles to the axis of the concave cylinder that it adds to.

The strengths found most generally useful in practice are the concave 0.50 D. spherical combined with the convex 1 D. cylindrical; the concave 0.25 D. spherical combined with the convex 0.5 D. cylindrical; and the concave 0.125 D. spherical combined with the convex 0.25 D. cylindrical. Of these three, the second is the most generally used. It is, however, best to have all of them and begin by using the strongest, unless vision equal to very nearly the full normal standard has been obtained by the combination first tried. Then, as the correction is made more and more accurate, the weaker lenses are to be employed in the same way.

Commonly, it is best to ascertain first that the strength of the spherical cannot be improved by any change; and then to use the crossed cylinder to fix the strength of the cylinder. But where the cylindrical portion of the lens is very strong, it may be better to reverse the order. First to ascertain, by turning slightly either way, where the cylinder in front of the eye gives the best vision, and then to use the crossed cylinder to correct its strength, before doing anything with the spherical part of the combination.

This matter may seem to be one of minute detail and small importance, but I have not known any one who had carefully tried it, who would be willing to work without the aid of such a lens, or who regarded it as a matter of little importance. This is its value even where the refraction of the eye is entirely constant under the influence of the mydriatic, but if one wishes to determine the strength of cylinder required without the use of the mydriatic, the crossed cylinder—indicating whether the cylinder supposed to be the proper one should be strengthened or weakened entirely independent of the accommodation of the eye, or at least of the regular accommodation of the eye—is quite invaluable.

Comment: Jackson's most important contribution to refraction was the perfection of the cross-cylinder. In the above article he proposed the cross-cylinder test for determining the precise amount of astigmatic error. In 1907 he announced the even more valuable cross-cylinder test for astigmatic axis, an application that was entirely original. Jackson's cross-cylinder was used quite differently from that first described by Stokes in 1849. Stokes noted that two cylinders of equal but opposite power neutralize each other when their axes are parallel; but if one cylinder is gradually rotated from this position, an astigmatic lens is formed of a power varying continuously from zero to twice the astigmatic power of either lens. After the cylinder is thus turned until it best suits the eye, a reference to a table gives the refractionist the information regarding the power of the indicated cylinder. The Stokes lens could only give an approximate measurement of well-marked astigmatic errors upon the basis of an axis previously established by other means as by the distortion noted in viewing a distant small circular light. The Stokes lens, as well as its later modification by Dennett, remained but a scientific curio except for its adaptation by Jackson as a malingering test. For this purpose Jackson placed in the trial frame a pair of 2.0 D. cylinders of opposite power with axes vertical over the admittedly good eye. Then while the subject, with both eyes open, viewed the chart, the outer cylinder was rapidly flipped 90 degrees. This created a lens equal to +2.00S/−4.00 C × 180 that reduced the vision of the good eye to less than 20/200, so that whatever was read registered the acuity of the other eye.

Jackson stressed that the cross-cylinder should be rotated while the subject was observing the smallest letters discernible through the instrument. The 0.25 D. cross cylinder is generally used, but the 0.12 D. or 0.50 D. cross-cylinder may be more useful when the acuity is above or below average

130

respectively. In aphakia, some use the 1.00 D. cross-cylinder. Though letters or figures are the usual test object, the accuracy of the test may be affected by the psychologic phenomenon that the distortion in which the vertical components are clear is preferred over the reverse. This difficulty is over-come by the concentric circles introduced by Verhoeff, now available in the Projectochart and in transilluminated near-vision slides. The examiner need but ask whether the circles are more perfectly round in the first or second position of the cross-cylinder. A highly accurate refinement in the determina-tion of axis is the Crisp-Stine test, used with the simple cross-dial in which the midpoint of one of the four arcs is marked by the apex of a small triangle. After the preliminary refraction, the eye is fogged 0.25 D. and both the trial cylinder and the triangular marker are placed at the presumed axis. The 0.12 D. cross-cylinder is applied, and the query is whether the cross-lines look more alike before or after the turn of the cross-cylinder. If the presumed axis was correct, the application of the cross-cylinder shows a contrast in the lines that is reversed on rotation of the instrument; if incor-rect; the axis of the trial cylinder is shifted towards that position of the cross-cylinder which makes the lines look more alike. With both the trial cylinder and the triangular marker at the same axis, the tests are repeated until the axis is precisely localized.

The cross-cylinder is absolutely indispensable to those familiar with its use. Nevertheless, the instrument is still but little known outside the United States.

References

Egan, J. A.: A resumé of cross cylinder application and theory. Surv. Ophth., *1:* 513–529, 1956.
Crisp, W. H.: Edward Jackson's place in the history of refraction. Am. J. Ophth., *28:* 1–12, 1945.

Biographical Note

Edward Jackson (1856–1942) was born in Chester County, Pennsylvania of Quaker ancestry, though he later became a Unitarian. After gradua-tion as civil engineer, he embarked on the study of medicine and received his medical degree from the University of Pennsylvania in 1878. While en-gaged in general practice, an attack of diphtheria, subsequently compli-cated by paralysis of ocular accommodation, shifted his interest to ophthal-mology. The background in engineering, as with Javal and Prentice, attracted him to physiologic optics. His writings, which included a book on Skiascopy (1905), contributed greatly to the perfection of refractive technique in America. In 1888 he was appointed Professor of Ophthalmology at the Phila-delphia Polyclinic at the age of 32; and in 1890 he became Surgeon at Wills Hospital. The advent of tuberculosis in his wife determined the departure of the Jackson family to Denver in 1894. After her demise two years later Jackson continued in Denver as he feared a predilection of his children to this dread disease.

Jackson was a leading figure in ophthalmologic societies and headed the Section of Ophthalmology, A. M. A., in 1894, the American Academy of Ophthalmology and Otolaryngology in 1903, and the American Ophthal-mological Society in 1912. Then, as now the optometrists were battling the medical refractionists, but with more reason. They pointed out that many physicians with little special training were doing refractions under legal sanction. To remedy this situation Jackson conceived a plan of extra-legal certification of ophthalmologists. His suggestions prompted the creation of the first such certifying agency, the American Board for Ophthalmic Examinations. The idea gradually spread to the other medical and surgical specialties so that a total of 20 examining boards are now functioning. Jackson devoted his life to the education of the American ophthalmologist. He was a founder of the Colorado Ophthalmological Society (1899), Professor of Ophthalmology at the University of Colorado (1905) and initiated in 1923 a two-week postgraduate course that became the prototype of similar enterprises all over the country. When Jackson became editor-in-chief of the present American Journal of Ophthalmology (third series) in 1918, he infused new life in the journal by combining with it the previously published Ophthalmic Record, Annals of Ophthalmology, Ophthalmology, and the Ophthalmic Yearbook and Literature which he had launched in 1904. An endless array of pointed editorials revealed his vast and brilliant erudition. Jackson was awarded the Lucien Howe Medal of the American Ophthalmological Society and was the first recipient of the Leslie Dana Medal for special achievement in the prevention of blindness. The instruction program of the American Academy of Ophthalmology and Otolaryngology was inspired by him. At the 1942 session in his 87th year he gave a course on office management, just 15 days before his death.

Reference

Crisp, W. H.: Edward Jackson, student and teacher. Am. J. Ophth., *26:* 1–12, 1943.

Mechanism of Accommodation*

ALLVAR GULLSTRAND, M.D.

Uppsala, Sweden

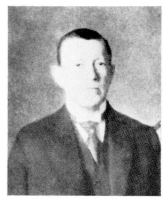

For a dioptric study of the accommodating lens it is necessary to know the nature of the changes in the form of its surfaces and of the increase of its thickness. The writer had the opportunity of examining repeatedly, over a long period of time, an intelligent young man, nineteen years old, who was an unusually good marksman and who could fixate well. The determination of the depth of the anterior chamber was made by Helmholtz's method. The radius of the anterior surface of the lens was measured directly with his ophthalmometer. Values between 0.3 and 0.4 mm were found for the displacement of the pole of the lens when the eye was accommodated for a needle placed 10 cm from the cornea. Results between 10.34 and 10.42 mm were found for the radius of the anterior surface of the lens with relaxed accommodation; and between 5.5 and 5.9 mm in case of accommodation for a point 10 cm away. Because of the difficulties of exact accommodation in the region of the near point the smaller value probably is the more correct. As yet there is no proof of a change of position of the posterior surface of the lens in accommodation. The curvature of the posterior surface of the lens increases in accommodation, though to a very slight extent. By an original method of his own, Gertz has come to the same conclusion. He found that the posterior pole of the lens exhibited no noticeable axial movement during accommodation.

In trying to construct a schematic accommodating lens, it appears to be best to represent the relations as they exist when the power of accommodation is greatest, that is, in youth. Accordingly, the writer has chosen the focusing for a point approximately 10 cm distant from the cornea. A symmetrical structure of the accommodating lens is probable. The choice of the definite value 5.33 for the radius of curvature was

* Appendix IV to Helmholtz's *Treatise on Physiological Optics*, Ed. 3, translated from German by J. C. Southall, Vol. I, pp. 382–415. Optical Society of America, Rochester, N.Y.

made because this number gives the value of the total index that corresponds to Matthiessen's law. The discrepancy between it and the value obtained by the writer's measurement is no more than might be due to the sources of error of the methods. For the refracting power of the lens an approximate value of about 33 D. is obtained. The refracting power of each surface of the lens is 9.375 D. The approximate value of 15 D. is found for the refracting power of the core lens. The forces operative in accommodation are too feeble to produce by compression any appreciable alteration of the volume or the indices of refraction of the various parts.

A comparison of the distribution of the iso-indicial surfaces in the passive and accommodating lens shows that the shifting of the individual parts in the direction of the axis is greatest in the equatorial plane, and that the parts lying nearer the axis of the lens are shifted more than those nearer the equator. As this might have been postulated from the anatomical structure of the lens, the conclusion is that the change of the total index accompanying accommodation is necessarily connected with the anatomical structure.

The lens fibers are attached both anteriorly and posteriorly, describing in their course arcs. When the points of attachment of the fibers are separated from one another by the increase of thickness of the lens, the arches must be spread, involving the greatest amount of dislocation of particles in the parts of the fibers farthest from the points of attachment. If the point of maximum centripetal shifting on each lens fiber were determined, and a surface passed through all these points, this surface of maximum accommodative shifting would coincide with the equatorial plane. But since the passive lens is asymmetrical, and the change of shape is particularly marked on the anterior surface, the surface of maximum accommodative shifting must be concave towards the front. Since the fibers of the posterior surface have their points of attachment situated more towards the periphery on the anterior surface, and towards the center on the posterior surface, and as these conditions are reversed in the case of the fibers of the anterior surface, the increase of curvature of the anterior surface of the lens during the accommodative change of form is accompanied by an axipetal shifting of the anterior point of attachment of the zonule. A necessary consequence of this accommodative change of the iso-indicial surfaces is the variation of the star-shaped appearance of a luminous point.

Thus, the dioptric investigation of the lens in accommodation has resulted in finding out the accommodative variations that occur in the substance of the lens. It appears that these changes, which may be grouped together under the name of the *intracapsular mechanism of accommodation,* are not only in complete agreement with the anatomical structure of the lens, but also establish the causal connection between this structure and the variation of the total index of the lens as proved by the change of refraction that occurs when the lens is removed or during the process of accommodation.

A comparison of the lens system of the exact schematic eye in the passive state and for maximum accommodation indicates the intracapsular mechanism of accommodation that was proved above. While this mechanism is known for the eyes of very young people, the best we can do in the case of the lens of people of middle age or older is to get an approximate idea of it, because the form of the surfaces of discontinuity in the lens is unknown. If the central portions become more homogeneous with advancing age, the mutability of form in the center of the lens begins to decrease, so that the maximum change of curvature of the surfaces of the lens cannot produce the same increase of the total index. Hence it follows that the amplitude of accommodation begins to decrease before the change of curvature of the surfaces of the lens influences the changes in the core. As soon as the central portion becomes less mobile, strains must arise during the changes of shape, and these lead to the formation of surfaces of discontinuity.

Anatomical and physiological investigations prove beyond doubt, that, with contraction of the ciliary muscle, the ciliary point of origin of the fibers of the zonule, particularly of those going to the anterior surface of the lens, is displaced towards the lens in the direction of the bundle; until, when the contraction is greatest, there is a relaxation of the zonule; and that this contraction is accompanied by an increase of the thickness of the lens and of the curvatures of its surfaces, especially of the anterior surface. Since the relaxation of the zonule does not begin until the contraction is greatest, it must be kept under tension during normal contraction by an axipetal movement of the points of insertion on the lens, especially of those on the anterior surface. Since there is only one force present which can maintain this tension, namely, the elasticity of the lens capsule, the extracapsular portion of the mechanism of accommodation consists essentially in an axipetal movement of the points of attachment of the zonule on the lens, especially on the anterior surface, this movement being due to the elasticity of the lens capsule. Modern investigations have established that the theory of the mechanism of accommodation remains just as Helmholtz, by a real inspiration of genius, conceived it.

The force that produces the change of form of the lens in accommodation is the weakest of the three that are present in the system, and, like all elastic forces, constantly diminishes during the development of its effect, so that the movement terminates without any jerk. The effect is promoted still more by the fact that, with increasing contraction of the ciliary muscle, the elastic resistance of the choroid is reduced by its stretching. In the relaxation of accommodation, the greatest force in producing the change of form depends on the elasticity of the choroid. When it is realized that opacities can originate in a previously entirely transparent lens of an older person as a result of an insignificant mechanical force, such as slight draining of the chamber, one is disposed not to underestimate the protective arrangement provided by the double antagonism of the forces acting in accommodation.

There has been quite a lot of discussion in ophthalmological literature of an astigmatic accommodation. It may simply be stated that no known facts indicate the possibility of a voluntary change of astigmatism by accommodation.

Comment: The mechanism of accommodation outlined by Helmholtz, though in general true, was incomplete and included some fallacious assumptions. Helmholtz postulated an elasticity of lens substance but Gullstrand showed that lens substance lacks resilience and is molded into the accommodative form by the highly elastic lens capsule. Helmholtz supposed that the refractive index of the lens remained constant; the calculations of Gullstrand showed that in accommodation only two-thirds of the increased power of the lens depended on the increase of surface curvature and that the remaining third was due to an augmented refractive difference between cortex and core. Hence two-thirds of the accommodative power is extracapsular, one-third intracapsular. The oscillations of refraction that frequently occur in diabetes are predominantly intracapsular. When the blood sugar is high, the nucleus of the lens becomes denser owing to withdrawal of water by osmosis and the eye becomes relatively myopic. After the blood sugar level is lowered by diet or insulin, the osmotic flow is reversed, and the nucleus becomes more hydrated, making the lens more homogenous and less refractive. Then, as the adsorbed sugar slowly leaves the lens, the hyperopia, thus induced, gradually diminishes to some extent.

The posterior surface of the lens fits the vitreous body so closely that only the anterior lens surface is free to deform when the zonule is relaxed. Spherical aberration diminishes during accommodation since accommodation causes the anterior surface of the lens to bulge at the center and flatten in the periphery. This accommodative anterior lenticonus, first noted by Tscherning, was verified by Fincham in 1925 who attributed the hyperbolic molding of the anterior surface of the lens to the thinness of the capsule at the anterior pole. The accompanying axial displacement of lens substance received clinical corroboration from slit-lamp microscopy when Vogt observed an axial shifting of a small subcapsular opacity during accommodation.

The blurred image in near fixation is the sensory stimulus for accommodation. The innervation supplied the eyes is consensually equal so that a normal individual accommodates simultaneously the same amount in each eye. The decrease in accommodating power with age is not caused by any weakening of the ciliary muscle but by a progressive hardening of lens substance which increasingly resists molding by the lens capsule. Since the loss of accommodative amplitude is apparently uniform each year up to age 60, the following equations are useful:

Probable binocular amplitude equals 18.5–0.3 (age)
Probable monocular amplitude equals 16.0–0.25 (age)

As the accommodative range is supplemented by a depth of focus averaging 0.5 D. an indicated increase in the presbyopic correction of 0.5 D. does not materially change one's near vision habits. An increase of 1.0 D. or more, however, produces an appreciable decrease in the near range which may require compensation by trifocals.

References

Duke-Elder, W. S.: *Text-Book of Ophthalmology*, Vol. 1. Mosby, St. Louis, 1938.
Morgan, W. M.: Accommodative changes in presbyopia. In *Vision of the Aging Patient*, edited by M. J. Hirsch and R. E. Wick. Chilton Co., New York, 1960.

Biographical Note

Allvar Gullstrand (1862–1930) was born at Landskrona in southern Sweden, the son of a prominent physician. He studied at the universities of Uppsala and Stockholm and received his medical degree in 1888. Because of his mathematical aptitude he was attracted to geometric and physiological optics in which he was self taught and earned his doctorate with a thesis on the theory of astigmatism. Appointed in 1891 docent in ophthalmology at the Caroline Institute in Stockholm, he proved to be an able surgeon, keen diagnostician, and excellent teacher. During this period he published clinical articles on conical cornea, lenticonus, and a new operation for symblepharon. In 1894, Gullstrand, then 32 years old, was called to the newly established chair of ophthalmology at Uppsala. He was the first to achieve the production of aspheric lenses and originated the punctal lens, the progenitor of the modern corrected curve spectacle lens. He invented a photometer for the light sense that permitted an exact measurement of the minimum perceptible. In 1900 he published a study of monochromatic aberrations and established the significance of light concentration and contrast to the retinal image. In 1908 he analyzed the intracapsular changes in the lens accompanying accommodation and produced a schematic eye with a cortex and core lens. In 1909 he edited and brought up to date the first volume of the third edition of Helmholtz's *Treatise on Physiological Optics* and added several appendices of his own. In 1910 he exhibited his large reflex-free ophthalmoscope in which a fundus image of incomparable clarity could be studied stereoscopically.

On August 3, 1911, he demonstrated a slit-lamp illuminating unit, the indispensable feature of the modern slit-lamp apparatus. In the same year he was awarded the Nobel Prize for his work on the dioptrics of the eye, the only ophthalmologist and the first Swede to be so honored. In 1914 he left the chair of ophthalmology to become professor of physical and physiological optics, a post especially created for him by the University of Uppsala. His international recognition was attested by membership in the Swedish Academy of Science and the German Ophthalmological Society and by honorary memberships in the ophthalmological societies of Jena, Vienna, Budapest, Dublin, United Kingdom, Mexico, Egypt, and Finland. In 1922, he visited America to attend the International Congress of Ophthalmology at Washington, D.C. In 1927, he retired at age 65 and received that year the von Graefe Medal awarded every ten years. Those previously honored were Helmholtz, Leber, Hering, and Carl von Hess. In 1930 he suffered a fatal cerebral hemorrhage and ophthalmology lost one of its truly great.

References

Ask, F.: Obituary. Acta Ophth., *8:* 247–252, 1930.
Blaauw, E. E.: Obituary. Arch. Ophth., *5:* 294–295, 1931.

Nature, Scope and Significance of Aniseikonia

WALTER B. LANCASTER, M.D.

Hanover, New Hampshire

ARCH. OPHTH., *28:* 767–775, 1942

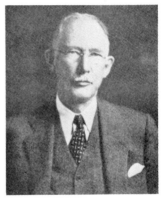

Aniseikonia is divided, for classification, into two types, normal and abnormal, or *anomalous,* as some ophthalmologists prefer to call it. Both types have long been recognized but not fully studied. As a result of Professor Ames's intensive researches, order is emerging from the chaos.

In the literature, normal aniseikonia is dealt with under the terms "disparity of the retinal images," which is simply the Latin for inequality of the retinal images, and "incongruity of the images," which means that the image of one eye does not exactly fit that of the other. Why does it not fit? Simply because the images are different in size and shape. Aniseikonia is merely a Greek word meaning images that are not equal, that differ in size and shape. It is probable that the term aniseikonia will more and more be used for *abnormal* differences in size and shape, *i.e.,* the anomalous incongruities, since a single word for such differences is convenient. Writers from the Dartmouth Eye Institute have used the word in this restricted sense.

What I wish to emphasize is that fundamentally the basis of binocular space perception is found in the normal differences in size and shape of the retinal images of objects in space by which one knows where they are—much about their relative size and shape and position—since these determine the size, shape and position of the retinal images. Normal aniseikonia, or retinal disparity, is the basis of stereoscopic depth perception, in which the two eyes, because of their lateral separation of 60 to 70 mm., get two different views of an object or of a group of objects (a field of view). The visual processes make use of this inequality, these differences between the two ocular images, for better perception

* Photograph by courtesy of Sight-Saving Review.

138

of the form and the spatial relations of the objects. These differences in the images are differences in size and shape, *i.e.* aniseikonia; for example, the relative position of points in the two images in a stereoscopic picture.

There are other normal forms of aniseikonia. One is the effect of nearness on the relative size of the image of an object on the nasal as compared with the temporal part of the retina, the significance of which Professor Ames has pointed out and permits me to quote. He has shown why a flat prism base-in will cause the nasal image of a nearby object in one eye to be larger than the temporal image of the same object in the other eye, thus explaining why prisms base in make objects appear nearer, although they cause divergence, which is associated with greater distance.

Another form of normal aniseikonia is seen in asymmetric convergence. Here the dioptric image of the object on the retina of the nearer eye (the abducted eye) will be larger than the image on the retina of the eye which is farther away (the adducted eye). The difference in size may easily be 5 to 10 per cent or even more, but it is "cheerfully borne" (Ludvigh). The reason is that ever since binocular vision began, the eyes have had to see that way, and they not only tolerate it, they take advantage of it to locate with greater precision the position in space of the object with reference to the observer. This is not surprising, since the difference in size is due to the position of the object.

In looking at nearby objects to right, to left, up or down—in any direction away from the primary position—since the two eyes are separated an appreciable distance, there will be differences in the images which depend on the geometric relation; *e.g.,* looking straight up will have a different effect than looking up to the right or up to the left and, of course, a very different effect from looking to the right or to the left or down. The amount and the kind of difference are the clues by which one knows in what direction the object is located. Formerly it was thought that knowledge of the direction of gaze was derived from proprioceptive sensations, but that is certainly a mistake. It is by the characteristic differences in size and in shape of the ocular images (*i.e.,* by the aniseikonia, the normal incongruities) that one locates objects in one's environment. Unless one grasps this conception, asymmetric convergence is an unsolved riddle.

Anomalous aniseikonia has been classified as: (1) meridional, axis 90 degrees; (2) meridional, axis 180 degrees; (3) over all, some magnification in all meridians; (4) cyclo type—(a) due to oblique cylinders and (b) due to cyclophoria—and (5) asymmetric type. Each type produces characteristic effects on spatial localization.

A rectangle of pasteboard about 30 by 50 cm. is held vertically 2 or 3 meters in front of the observer in the midline in his frontal plane. The images of this rectangle as seen by the two eyes are equal.

1. Rotate the rectangle around its vertical axis, and the image as seen by the right eye is different from that seen by the left.

2. Rotate the rectangle around its horizontal axis.

3. Move the rectangle in its same plane to the right or to the left or up or down.

4. Bend the rectangle so that it is convex or concave toward the observer.

With each of these procedures the normal aniseikonia gives the clue to the observer as to the position of the rectangle. With the rectangle in its original position, suitable lenses could be placed before the eyes to make the rectangle appear in any one of these different positions (artificial aniseikonia).

How Abnormal Aniseikonia Is Dealt with by the Visual Processes

By analogy with refractive errors and defects of motility, it might be expected that some compensatory mechanism would correct the difference in size of the images.

There is no evidence of the existence of such a corrective mechanism, much less any knowledge of how it might operate. It must be concluded that the difference is dealt with in some entirely different way. Nature's favorite way of dealing with a difficult or an intolerable situation is by suppression, or inhibition, as the physiologists prefer to call it. For example, in certain defects of motility, when the compensatory mechanism fails, causing diplopia, the situation is met by suppression of the vision of one eye. This may result in amblyopia of one eye from persistent inhibition (ex anopsia), or it may result in an inhibition so nicely adjusted that when either eye fixates, the vision of the other eye is suppressed temporarily (alternating strabismus). Moreover, the suppression may effect only a limited part of the retina, allowing it to escape the unwanted effect but preserving its activity for other situations.

Suppression is by no means limited to the visual processes. It is a generally utilized device, for example in hearing and other sensory activities; in fact, civilization and etiquette depend on inhibition of instinctive impulses.

To understand how inhibition is made use of in dealing with abnormal aniseikonia, consider what abnormal aniseikonia does and what conflicts and frustrations it may excite. The binocular clues, though in many cases the most perfect means of spatial localization, are not the only ones. Very important are the monocular clues based on perspective, overlapping, shadows, knowledge of size and of form and previous experience.

Thus in a given situation one receives information from monocular clues, as well as from binocular clues, and what one makes of it is not determined solely by the physical stimuli but, although primarily excited by them, is modified by some mechanism at a higher level. "The image awakens unconscious reproductions or memories of past experiences which modify it so that the ultimate perception does not correspond with the immediate stimulus but conforms with the background provided by experience." For example, a tilted circle gives a retinal image which is an ellipse, but if it is known to be a ring, it gives the impression of a circle in a particular position. One's impression of the size of a well known object and of its shape do not depend solely on the size and the form of its retinal image. The phenomena of "color constancy" and "memory colors" and the effect of different conditions of light intensity and quality on color perceptions are good examples of how the visual processes put two and two and two and two together and make seven or eight or nine, as the conditions seem to warrant. The pattern that emerges must have meaning, must make sense, must conform to experience.

This is exactly what takes place in the locating of objects in space. There are clues from monocular vision, clues from binocular vision (if affected by abnormal aniseikonia they may be false or misleading clues), clues from memory, clues from past experiences and clues from other sensory sources. It is in the presence of such clues that the "interplay of the psychic processes" produces a consistent, coherent, harmonious result, a perception that makes sense, that satisfies one's comprehension. To quote Duke-Elder:

> It is impossible to experience a pure isolated sensation. Even the simplest and most elementary perceptual process comprises a synthesis of many types of different impressions; and to add to the complexity, the synthesized product is moulded upon and influenced by a substratum of past experience and inherited dispositions, to assess which is beyond our knowledge, while its nature is continually undergoing alterations impressed upon it by the higher centers, more especially with regard to the distribution of the psychological factors of attention and interest.

In interpreting a field of view, the visual processes throw into the discard (*i.e.*, suppress) such clues as do not contribute to the consistent, coherent, harmonious result. One must picture to oneself a conflict going on between different factors. When correcting clues are scanty, faulty clues tend to predominate. Habit greatly facilitates the correct interpretation. Thus a person with abnormal aniseikonia (natural or induced by size lenses) will under certain conditions show no apparent defect in his spatial localization (though he may show premature fatigue from the struggle and frustration, which of course are entirely subconscious). Under other conditions (absence of correcting clues, including lack of previous experience with the environment), his orientation is faulty and confusing.

I have dwelt at some length on the psychologic aspect of the subject because it is the key to an understanding of certain questions that are sure to arise in one's mind when one gives thought to the subject: (1) Why is it that if abnormal aniseikonia is such a factor in spatial localization so few persons are aware of or show disturbed orientation? (2) How is it that aniseikonia causes symptoms of eyestrain?

1. Persons who for experimental purposes continuously wear size lenses to produce an artificial abnormal aniseikonia soon acquire a certain degree of adaptation to them (Dr. Burian has shown this and permits me to quote him). However, as soon as such a person finds himself in an environment where monocular clues and clues from memory are meager or absent, he manifests the signs and symptoms of abnormal spatial localization, no matter how long he has worn the size lenses or how fully he seems to be adapted. All this will be set forth with a wealth of detail and full experimental demonstration by Dr. Burian. In the same way, a person with natural abnormal aniseikonia (*i.e.*, not induced artificially by wearing size lenses) shows a pronounced degree of adaptation in his daily life. However, when such a subject is placed in an environment devoid of clues from sources other than binocular vision, such as monocular clues, especially rectilinear clues and clues from knowledge of the environment, memory and past experience, he always shows that the underlying misleading clues are there. For example, a test with the horopter or with the leaf room would show their presence.

2. The question, "How is it that aniseikonia causes the symptoms of eyestrain?" is not easily answered; in fact, the answers to the questions of how errors of refraction and of motility cause the symptoms of eyestrain are far from satisfactory. The identity of the symptoms shows that they must have something in common. It has been commonly assumed that the symptoms of heterophoria are due to fatigue of a weak muscle. There are two objections to this assumption. The first is that the symptoms are not such as would be likely to result from fatigue of a muscle; the second is that the external ocular muscles are so strong that they

are not likely to become fatigued and there is no satisfactory evidence that they do. In myasthenia gravis the muscles show weakness and great fatigability, but the symptoms are not those of eyestrain. The evidence that the symptoms of eyestrain in hypermetropia with astigmatism are due to fatigue of the ciliary muscle is also unsatisfactory. In the case of abnormal aniseikonia, there is no known muscular mechanism for compensating for it, and so one is forced to seek elsewhere.

Aniseikonia interferes with the smooth functioning of the visual apparatus. Poor illumination, reading poor print or reading on a train or other moving vehicle embarrass the visual apparatus and so throw added burdens on it. These factors compel greater efforts on the part of the adjusting mechanisms to secure improved seeing, thus causing eyestrain. Similarly, aniseikonia throws an added burden on the visual apparatus by interfering with its smooth functioning.

It is an important fact that the eyes do not in ordinary easy activities make the most perfect adjustments of which they are capable. Focusing is not as exact as the eyes are capable of. On the contrary, the eyes take advantage of their depth of focus and when looking at distant objects may be focused anywhere within 0.25 to 0.50 D. of infinity. When looking at a near object, for example, a book, they often find it near enough for practical purposes to focus 0.50 D. beyond the object, or the book.

The fixation apparatus does not fixate each word, much less each letter, as the eyes skip across the page in ordinary easy reading. But when a difficult passage, perhaps poorly printed, in a foreign language or dimly lighted, is encountered, then the mechanism for fixation has to perform a much more exacting task. Similarly, the fusion apparatus demands adjustment of the visual axes of the two eyes so that images fall, not on exactly corresponding points, but only on corresponding areas. However, when the demand arises, when the presence of difficulties calls for greater efforts to secure more perfect seeing, then the eyes are whipped up to more accurate focusing, fixation and fusion, thus taxing the adjusting mechanism far more than when the visual apparatus is functioning smoothly and easily, well within its capacity.

In the case of aniseikonia there is another obvious factor to be reckoned with. The adjustments call for inhibition, for selections among conflicting clues, for dealing with frustrations—a series of adjustments on a higher level than those which deal with focusing and fixation. These are cortical, psychic and mental, though mostly subconscious. Psychiatrists are keen about the strains due to frustrations. Thus on this higher level there are adequate causes for symptoms of eyestrain.

I submit, as further food for thought, that the precise similarity of symptoms of eyestrain from the various causes (refractive errors, heterophoria, poor lighting, aniseikonia) shows that these symptoms are traceable to fundamental causes common to all. On the one hand, aniseikonia makes demands not only on the psychic adjustments but on the adjusting mechanisms of accommodation, fixation and fusion; and, on the other hand, errors of refraction and phoria make demands not alone on the lower mechanisms but on the higher psychic activities of inhibition, mental adjustments and frustrations. The visual function is so complex but so integrated that all these factors I have mentioned work together in producing eyestrain.

Comment: Lancaster coined the word "aniseikonia" in 1938. The difference in retinal image size due to the spectacle correction of anisometropia was noted by Donders (1846) and abnormal aniseikonia is still most commonly associated with anisometropia. The first intensive research on aniseikonia was undertaken by Ames and his coworkers during a 15-year period (1932 to 1947). Since anisometropia is partly refractive, partly axial in origin, an estimate of 1 per cent image size difference per diopter of anisometropia is a fair approximation. In the eye with the smaller image, appropriate magnification can be secured most simply by increasing the curvature and thickness of its lens and changing the distance from the lens to the eye (an increase for plus lenses, a decrease for minus). For myopic corrections greater than −2 D. no increase in magnification is obtained by increasing the curvature, since its magnifying effect is then compensated by the further displacement of the vertex of the correcting lens away from the eye. Zoubek and Polasek of Prague have experimented with an equidistant spectacles as an economical solution (1962). A magnifying lens of zero power has a base-up prismatic action at the reading point similar to a slab off— a magnification of 2 per cent producing a prismatic action of 0.7 prism diopter. Friedenwald advocated this method to reduce anisophoria (1936).

Lawrence T. Post dispensed 1500 aniseikonic corrections over a 12-year period at Washington University. The aniseikonia was measured accurately with the space eikonometer. The basic errors of ametropia and heterophoria had been meticulously corrected. Questionnaires indicated that 80 per cent were significantly or completely relieved of their symptoms. Most of the patients were neurasthenics and many had consulted previously numerous ophthalmologists. He considered that aniseikonia was directly responsible for symptoms in only a small group with the largest amounts of aniseikonia, and that the average ophthalmologist would encounter too few such cases to warrant the time, energy and expensive equipment required for measurement. Post advocated a few central stations instead, where an unhurried examination would be given by a conscientious, psychiatrically trained ophthalmologist. Several days should be allowed for the tests, "because here, if ever, a thorough study of the patient is needed."

Adelbert Ames, Jr., who inspired the renewed interest in aniseikonia, was not a scientist primarily. He was educated as a lawyer and then turned to art. Ames became interested in visual imagery when he noted the differences in the paintings of the same scene by him and by his sister. This led him to establish a department for research in physiologic optics at Dartmouth

College in 1919. In 1932 he published a series of papers on what was later known as aniseikonia. In 1937 the Dartmouth Eye Institute was instituted, with Bielschowsky as director till his death in 1940; Lancaster then became chief until his resignation in 1942, after which Burian carried on till 1945. In the meantime Ames had become increasingly apathetic to the drift toward clinical ophthalmology and closed the Dartmouth Eye Institute in May 1947.

References

Burian, H. M.: The history of the Dartmouth Eye Institute. Arch. Ophth., *40:* 163–175, 1948.
Berens, C., and Bannon, R. E.: Aniseikonia. Arch. Ophth., *70:* 181–188, 1963.

Biographical Note

Walter Brackett Lancaster (1863–1951) was born in Newton, Massachusetts, with the distinction that both his father and mother traced their ancestry to the Mayflower pilgrims. He was a brilliant student and graduated from Harvard College *magna cum laude* in 1884, and from Harvard Medical School in 1889. Several years of postgraduate study in Europe followed; he was particularly influenced by Prof. Ludwig Mauthner of Vienna, who inspired in him a lifelong interest in physiologic optics and related problems. After returning to Boston, Lancaster gave postgraduate courses in physiologic optics at the Harvard Medical School, which he continued for over 40 years. He joined the staff of the Massachusetts Eye and Ear Infirmary in 1897, becoming "surgeon" in 1920, and also served as Attending Ophthalmologist at the Boston City Hospital. He was deeply concerned with the postgraduate training of American ophthalmologists, first writing on the subject in 1913. Lancaster was an original member of the American Board of Ophthalmology, founded in 1916, and as its first secretary made the plans for the examinations. Because of poor health at the beginning of his career, due to chronic appendicitis which was not diagnosed and operated till 1910, his most active work began in later life. He was a skillful ophthalmic surgeon and his techniques in cataract extraction and ocular muscle surgery were widely adopted. His model of the electromagnet is still most popular. His zeal for physiologic optics never abated; he revived the use of astigmatic dials (1916), devised a new method for demonstrating disturbances of ocular motility (1937), established a summer course for orthoptic technicians (1948) and was sympathetic to the iseikonic research of Ames at Dartmouth College. At his instigation Bielschowsky was invited to head the Dartmouth Eye Institute, and after his death, Lancaster served as chief there from 1940 to 1942. In 1946, at age 83, Lancaster inaugurated an annual summer course in the basic sciences of ophthalmology for the medical officers returning from World War II, which still continues as "the Lancaster course," a fitting memorial to a dedicated educator in ophthalmology. Lancaster received practically all the honors awarded by American ophthalmology. He was at various times president of the American Board of Ophthalmology, American Ophthalmological Society, American Academy of Ophthalmology and Otolaryngology, Section of Ophthalmology of the American Medical Association, and the New England Ophthalmological Society. He received the Knapp Research Medal (1914), the Leslie Dana Gold Medal (1943) and the Lucien Howe Medal (1945). He was a director of the National Society for the Prevention of Blindness, helped to found the Boston

146

Nursery for Blind Babies, and was associate editor of the *Optical Journal of America*. Active to the last, Lancaster completed his book, *Refraction and Motility* just before his death at age 88.

*References**References*

Burian, H. M.: Obituary. Arch. Ophth., *47:* 116–119, 1952.
Dunphy, E. B.: Obituary. Am. J. Ophth., *35:* 427–431, 1952.

Part Five
Anatomy

On the Anatomy and Pathology of Certain Structures in the Orbit not Previously Described

J. M. FERRALL, M.D.*

Dublin

THE DUBLIN JOURNAL OF MEDICAL SCIENCE, *19:* 329–356, JULY, 1841

Anatomy of the Tunica Vaginalis Oculi, and Muscles of the Eye

Having separated the divided conjunctiva, we expose, not as has been described by anatomists, a cushion of adipose tissue, but a distinct tunic of a yellowish white colour, and fibrous consistence, continuous in front with the posterior margin of the tarsal cartilage, and extending backwards to the bottom or apex of the orbit, where its consistence becomes less strongly marked. By proceeding in the manner I

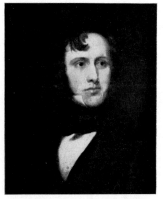

have mentioned, the parts are displayed without any elaborate dissection. The sharp end of a probe, or director, will be sufficient to separate the ball of the eye from the new organ, by breaking gently the fine cellular tissue which connects them. Its colour is totally different from that belonging to its external surface, and it is here perfectly smooth,

*Portrait from an oil painting at St. Vincent's Hospital, Dublin. By courtesy of the Mother Rectress.

where the eye glides over it in its movements. The muscular substance of the recti muscles is no where visible; they lie on the outside of this tunic, which insulates and protects the eye in the most perfect manner.

The most beautiful portion of this mechanism, however, remains to be described. In the concavity of this tunic, and about half an inch posterior to its anterior or orbital margin, are to be found six well-defined openings, through which the tendons of the muscles emerge in passing to their insertion in the sclerotic coat, and over which they play, as over pulleys, in their course. The tendons are loosely connected to the edges of those apertures by fine cellular tissue, which opposes no obstacle to their gliding movements. The annexed sketches from original drawings made by Mr. Neilan, in April, 1840, will illustrate the parts.

Fig. 1 represents the eyelids divided and thrown back, and the tunica vaginalis exposed by opening the conjunctiva in the situation of its fold. The tendon of the internal rectus muscle is seen passing over the pulley in the tunic to reach the sclerotic coat of the eye.

Fig. 2 shows the same preparation. The ball of the eye is drawn downwards in order to expose the superior rectus, and superior oblique muscles. The superior oblique muscle having passed through the pulley attached to the frontal bone, is concealed by the tunic, from which it emerges close to the point of exit for the superior rectus.

The physiology of this tunic, which I have ventured to term the *Tunica Vaginalis Oculi*, will be conveniently considered in relation to each of its separate offices, namely, as an investment and protector of the globe of the eye, and as regulating the direction in which the muscles of the eye are to exert their force. In either of those capacities, this new and beautiful apparatus (independent of its pathological importance) appears to possess a physiological interest, entitling it to a high place among the many evidences of design, with which the animal frame abounds.

The uses of this tunic, as a covering, will be obvious from a brief consideration of the inconveniences to which, without this protection, the eye would be subjected during the action of its muscles. These muscles, it has been invariably taught, were in close contact with the globe of the eye, on their passage to their insertion, the interspaces being occupied by the fat of the orbit. This description of the parts, which is to be found in the works of the best authors, implies, that during the frequent action of its muscles, the eye must sustain a pressure as great and as suddenly applied, as the movements of the organ are rapid and energetic. Yet this could hardly have occurred without producing some phenomena capable of exciting our attention.

Every person is familiar with the effects of a slight blow on the eye. A flash is perceived at the moment; and sometimes from a shock so slight, as when the corner of a handkerchief is blown by the wind into the eye, that I am inclined to believe, the coruscation is occasionally produced by the protective action of the orbicularis muscle alone. To this cause Sir Charles Bell attributes the flash perceived in the act of sneezing, and I think, he has succeeded in establishing his opinion.

Certainly, if the tunica vaginalis had no existence, it would be difficult to imagine how the recti muscles could communicate the rotatory movements to the eye, without, in a greater degree, exerting a retracting power; and if more than one muscle were in action at the same time, it is manifest that the latter force must predominate. It is certain that the human eye has never been observed to have been retracted within the orbit; but why the muscles were prevented from communicating this movement, has never been hitherto explained.

Retraction is known to take place in some of the lower classes of animals; but in them an additional muscular apparatus is provided for the purpose. The strong retractor muscle, or bundle of muscles, is inserted into the globe of the eye at its posterior part, near the entrance of the optic nerve, and cannot, therefore, exercise any injurious pressure on the organ. In certain animals, in which I have found the tunica vaginalis developed, the recti muscles appear to me to antagonize the proper retractor, by the passage of their tendons over the trochleae described. This may be made obvious by pulling the retractor, and consequently the globe of the eye backwards into the orbit, when the tendons of the recti muscles will be drawn backwards along with the eyeball, and made to play freely over the pulleys in the tunic. I am inclined to believe, therefore, that in those animals the eye is brought back into its proper position, by the recti muscles, when the retractor ceases to act.

There can be no doubt, then, that the force exerted by the recti muscles of the human eye, acquires a new direction by the passage of their tendons over the trochleae in the tunica vaginalis. They are enabled by this contrivance to act as if they arose from the sides instead of the bottom or apex of the orbit, while they possess a range or extent of motion greater than in that case could belong to them. They enjoy the extent of motion which is the property of length of fibre in muscle; while a suitable direction is given to their action by the mode in which their tendons are conducted to the eye. Many additional observations might be made in reference to the offices of these structures. Enough, however, has been advanced to show, that the received anatomy, and known functions of the parts, involved a series of physiological contradictions, which a knowledge of this new and beautiful mechanism at once reconciles and explains.

Extirpation of the Globe

Should extirpation be determined on, in a case where the disease was in an early stage, or should the appearances render it probable that it was confined to the globe of the eye, a very simple operation will accomplish the object.

In Mr. Traver's case, where the head symptoms were urgent, and haemorrhagic oozings took place from a fungus protruding through the cornea, the operation succeeded in curing the patient. The morbid growth originated within the globe of the eye, and had not contaminated the optic nerve or orbital appendages. Where both are healthy, an operation might be performed which would secure the patient against the most formidable incidents to the usual proceeding. The vessels, nerves, and muscles of the orbit might be spared by operating within the tunic—haemorrhage would be avoided—and the orbital parietes, thus retaining their covering of periosteum and cellular tissue, &c., would be guarded against inflammation, which sometimes extends into the cranium.

The comparative safety of an operation limited by this fibrous tunic is obvious, but an additional recommendation will be, the facility of its performance. The conjunctiva being freely divided, the six tendons may be snipped across with a scissors one after another, where they emerge from the tunic. The eyeball will then be easily detached by a probe or director passed freely around it; when one step alone would remain—the division of the optic nerve. When we recollect that the roof of the orbit is occasionally found to be as thin as paper in some parts, it will appear most desirable to avoid stripping it of its coverings, by operating within this second orbit, or proper fibrous socket of the eye.

The reflections suggested by a review of the cases which led to the present inquiry, as well as of this new and curious mechanism itself, may be reduced to the following propositions:

1st. That the description of anatomists, which places the globe of the eye in contact with the fat and muscles of the orbit, is erroneous.

2nd. That there exists a fibrous tunic, investing and insulating the eyeball, and separating it from all the other structures in the orbit.

3rd. That the uses of this tunica vaginalis oculi are, to present a smooth surface, facilitating the movements of the eye; and by its density and tension, to protect it from the pressure incidental to the swelling of its muscles during their action.

4th. That the openings in this tunic perform the office of pulleys, giving a proper direction to the force exerted by the muscles—securing the motions of rotation, and opposing those of retraction, which would otherwise predominate.

5th. That certain cases of disease within the orbit, accompanied by protrusion of the eyeball, are to be explained, only by reference to the tunica vaginalis oculi, and the other fibrous tissues now described.

6th. That a correct knowledge of the anatomy of the orbit and of the fibrous structures alluded to, is essential to the operating surgeon, in dealing with abscesses and tumours, in extirpation of the eyeball, in the operation for strabismus, and all operations on that cavity.

Comment: The fascia bulbi (Tenon's capsule) was first carefully described by Jacques René Tenon (1724–1816), a Parisian ophthalmologist, in 1802. His findings were ignored until the strabismus operation, originated by Dieffenbach in 1839, gave a practical interest to the precise anatomy of the ocular muscles and their vestments. In 1841 Amédée Bonnet of Lyons and Joseph Ferrall of Dublin, both unaware of Tenon's discoveries, independently perfected the description of the fascia bulbi and pointed out its surgical significance in the removal of the eye. Tenon's capsule is a fibrous membrane that envelops the scleral part of the globe. Anteriorly it fuses with the conjunctiva 2 mm. from the corneal limbus, posteriorly it fuses with the sclera and the external sheath of the optic nerve, and in between it is connected with the sclera by loose connective tissue. The fascia bulbi has four principal subdivisions:

(1) Muscle sheaths. On entering the fascia bulbi, a reflection of the capsule ensheaths each muscle like a finger in a glove. These muscle sheaths extend nearly to the muscle origins. Since the muscles are firmly connected with the openings through which they enter the capsule and the sheaths are adherent to the muscle fibers, the cutting of a muscle tendon at its insertion causes the muscle to retract but 3 to 5 mm.

(2) Intermuscular fascial membrane. Anterior to the equator of the globe an expansion of the sheaths between adjacent margins of the recti muscles connect to form a girdlelike structure anchored at the tendon insertions to the main body of the fascia bulbi. The maximum effect of a recession operation is obtained only if all the fascial connections of the muscle sheath are scrupulously severed. After operations for strabismus or retinal detachment the cut edges of the fascia bulbi should be approximated separately from the conjunctiva with 5–0 plain catgut sutures to minimize scar tissue formation as excessive scarring may limit ocular rotation.

(3) Check ligaments. The outer surface of each muscle sheath gives off one or more attachments to the orbital wall which serve to check excessive movement of an ocular muscle. Check ligaments of the lateral and medial recti are also inserted, respectively, into the lateral and medial palpebral ligaments and the lacrimal caruncle. The outer surface of the fascia bulbi is firmly connected posteriorly with the orbital fatty reticulum. This relation exerts a further check action on the extraocular muscles and promotes their smooth action. Because of the firm pericorneal attachment of Tenon's

capsule to the globe, the two move together on the cushion of fat behind them. Scobee held that anomalous development of the fascia was a frequent factor in underaction of a muscle, and found such anomalies in half of the patients operated for esotropia.

(4) Suspensory ligament of Lockwood. Where the inferior rectus and the inferior oblique muscles meet, the sheaths of the muscles fuse with one another and the main body of the fascia bulbi to form a hammock that supports the globe, an extension of which to the lower tarsal plate and cul-de-sac helps to hold them in place. Similarly, the fascial sheaths of the levator and the superior rectus fuse and an extension of this fibroelastic tissue is attached to the upper cul-de-sac.

Before the anatomy of the fascia bulbi was understood, eyes were removed by extirpation, a butcher-like operation introduced by George Bartisch in 1583. This brutal procedure was used only for tumors and then rarely. Bowman reported that but four extirpations were done at the Royal Ophthalmic Hospital in nine years. Ferrall conceived the modern technique of enucleation through a fortuitous circumstance. It happened that a patient of his had an enormous orbital tumor which pushed the globe entirely out of the socket so that Ferrall easily delivered the eyeball after merely cutting the ocular muscles and optic nerve. His subsequent studies on the fascia bulbi led him to conclude: "The comparative safety of an operation limited by this fibrous tissue is obvious, but an additional recommendation will be the facility of its performance." For the following 15 years enucleation like extirpation was used almost exclusively for malignant growths. To Critchett belongs the credit of widening the indications for enucleation to its present scope. In 1855 he advocated enucleation for painful blind eyes, injured eyes in danger of sympathetic ophthalmia, staphyloma and intraocular foreign bodies. The Ferrall-Bonnet operation left the patient with a large empty socket that gave no support to the lids or to an artificial eye. In 1886 Frost proposed the insertion of a hollow glass ball in Tenon's capsule. This procedure, as modified by Lang, rapidly became standard practice. The Frost-Lang method is still in general use except that the lighter and more durable plastic implant has been substituted.

Reference

W. H. Fink: *Surgery of the Oblique Muscles of the Eye,* pp. 335–343. St. Louis, C. V. Mosby Co., 1951.

Biographical Note

Joseph Michael Ferrall (1790–1877), otherwise known as O'Ferrall, was of lowly lineage and did not begin the study of medicine until he was 25 years old. His father had died while he was a child and as the eldest son he worked for years as a clerk to support the family. He received his medical degree in 1821; among his instructors were Colles and Cheyne. In 1834 the Sisters of Charity opened St. Vincent's Hospital with Ferrall in charge. For 10 years Ferrall worked there assiduously, making autopsies on nearly every fatal case. He fervently insisted on the indivisibility of medicine and surgery. He wrote 109 papers, a testimonial to his amazing industry. His most important contribution was the introduction of enucleation. In this, his priority over Bonnet was proved by Hildige (Dublin Hospital Gazette,

1859), who showed that Ferrall anticipated the French surgeon by more than a year. Ferrall's eyesight became seriously deteriorated from glaucoma in 1859, but by means of a reading slit he would read line after line of print very slowly. In 1867, his fatal ailment began with a painful palsy of the right leg. The large fortune that he had accumulated was given to St. Vincent's Hospital and his sister bestowed a portrait of the hospital's great surgeon and benefactor.

References

E. D. Mapother: The lives and writings of O'Ferrall and Bellingham. Dublin J. Med. Sc., *64:* 461–475, 1877.

A Century of Service, 1834–1934, St. Vincent's Hospital, pp. 57–59.

Observations on the Contractile Tissue of the Iris

JOSEPH LISTER, M.D.

London, England

QUARTERLY JOURNAL OF MIRCOSCOPICAL SCIENCE, 1853, *1:* 8–17

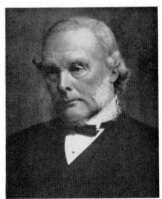

An operation for artificial pupil, by excision, performed by Mr. Wharton Jones, at University College Hospital, on the 11th of August of the present year (1852), placed in my possession a perfectly fresh portion of a human iris, and I proceeded to avail myself of this somewhat rare opportunity of investigating the muscular tissue of the human iris. On placing under the microscope, 4 hours after the operation, portions of the tissue carefully teased out in water with needles, I found that some of the muscular fibre-cells had become isolated, and presented very characteristic appearances. I accordingly made camera lucida sketches of the finest specimens.

Having thus satisfactorily verified the fact of the existence in the iris of tissue identical with ordinary unstriped muscle, I was naturally led to inquire into its distribution in the organ: and, as this is a subject of great interest, and one about which much difference of opinion has prevailed, I may mention here the facts which I have hitherto observed, although there be not very much of actual novelty in them.

My experience, I must confess, accords with that of Kölliker, viz. that the sphincter is readily seen, while the dilator is that whose investigation alone presents very serious difficulty. In the first iris that I examined with a view to the distribution of the muscular tissue, I was struck, after removing the usual pigment, with the appearance of a band on the posterior surface of the iris, near the pupil and parallel to its margin, quite evident to the naked eye, elastic and highly extensible. This proved to be the thickest part of the sphincter pupillae. I have examined six human irides with reference to the distribution of the muscular tissue, but in none have I had any difficulty in recognising the sphincter, which, I have also found equally distinct in some of the lower animals, viz. in the rabbit, the guinea-pig, and the horse. In man I find it about 1-30th of an inch in width, thickest towards its outer part, where it lies nearer the posterior surface of the iris than the anterior, and thinning off towards the pupil, where it forms a sharp margin, covered apparently on its anterior aspect only by some vessels and nervous threads and a delicate epitheliated membrane, which is thrown into beautiful folds when the pupil is contracted. The fibres of the sphincter are not absolutely parallel, and this deviation is probably produced in part by the dilating fasciculi sweeping in at various parts in a curved manner, and becoming blended with the sphincter. The reason for this supposition will appear hereafter. By teasing out under the microscope a portion of the actual pupillary margin, I found the sphincter to consist at this part of apparently unmixed muscular fibre-cells, without any connecting cellular tissue. Indeed, the great facility with which the tissue may be thus broken up appears opposed to the idea of the fibre-cells being united end to end into fibres, as the descriptions formerly given of unstriped muscle would lead one to suppose. The ends appear to separate as readily as the edges and surfaces, and it would rather seem as if the fibre-cells of a fasciculus were placed with their long axis in one direction, cohering generally to one another, but without the formation of longer fibres than each cell itself constitutes. I may here mention incidentally that in the circular coat of the aorta of the sheep, where the muscular tissue is disposed in thin layers among the elastic tissue, I have observed a distinctly alternate arrangement of the fibre-cells without any formation of fibres. A portion of the outer and thicker part of the human sphincter pupillae proved also extremely rich in muscular fibre-cells. In the rabbit and guinea-pig the sphincter has much the same appearance as in man, whereas in the horse it forms a wide but very flat band.

The dilating fibres of the iris present a very difficult subject of investigation.

And here I must express my belief—a belief the result of repeated and very careful observations—that the fibres described by Mr. Bowman as probably the contractile fibres of the iris are in reality the outer cellular coats of the vessels. The outer coat is very abundant in the vessels of the iris, and indeed even in the blue eye towards the sphincter quite obscures the bore of many of the vessels, and prevents the recognition of their vascular character, which can only be determined by tracing them to their more external and more obviously vascular trunks. The distribution of these vessels, radiating between the sphincter and the circumference of the iris, and forming in the

156

region of the sphincter a close and knotted plexus, corresponds accurately with Mr. Bowman's description of the distribution of the fibres of the iris. His account of the tissue of these fibres, which he considers as probably contractile, harmonises with the characters of the cellular tissue that clothes the vessels. This is peculiar; consisting of very soft-looking fibres, whose fasciculi often require the best aid of a first-rate glass to resolve them into their constituent elements; destitute apparently of yellow elastic fibres, as in the case of the cellular tissue of the uterus, but, like this, containing abundance of free nuclei, of roundish or elongated form. The fibres are completely gelatinised by acetic acid. Now such a tissue can hardly, in the present state of our knowledge, be regarded as contractile; at any rate, if we can find any ordinary muscular tissue to account for the dilating action. On teasing out portions of the outer part of the human iris, I have found long delicate fasciculi, whose faint outline, absence of fibrous character, and possession of well-marked elongated nuclei parallel to the direction of the fasciculus, left no doubt in my mind that they were plain muscular tissue.

So far my observations regarding the dilator agree with Kölliker's, but whether or not these fasciculi are connected with the cellular coat of the vessels I have hitherto been unable to determine.

Among the lower animals the albino rabbit and guinea-pig appeared but little suited for the elucidation of this point. I have been most successful with the eyes of a horse, where, from the thickness of the iris and the abundance of pigment (for the eyes were black ones), I anticipated but little result from my examination. Having removed the uveal pigment from behind, I found that I was also able to strip off from the anterior surface a tough membrane, a portion of which, put under the microscope, appeared to be made up of peculiar short felt-like fibres, which were gelatinised by acetic acid. At and near the pupillary margin this membrane comes off in a continuous layer, leaving a delicate reticular structure, which contains the muscular tissue. It also contains vessels, as I proved by injection, and a black network, which consists of fine fibres, yellow, and highly refracting, more or less encrusted with pigment. I am uncertain whether or not this be a network of divided nerve-tubes with adhering pigment; in some spots the pigmental crust was absent from a considerable length of the fibres. The sphincter pupillae is beautifully seen as a broad flat band, of extremely well-marked, unmixed, muscular fibre-cells; but crossing this at right angles are found, here and there, other flat bands of fibre-cells, which are in so thin a layer that without isolation the width of the individual cells cannot be seen, and they are evidently of similar dimensions to those of the sphincter. On addition of acetic acid their nuclei are also seen to be exactly like those of the sphincter. These bands divide in their course towards the pupil into several fasciculi, some of which cross over the sphincter at right angles till very near to its pupillary margin, and then seem to blend with the sphincter by making a slight curve. Most of the fasciculi, however, arch away earlier from their first course and join the sphincter in more or less oblique lines. The bands from which these fasciculi diverge may be traced away from the pupil for some distance, continuing their course at right angles to the sphincter till they are obscured by other tissues. Hence I think the inference may fairly be drawn that these are the insertions of the dilating muscular bundles. In the horse, then, the dilating fasciculi appear to consist of precisely the same tissue as the sphincter, and to blend with it in their insertion. The flat bands of muscular tissue above spoken of seemed to have no special relation to the vessels, some of which were filled with injection. In the outer part of the iris of the same horse I found a delicate muscular fasciculus lying near but not intimately connected with one of the radiating vessels of this part. In the human iris I have seen a muscular fasciculus, as it appeared from the nuclei it contained, crossing the sphincter at right angles for a short distance; this observation, so far as it goes, seems to imply that the same mode of insertion of the dilator occurs in man as in the horse.

The fibre-cells of the dilator appear to be held together much more closely than those of the sphincter, at least in the outer part of the iris; for I have never been able to define the individual fibre-cells in a perfectly satisfactory manner in the dilator, though I have often teased out portions of the outer part of the iris. The dilating muscular tissue is also probably less abundant than the muscular tissue of the sphincter; and this, if the fact, will help to account for the comparative difficulty in discovering it. I may here mention that both in the cat and in the rabbit, soon after death, dilatation of the pupils being present, exposure of one iris to the air caused it to contract at once, while the pupil continued dilated in the other eye, which was untouched. I do not know if this fact has been observed before, but it is interesting in two ways— first, as showing that the muscular tissue of the iris, like other muscular tissue, is obedient to the stimulus of exposure; and, second, as proving either that the sphincter is in these animals a decidedly more powerful muscle than the dilator, which is equally exposed to the stimulus; or else that the fibres of these two muscles have different endowments, as has been shown by Mr. Wharton Jones to be the case with the muscular tissue of the arteries and veins of the bat's wing; where, although the veins are muscular, and even contract rhythmically, yet the arteries alone exhibit tonic contraction when irritated by mechanical stimulus.

A rich network of extremely fine fibres, seen readily in the blue

158

human iris viewed from the anterior aspect, appears to represent the nerves of the organ. The fibres are of a yellowish colour, and are possessed of pretty high refractive power; they present, if really nervous, a good illustration of the division and anastomosis of ultimate nerve-fibres; the smallest divisions visible under a high power are seen only as fine lines.

Comment: Galen believed that the iris enlarged and contracted by the to and fro surge of blood like erectile tissue. This view was likewise held by the physiologist Haller (1756). Microscopic study established the presence of the sphincter (Meckel, 1820). As late as 1893, Günhagen maintained that the pupil dilated by virtue of its own elasticity. In 1849, Brown Séquard showed by injecting the blood vessels that the erectile theory could not account adequately for the play of the pupil. According to Duke-Elder, the first person to establish the true nature of the longitudinal fibers was Joseph Lister in 1853. This was his first piece of research. He studied the muscle fibers derived from the teased-out fresh tissue of a patient on whom the operation of optical iridectomy had been performed by Wharton Jones. Physiologic experiments previously had indicated the existence of a dilator muscle. Petit in 1727 discovered that section of the cervical sympathetic paralyzed dilation. Langley and Anderson later demonstrated, in 1892, that this action was independent of inhibition by the sphincter. Final clarification followed embryologic investigations (1898–1902), which revealed that both the sphincter and dilator muscles of the iris are derived from the anterior prolongation of the pigment layer of the retina. The epithelial cells that produce the sphincter are completely transformed into plain muscle fibers, but with the dilator the transformation is incomplete and myoglial fibers or myoepithelial cells result. The spindle-shaped cell bodies of the dilator tail off at one or both poles into long fiber-like processes that stain like muscle tissue. These fibers run radially in a single sheet anterior to their cells between the stroma and the pigment layer. The dilator muscle sends out prolongations at its ciliary margin that run obliquely into the ciliary muscle and into the pectinate ligament, thus providing the muscle with a fixed attachment. Though the dilator muscle is apparently tenuous, its total bulk is three times that of the sphincter. The poor development of the dilator at birth explains the difficulty in dilating the pupil of a newborn with a mydriatic.

Reference

W. S. Duke-Elder and K. C. Wybar: *System of Ophthalmology. Anatomy of the Visual System,* Vol. II, pp. 178–184, C. V. Mosby Co., St. Louis, 1961.

Biographical Note

Joseph Lister (1827–1912), the founder of antiseptic surgery, was born 5 miles east of the heart of London. Lister owed to his Quaker upbringing the placid manner and deep human sympathy that endeared him to patients and students. His father, a wine merchant, was fascinated by optics and his experiments led to the development of the achromatic microscope for which he was elected to the Royal Society in 1832. Lister received his medical degree from University College, London, in 1852. His professor of ophthalmology was Wharton Jones, a man of wide culture, who stimulated Lister to undertake his classic study of the contractile tissue of the iris. His professor of physiology, William Sharpe, advised Lister to work with Professor James Syme of Edinburgh, the leading surgeon of his day. Lister became successively his assistant, house surgeon and, in 1856, his son-in-law. In 1857 Lister presented his important paper on "The Early Signs of Inflammation" before the Royal Society of London. In 1860 he was appointed to the chair of surgery at Glasgow University and in 1863 he gave the Croonian Lecture on the coagulation of the blood. Lister was troubled by the disastrous toll of postsurgical infections and their complications— septicemia, pyemia, erysipelas, hospital gangrene and tetanus. One-third of amputations died. In 1865, a reading of Pasteur's writings inspired the idea that putrefaction in wounds might well arise from the same cause as fermentation in wine. Since carbolic acid had proved effective in purifying sewage, Lister introduced this antiseptic in the treatment of compound fractures, applying pure carbolic acid to all parts of the wound. In 1870 he substituted 5 per cent aqueous solution of phenol. Lister introduced also sulphochrome catgut sutures, as a ligature for arresting hemorrhage. His bacteriologic investigations led him to discover the microorganism responsible for the souring of milk which he named *Bacterium lactis*. In 1869 Lister succeeded Syme in the chair of clinical surgery at Edinburgh, and in 1877 he accepted the chair at King's College, London, which he held for 15 years. In 1876, Lister visited America to attend the International Medical Congress at Philadelphia. Thanks to Lister, von Bergmann, and others the incidence of infection in clean surgical wounds was reduced to a low of 0.25 per cent. At the International Medical Congress meeting in Amsterdam in 1879, Professor Donders, the president, acclaimed: "It is not only our admiration which we offer you, it is our gratitude." Lister became a baronet in 1883 and a peer in 1897, the first medical man to be so honored. In 1895, he succeeded Lord Kelvin as president of the Royal Society. The Lister Institute of Preventive Medicine in London, modeled on the Pasteur Institute, was in 1903 fittingly named in his honor.

References

D. Guthrie: *Lord Lister, His Life and Doctrine,* The Williams & Wilkins Co., Baltimore, 1949; R. Adams and B. Fahlman: Sterility in Operating Rooms. Surg. Gynec. & Obst., *110:* 367, 1960.
Lebensohn, J. E.: Homage to Lister. Am. J. Ophth. *64:* 322–323, (Aug.) 1967.

The Anatomy of the Muscles, Ligaments, and Fasciae of the Orbit, Including an Account of the Capsule of Tenon, the Check Ligaments of the Recti, and of the Suspensory Ligament of the Eye

C. B. LOCKWOOD, M.D.

J. OF ANAT. AND PHYSIOL., 1885, 20: 1–25

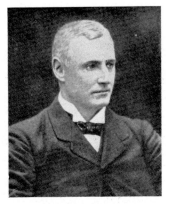

The capsule of Tenon and insertions of the ocular muscles. The insertions of the ocular muscles are so intimately related to to the aponeurosis which surrounds the sclerotic that it will be best to consider these insertions and the aponeurosis together. When the levator palpebrae has been divided, the structure is quite easily separated from the orbital fat. When this has been done, three parts will be found to demand attention: (1) A central part which surrounds the globe; (2) the prolongations which this sends along the muscles of the eye; and (3) its connections with the walls of the orbit.

The central portion of the capsule of Tenon is perceived to be a fibrous capsule which surrounds the globe from the ciliary margin of the cornea backwards to the entrance of the optic nerve; its anterior third is intimately related to the back of the conjunctiva; its middle third sends prolongations to the muscles of the eye; its posterior third is in contact with and loosely adherent to the orbital fat. Its thickness is not the same in any part, for it is strengthened by various fibrous bands, and it is easy to see that it becomes thinner posteriorly, and is continuous with the sheath of the optic nerve, both structures being fastened to the sclerotic.

The thin membrane which the union of the conjunctiva and capsule forms may easily be separated to within an eighth of an inch of the margin of the cornea, but any further endeavor entails laceration.

Relation of the inferior rectus of the capsule of Tenon, inferior oblique, and lower eyelid. In general characteristics the sheath of the inferior rectus is the same as the others. Its upper part has no peculiarity. The under part of its sheath may be said to consist of two superimposed layers—a superior and inferior. The superior layer keeps in contact with the under surface of the muscle, and is continuous with that part of the capsule of Tenon which supports the anterior hemisphere of the eye; the inferior layer is inserted into the posterior border of the sheath of the inferior oblique. Further, by means of the lower part of its sheath, the inferior rectus forms connections with a structure, which probably has a very important influence upon its action, and which will now be described as follows:

The suspensory ligament of the eye. The suspensory ligament is a band of fibrous tissue, stretched, like a sling, from one side of the orbit to the other. The fibers which compose it converge at each end to be inserted into the malar and lachrymal bones; in the middle they diverge to form a shallow cup upon which the eye rests. The widest part of the suspensory ligament is intimately woven with the capsule of Tenon, but not to such an extent as to conceal the identity of its fibers. In order to ascertain this, the lower eyelid should be removed layer by layer to the tarsal cartilage and conjunctiva. After a little fat has been taken away from the neighborhood of the inferior oblique muscle, many of the fibers of the ligament are easily seen crossing in front of the muscle. A more correct opinion of the relations of this ligament to adjoining parts, and especially to the globe, may be derived from a vertical section made through the long axis of the eye. In this the lower part of the capsule of Tenon will be found notably thickened, and the extent of this thickening may be indicated by saying that the lower quarter of the circumference of the globe rests upon it. The thickened portion of the capsule of Tenon is divided by an aperture through which the inferior rectus passes. The posterior part, and this is a very significant point, is thickest just behind this opening, but it gradually becomes thinner as it passes round the eye; whilst the anterior part looks crescentic, and send a long thin horn backwards beneath the inferior rectus, forming the upper layer of the under part of its sheath, and another forwards to become continuous with the ocular conjunctiva and inferior tarsal cartilage. It is united to the latter by a short thick process which it gives off in front. In the hollow of the crescent lies the sclerotic; in contact with its lower surface is the sheath of the inferior oblique. At its largest part, which is in close proximity to the conjunctiva the crescent is at least a tenth of an inch thick, more than twice the bulk of the rest of the capsule of Tenon. This thickening is due to the suspensory ligament.

By far the clearest idea of the suspensory ligament may be obtained from horizontal sections. These should be made on a level with the canthi. The insertions of the ligament into the malar and lachrymal bones are very distinct; each is about an eighth of an inch thick, and is attached vertically for at least half an inch. They are opposite the equator of the eye, and are about on a level with its lower half. The lowest parts of these bony insertions approach the floor of the orbit. The inner one is fastened to the periosteum which covers the lachrymal crest; in front its fibers pass over the lachrymal sac; behind it is continuous with the periosteum of the orbit and the lowest part of the check ligament of the internal rectus. As the ligament approaches the eye, it spreads out, and is continuous with the capsule of Tenon. The outer insertion of the suspensory ligament adheres to the periosteum of the malar bone just behind the external edge of the orbit, and at this point its posterior surface receives fibers from the check ligament of the external rectus. It is important to note that its under surface is fastened to the floor of the orbit by numerous irregular fibrous fasciculi; and it is further attached to the orbit through its connections with the sheath of the inferior oblique.

Uses of the suspensory ligament. The most important duty of the suspensory ligament, to support the eye, is obvious. When the eye has been removed from its upper surface, considerable pressure may be made upon the upper surface of the ligament without doing more than stretch it. It is a matter of common observation that immediately after excision of the superior maxilla, the eye maintains its position. The presence of the suspensory ligament offers a ready explanation of this circumstance. The expression "immediately" is used, because at later periods the globe may be drawn out of place by cicatrization. Another qualification is also needed, for I am informed that when the inner and outer walls of the orbit are very freely taken away during the performance of the operation, the eye may drop so much as to entail its removal. Under these circumstances, the orbital insertions of the suspensory ligament have been destroyed. This accident is likely to occur whenever incisions are carried above the level of the canthi.

In addition to the function which has just been mentioned, the suspensory ligament seems to perform another, which depends upon its connection with the inferior rectus and inferior tarsal cartilage. When the muscle is in action, it swings the suspensory ligament backwards, and owing to the intimate union of the latter with the inferior tarsal cartilage, the lid also moves. Its range sems to be so limited that it is able to control the contraction of the muscle, and so act as a check ligament.

Comment: The suspensory ligament seems to be not too effective in preventing the globe from sagging. In fracture of the floor of the orbit the globe sinks down and backwards causing a sequential enophthalmos. Exophthalmos due to orbital cellulitis and endangering the optic nerve has been decompressed successfully by removal of the orbital floor through the maxillary sinus.

Since the inferior rectus and the inferior oblique are joined by the suspensory ligament, the operator must make certain when the inferior oblique is picked up on a muscle hook that the inferior rectus is not included. The attachments of the sheaths of the inferior rectus and inferior oblique to the suspensory ligament vary tremendously in density and this variability explains the uncertain results of myectomy of the inferior oblique near its origin. After such a myectomy the inferior oblique continues to act on the globe to a greater or less degree depending upon whether its union with the suspensory ligament is firm or loose.

The attachments of the ligamentous expansions of Tenon's capsule to the margin of the orbit keep the eyeball from being retracted into the orbit when the recti contract or from being pulled forward by the contraction of the obliques.

References

Scobee, R. G.: The fascia of the orbit. Am. J. Ophth., *31:* 1539, 1948.
Adler, F. H.: *Physiology of the Eye,* Ed. 2 Ch. X. C. V. Mosby Co., St. Louis, 1953.

Biographical Note

Charles Barrett Lockwood (1856–1914) was born in Stockton, England; he was graduated from the medical school of St. Bartholomew's Hospital in 1878, and was attached thereafter to the teaching and surgical staff of this institution. From 1882 to 1892 he was a demonstrator in anatomy and in 1887 he founded with Humphry the British Anatomical Society. From long service in the dissecting room he attained a profound anatomical knowledge, the foundation of his later surgical dexterity and confidence. At the beginning of his career he was much interested in the eye and became clinical assistant to Tay at the Royal London Ophthalmic Hospital. Indeed, his first important paper was "The anatomy of the muscles, ligaments and fasciae of the orbit." Unfortunately for ophthalmology he subsequently devoted himself to general surgery and his surgical writings were standard works in his day. Though extremely reserved personally, he loved teaching as it served to clarify his ideas. He was wont to say: "It is one thing to know, and another thing to impart your knowledge to others." Lockwood placed extreme emphasis on asepsis. In 1904 he lectured before the Medical Society of London on this subject and in his last three years gave classes also in bacteriology. During an operation for appendicular peritonitis he pricked his finger and tragically fell himself a victim to septicemia.

Reference

Obituary. St. Bartholomew's Hospital Reports, *50:* 101, 1914.

Part Six

Cataract

The Couching Operation for Cataract

BENEVENUTUS GRASSUS

Montpellier, France

DE OCULIS, PP. 33–36, FERRARA, 1474.*

A proper cure begins with a purgative, using my Jerusalem pills, compounded only by me. The formula of these is spurge, half an ounce, hepatic aloes, five ounces, to be ground with sugar of roses. After purgation, at the third hour, the patient should be placed astraddle a bench, as if on horseback. Now be seated on the same bench face to face with the patient, who will keep one eye closed. So begins the operation in the name of our Saviour Jesus Christ.

With one hand raise the upper lid, and with the other hold a silver needle and direct it toward the outer lacrimal region. Then perforate the eye coats, pushing and turning the instrument around with the fingers until you touch the diseased matter, which the Saracens and Arabs call *linzaret* (but which we call cataract), with the point of the needle, and dislodge it from its position in front of the pupil. Then push it well below, holding it there until you have said four *pater nosters*. Then carefully and slowly turn the needle back to its first position in front of the eye. If the cataract follows the instrument and shows itself in front, you must again depress it, pushing it this time as much as possible toward the ear. Then withdraw the needle in the same manner that it was inserted. And note well that having entered the instrument you must not withdraw it until you are convinced that you have depressed the cataract in the manner just described.

* Excerpt from the Translation by Casey A. Wood, M.D.

After the operation the patient's eye must be closed, and he should be kept in bed on his back in a shady part of the house. He must not be moved nor allowed to look at a light for eight days, during which period the eye operated on must be dressed with white of egg twice a day and twice during the night. His diet should be soft, fresh eggs with bread. If the patient is young, let him drink water; if old, he may drink a little wine well diluted with water. Many (physicians) allow such patients the meat of chicken, but I prohibit it as being too heavy. That sort of diet causes a rush of blood to the eyes and interferes with natural healing. Finally, after eight or nine days, let the patient make the sign of the Cross and leave his bed. He may now bathe in cold water and so accustom himself to that practice.

Such is the procedure with all curable cataracts, whether they be chalk-white, bluish, blue, or yellowish. Pay no attention to any kind of treatment except that given in our book. We call the operation *acocee*, or reclination of the cataract with a needle. It is also called *alglugal* for the same reason.

The needle should be made of gold or silver. I am opposed to the use of steel, which has at least three disadvantages: First, it is much harder than silver and on that account injures every part it touches; and remember that the cataract is also hard, and in operating the point of a steel needle might break off and remain in the eye. In that case the whole eye might be destroyed by the pain that results; for severe pain may bring on cold abscess and an obstinate and continuous flow of tears unfavorable to a cure of the cataract. A steel instrument is also very heavy, and the patient experiences more pain in its use because of its weight and hardness than if it were made of gold or silver, that are less harmful on account of their purity and softness. Take note, also, that a gold instrument especially clarifies objects with which it comes in contact because of its inherent power over cold and dampness.

You have heard the causes, varieties, accidents, and treatment of curable cataract. Now listen to the differences between them as regards a restoration of that light which improves the vision. For example, the first variety—white like the purest chalk and produced by a blow on the eye—is easy to cure unless the patient does not perceive lights as the result of the injury, in which case the humors of the eye were involved, just as the corporeal humors in other parts are dissolved by a blow.

Comment: The first description of the couching operation in European literature is that by Celsus at about the beginning of the Christian era. Since the Hippocratic writings say nothing of the subject, Celsus must have derived his knowledge from the Alexandrians and it is probable that they were indebted to the Hindus. Couching for cataract is described in the Ayur-Veda (The Science of Life) by Susruta, who probably flourished during the Buddhist ascendency (sixth century, B. C.). In Europe the couching operation was left for the most part to itinerant practitioners since the contemporary physicians shunned all surgery and particularly that of the eye. Guy de Chauliac (1300–1368), the star of the University of Montpellier, was one of the first to take the operation of couching out of the hands of travelling quacks. He acknowledged the great influence of the writings of Grassus. For more than a century after Daviel demonstrated the feasibility of cataract extraction in 1747 the pros and cons of couching versus extraction were ardently debated. In 1722 Percival Pott, a proponent of couching, gained the conception of discission as a distinctive method of dealing with soft cataracts. In 1785, Von Willburg gave couching a new lease of life by changing the maneuver from depression to reclination. Reclination was advocated by Argyll Robertson, Delafield, founder of the New York Eye and Ear Infirmary, Edward Reynolds, co-founder of the Massachusetts Eye and Ear Infirmary, and many others of eminence. Reynolds, who had studied under Lawrence, was the first in America to couch a cataract. On his return home he found that his father was blind from bilateral senile cataracts and the son successfully couched both lenses at one sitting in 1818. Von Graefe, whose skill and insight were universally respected, rekindled interest in extraction and secured its definitive acceptance.

Reference

Lebensohn, J. E.: The bicentennial of cataract extraction. Am. J. Ophth., *30:* 922–923, 1947.

Biographical Note

The available data regarding Grassus are meager and conflicting. Casey Wood concludes that Grassus was a Hebrew born in Judea sometime during the 11th century, that he read and spoke Hebrew, Arabic, Italian and Provençal, that he was educated at the medical school of Salerno, that he practiced in the Near East and in several southern European cities, and that he settled in Montpellier after acquiring a wide reputation as a skillful operator on cataracts. Here, free from persecution and welcomed as a teacher and physician, he wrote his book and taught his art. His book, variously entitled *Practica Oculorum* or *De Oculis* was for more than 500 years the most popular ophthalmic manual of the Middle Ages, and became the first incunable on the eye. The second printed work on the eye was the compend of Johannes de Peckham, Archbishop of Canterbury. More than two dozen codices of the Grassus manuscript are extant in Hebrew, Latin, French, Provençal and English. In these the author's name has the following diversification: Raffe, Graffe, Grasse, Grassus, Grapheus, Grafton and Benevenutus Hierosolimitans (Benevenutus of Jerusalem). His Hebrew name was undoubtedly ha-Rafee, the physician. The earliest codex of Grassus still extant is of the thirteenth century and now rests in the library of the University of Basel. Casey Wood considers that the Christian formulas incorporated in the text were the act of a prudent printer-publisher. But does not the modern ophthalmic surgeon begin and end his operations with a silent prayer! Grassus was proud of the large fees that rewarded his surgery, but stated "have always compassion for the poor, so that God may grant you the favor of successful operations!"

Reference

Sobotka, H.: Ophthalmology during the Middle Ages. A. M. A. Arch. Ophth., *57:* 366–375, 1957.

A Mew Method of Curing Cataract by Extraction of the Lens

JACQUES DAVIEL, M.D.

Paris, France

Memories de l'Académie Royale de Chirurgie, Paris, 1753, 2: 337–354*

The ancients believed that a cataract consists in a kind of membrane, and that this membrane is formed by an inspissation of the aqueous humor. But now we know that a cataract consists in a clouding of the crystalline lens. That is a truth which everybody knows and nobody contests. Therefore I will waste no time in adducing new proofs. We are chiefly indebted for the discovery in question to the famous Lasnier, fellow of the College of Surgeons at Paris, who had knowledge of the matter very long before Maître-Jan and Brisseau; but the true proposition was essentially confirmed by these two later men.

The true cataract is a clouding of the lens, either of the whole or of a part; without the accompaniment of any other ocular affection.

It is not the color which declares the favorable variety; but the eye must be otherwise sound, the pupil must dilate (by ½, ⅓, ¼) and the patient must be able to distinguish light from darkness.

The false cataract, that of the bad variety, consists of a clouding of the crystal, combined with immobility of the pupil, which is either too markedly dilated or contracted. The patient cannot descry the shadow of an object. These signs sufficiently often indicate amaurosis. Then there may be also severe headaches, a stubborn ocular inflammation, and the like.

The ancients who regarded a cataract always as a membrane, invented ways and means of depressing it in correspondence with that view. Some made use of round needles, with a view to rolling up the membrane like a ribbon; others, of needles that were sharply pointed, the less to injure the sclera; a few employed cutting needles in order to sever the thread, which, according to their view, affixed the cataract to the ciliary processes; at length Freytag invented a spring-pincette, ending

* Based on the translation by Thomas Hall Shastid, M.D., Superior, Wisconsin, American Encyclopedia of Ophthalmology, Cleveland Press, 1914, 5: 3755–3767.

in needles with which he designed to draw the membranous cataract out of the eye.

In 1745, at Marseilles, in the conviction that sharp and incisive needles produce those accidents which often enough are seen subsequent to the ordinary operation, I invented a flat and blunt needle with a spatula-shaped extremity, with which I believed that I could depress a cataract more successfully after I had made the puncture with an ordinary needle. But experience has convinced me of the contrary, and the operation which I am soon to describe has not a little contributed to awaken in me the considerations to which I owe the procedure which I now am practicing.

A hermit of Aiguilles, in Provence, who had already undergone an unsuccessful operation on his right eye, came to me at Marseilles, requesting that I try the second eye. I was, unhappily, no more fortunate than was my predecessor. By means of the ordinary needle, cutting on the side, I was in no position to depress the cataract. Indeed it came to this, that several fragments of the broken up cataract arrived in the anterior chamber. I saw this chamber filling up with blood until my needle was no longer visible, and I had to withdraw my instrument from the eye before completing the operation. This accident decided me, after the example of M. Petit, to open the transparent cornea for the purpose of removing the blood and the fragments of the cataract from the anterior chamber. I introduced a half-curved needle, and enlarged the first opening in the cornea with small curved scissors; thereupon came out all that had been in the anterior chamber, the pupil became clear, the patient distinguished at once all objects held before him. But, as his eye had been too greatly weakened by the first operation, the second unfortunately remained without success and was followed in two days by suppuration of the organ. These accidents were, without doubt, occasioned by the traction on the internal membranes and by the dilaceration of the vitreous body.

This case, which accident had brought before me, occasioned me to decide that, thereafter, I would only operate in that very way in which I had carried out the procedure for the hermit, through an opening of the cornea to go in quest of the lens in its capsule, to bring it through the pupil into the anterior chamber and to extract it from the eye. I did this operation for the first time for a woman. I opened the cornea in the way mentioned, brought the little spatula, which I have already described, upon the upper portion of the cataract, made it free and drew it piecemeal from the eye by the aid of this instrument. The pupil was clear, the patient had not the slightest accident, and, fourteen days late, was completely cured.

Encouraged by this success, I carried out this procedure on four other patients in order at least to institute a comparison of these difficult methods and to try whether I might find one which should be free from the all-too-frequent accidents.

I determined to perform the cataract depression with two instruments. The one, of steel, was a small, straight knife, for the purpose of opening the scleral membrane at the customary place. Through this opening I at once passed the little spatula against the highest portion of the cataract, between the latter and the posterior surface of the iris, and thus completed the depression of the cataract with ease and safety.

After a large number of operations, performed in accordance with this method, some in the presence of the most distinguished masters of the art, had produced remarkable results; I believed I might dare to conclude that this method was preferable to the other.

I was in a position personally to compare all that had been until that time invented, especially instruments and methods.

All sorts of needles have been employed by me. I have also performed the operation in various manners, inasmuch as I now brought the needle behind the crystalline, in order to break through the posterior lamella of the capsule, and now sought to open the capsule at its under part in order to cast the lens into the vitreous via this opening. But I have observed that the operation, when performed by the last-named method, only succeeds exactly when the lens-capsule is very thin and delicate. Then the lens, when it has been cast beneath the vitreous, does not rise again so easily, and there follow only a few accidents which are common to all sorts of operations. However, it is very different when one strikes a firm capsule, a soft cataract and a rather thick vitreous; then the irritation of the membranes by the needle and the necessary splitting of the vitreous, sometimes occasion very considerable complications, now and then even suppuration of the eyeball and wasting of this organ. Although I had used, as one might say, every sort and kind of cataract operation, still I was not satisfied with the results, and instituted new investigations, in order to determine with exactness what disturbance of the inner portions of the eye must of necessity follow the operation with a proper needle. The results of the operation were very various. Truly, in a few happy experiments, the pupil was found clear and the lens at the bottom of the vitreous, without any sort or kind of disturbance of the inner parts. But, in cases, the pieces of the lens which had been broken up by the needle, arrived in the anterior chamber; the more I moved, or stirred, the needle in the eye in these cases, the less did the eye become clear. Sometimes I found the greatest difficulty in removing the lens from its capsule, and finally it happened to me to find it between the retina and the choroid, and both of these membranes torn in different places.

I doubted then no longer that the disturbance of the different parts, which I had witnessed in cadavers' eyes, and which exhibited a very great variety, was the cause of those disorders whose unhappy effects made themselves only too perceptible in the living. I must therefore believe that those disorders depend not only on the introduction of the needle into the eye, of whatsoever kind that instrument may be, but also on the resistance of the membranes, and, before all, of the lens, according to the place in which it came perchance to lie after the depression.

Indeed, if one only considers a little the form of the different needles, one immediately perceives that those which are thin and pointed only stick, or pierce, and, as they do not present a sufficient surface, often enough they cannot press upon the cataract sufficiently to depress it into the depth of the vitreous, or, at the least, that they must occasion those accidents which accompany the wound of puncture.

The cutting needles sever the blood vessels, and often occasion hemorrhages into the ocular interior, which hinder the completion of the operation.

Those which are flat, blunt, and rounded off, may contuse and lacerate the inner membranes of the eye, and, by consequence, occasion disagreeable accidents.

Aside from the accidents which must be attributed to the needles, the lens itself may, of course, by its mere presence, injure the different portions of the eye—a fact which, as above remarked, depends upon the different situations which it may assume subsequent to the depression. I pass over the accidents which the most careful operator cannot entirely avoid, though he be as careful as he may.

Despite these various unfortunate matters, I believed that I might employ my last procedure, by preference, still more widely—a procedure which consists in this: first, to employ a cutting instrument, and afterwards a flattened needle, for the purpose of depressing the cataract until the idea which I had won from the operation on the hermit had attained in my mind to a certain ripeness. But the occurrence of which I am about to speak, gave to my conviction its final completion.

On the 8th day of April, 1747, I was called to a private person whose cataract appeared to be very favorable and the eye, also, in good condition for an operation. I began to operate on the left eye, whose cataract appeared to me to be the more solid. However, it was not possible for me to depress it. The pupil remained clouded after the operation, and the patient saw absolutely nothing. I then passed over to the right eye, with which I also had much trouble. Inasmuch as I could by no means depress the cataract in this eye, I decided then to open the cornea, as I had done in the case of the hermit. I enlarged the opening, then with a small pincette held the cornea well up and passed through the pupil my small spatula, with which I extracted from the posterior chamber the entire lens, which had divided and then been broken into pieces by the first operation which I had made already on this eye. The extraction was followed by the exit of a part of the vitreous, which, in fact, had also been divided by the earlier operation. But in spite of this disturbance, the patient distinguished objects very well after the operation. The latter had no bad results. The patient was well a very short time afterward.

After this time and during the three following years I performed this operation several times upon the living, in order to get accustomed to it gradually. But, for the first time, while on a journey to Mannheim for the purpose of treating the Electoress of Zweibrücken for an old affection of her left eye, I came to a firm decision in the future to operate for cataract only by extraction of the lens.

I had occasion to pass through Lüttich and to stay there for a time. There I performed six operations in accordance with this method and all with the greatest success. One which I performed at Cologne on a priest of a religious order, yielded a very surprising result, inasmuch as the cataract was as soft as jelly. In spite of that fact, the priest was able, fourteen days later, to read the Mass.

Herr con Vermale, corresponding member of the Academy and surgeon-in-chief to the Elector of the Palatinate, has reported the operations which he saw me perform at Mannheim in a letter which he caused to be printed, and which he addressed to M. Chicoyneau, first physician to the King. Since that time I have used this operation further in different places, and reckon up to this time (Nov. 15, 1752) 206 operations, of which 182 were successful. That means, I think, that one can infer a decided advantage from an operation which has only just now been invented. Hereunder I give a description of the details.

When a diagnosis has been made of cataract, then questions do not arise, for this method, as to the condition of the cataract, its age, softness, hardness, or color. The operation will be equally successful, provided the eye is otherwise sound. For the chief purpose of my operation is the extraction of the cataractous lens from its bed. That is very easily attained under the precautions of which I shall shortly speak.

The preparation of the patient I carry out in the usual well known manner. On the day selected for the operation, I place the appurtenances in order; these consist of bandages, compresses, tiny bits of linen, lead plaster cut egg-shaped, pledgets of cotton, warm water and wine.

The instruments which I employ are: 1. A needle, sharpened to a point in front, cutting on the side, somewhat curved, and lance-shaped, for the first opening. 2. A needle blunted off in front, cutting on the side, also curved, for the purpose of enlarging the first opening. 3. Two curved, convex scissors. 4. A small spatula, of gold, silver, or steel, slightly curved, for the purpose of lifting the cornea. 5. Another small needle, sharp forward and cutting on both sides, for the purpose of opening the anterior capsule of the lens. 6. A small spoon of gold, silver, or steel, in order to facilitate now and then the exit of the lens or to extract pieces of its substance when these remain behind in the pupil. 7. A small pincette, for the purpose of removing bits of membrane, which may perchance be present.

All these instruments are arranged in order upon a plate, and entrusted to an assistant whose business it is to reach them to the surgeon as needed.

When all is thus arranged, the patient is brought into a room of only moderate brightness, in order that a too strong light may not contract the pupil and enter the eye too abundantly subsequent to operation, which may produce dazzling.

The patient is set on a rather low stool, or on a chair without any back. The operator sits upon a higher chair, in front of the patient and facing him, so that the former, while he operates, can support his elbow on his knees.

He covers the other eye with a bandage. Then an assistant, standing behind the patient, lays one hand upon his forehead, lifting the upper lid with two fingers, while the second hand is laid beneath the patient's chin.

The surgeon draws down the lower lid, seizes the first needle, sinks it into the anterior chamber, close to the sclera, while he avoids all injury to the iris, and passes it higher than the pupil, then he draws the needle very gently out again, takes up the blunt-pointed needle, and enlarges therewith the incision already begun, drawing the instrument to right and left, in order to open the cornea in the form of a half-moon, corresponding to its curvature.

But, as the cornea is then a little flaccid, the surgeon takes up the curved, convex scissors, brings its blunt arm between cornea and iris, and completes the incision first upon the one, then on the other, side in order to bring it on each side a little above the pupil.

One should, of course, observed that the convexity of the scissors must be directed toward the eye. With respect to the curvature-on-the-flat, therefore, two pairs of scissors are essential, which fit the curvature of the cornea as well on the nasal as on the temporal side.

The surgeon takes then the small spatula, raises with it gently the separated portion of the cornea and incises with the little edged and pointed needle the capsule of the lens. Sometimes one has to cut this membrane all around and remove it in its entirety, when it is thickened and folded; and then it can be drawn out, when well cut round, with the tiny forceps.

When one has circumcised the membrane which enclosed the lens, then he must carefully introduce the small spatula between the body of the lens and the iris, in order to make the cataract entirely free and to facilitate its exit. Now the surgeon needs all his foresight. He is about to remove the veil that covers the light. To this end he presses very gently on the ball, avoiding even the slightest pain. Thus the operator avoids rupturing the posterior capsule of the lens, which acts like a dam to prevent the exit of the vitreous humor. With delight is seen the gradual dilation of the pupil, and the soft gliding hither of the lens (which first allows its margin to appear) in the anterior chamber and from there upon the cheek. At once the pupil is clear; the cloud which covered the eye has been dissipated; the patient, who before was plunged in darkness, glimpses the day with astonishment and satisfaction.

Now one sets in order the pupil, which sometimes, through the exit of the cataract, especially when it is hard and firm and very large, loses its regular shape. When the operation is complete, the patient is bandaged, in order to guard against the effects of excessive light.

Should it happen that the cataract is soft and tough, so that it breaks in pieces, then the fragments can be removed by means of the tiny spoon, which the surgeon passes into the pupil as often as necessary. Then the corneal cap is accurately replaced, the eye is wiped gently with a soft and delicate sponge, dipped in lukewarm warm (in which have been mingled a few drops of alcohol) or else in some sort of collyrium. The plaster is laid on the eye, on that a little cotton in pledgets, and the whole is fastened with a bandage, but without any pressure. One covers the head with a linen cloth, has the patient lie down in a dark room, if possible on the back, and in a bed surrounded by curtains.

The eye is bathed in a softening and solvent decoction, twice or thrice a day, and as often as seems to be necessary. One should not forget blood-letting and a correct mode of life. The patient is, besides, treated on general principles.

Howsoever strongly convinced I may be of the advantages of this operative procedure. yet I cannot deny that it is also liable to its own peculiar accidents. Yet these are of such a kind that one can easily remedy them, indeed a few can be prevented. During the performance of the operation, for example, a part of the vitreous can come out from the eye; but this can be avoided well-nigh to a certainty, by only pressing gently on the eyeball, when causing the lens to come forth.

There are indeed cases in which it seems to be necessary to employ a heavier pressure. If the capsule of the lens is adherent to the iris, the union must be separated with the small spatula; then the pupil slowly yields for the exit of the lens.

If, because of injury to the iris, blood is once effused into the anterior chamber, it will quickly run out of itself through the corneal incision; it in no wise hinders the operation. This accident recently occurred to me in the presence of Mm. Dran, Morand, la Faye, and a few others; the eye received no harm from it, the patient sees just as well with it as with the other, which was operated upon immediately after its fellow.

That all the aqueous humor is lost at once, is a necessary, but harmless, unpleasantness. If, however, one withdraws too rapidly the needle used for opening the cornea, the iris may follow the aqueous: it is then caught betwixt the lips of the little wound. However, it is easily freed by lifting the cornea very gently with the tiny scalpel. Sometimes merely the natural movements of the eye result in the reposition of the iris.

In the course of the treatment the iris may again prolapse, and form a staphyloma. But this is easily remedied by shoving the iris back. Prolapse can also almost certainly be prevented by taking care when binding up the eye not to do the bandaging too tightly, for the accident in question is almost always caused by too great pressure.

I believe it will be admitted without further remark that these accidents signify little in comparison with those which may occur after the customary methods. But these are not the only advantages of my procedure. A comparison with other methods brings out plainly much more considerable points of superiority.

1. If a person operates according to the old procedure, he has to wait until the cataract is ripe.

2. When a cataract is depressed, it may, no matter how fast it is, once more arise. One cannot deny that this accident now and then occurs. Here, on the contrary, one is perfectly certain that a cataract extracted from the eye will never arise again.

3. After the usual procedure, the cataract sometimes arrives, either wholly or in part, in the anterior chamber; that occurs sometimes in the course of the operation, and further, as is well known, several years thereafter. As the cornea is not opened, the cataract plays the

176

role of a foreign body in the anterior chamber, and its movements may be very disagreeable; indeed it may even occasion the loss of the eye, or, at all events, render necessary a second operation. By my method I remove the cataract absolutely and completely from the eye, after bringing it (advantageously) through the aperture of the pupil.

4. If a person operates in the customary manner on a soft cataract, the operation often remains uncompleted because of the bits of torn-up capsule, laden with tough fragments of lens, which may close the pupil, and, thereby, offer to the rays of light the same obstruction as an entire cataract. By my procedure I have extracted also soft cataracts; I have removed a few that resembled bladders filled with water; I have loosened some that had become adherent.

5. In order to depress the cataract according to the old procedure, one must press through the vitreous body and cut into its branches, which sometimes, by the more or less frequent motions of the needle, are wholly torn up. That cannot occur without decided consequences, and cannot be wholly avoided by the use of needles devoid of point and edge. It is easy to perceive that this accident cannot occur by my procedure.

I believe that I have now said enough to prove the superiority of this procedure, and the preference it deserves over the others. It has won the suffrages of those masters of our art before whom I have been able to operate; a number have already adopted it. It remains only for me to prove further that I am the inventor of this operation, whose discovery by me has been disputed—I know not from what motives.

Comment: Brisseau demonstrated in 1705 that the mysterious cataract was simply an opacity of the crystalline lens. The lens had been assumed to be the seat of vision previously, which idea is implied in the Biblical phrase "precious as the apple of the eye." Daviel stressed that his cataract operation logically stemmed from knowing the true nature of cataract. His first deliberate extraction occurred in 1747 as a surgical emergency following a vain attempt to couch either lens in a man with bilateral cataracts. Three years later Daviel decided definitely to operate for cataract by this method only. Daviel's operation was supported enthusiastically by the elder Baron Wenzel who admitted destroying a hatful of eyes before achieving the requisite skill.

For the following century the pros and cons of couching and extraction were ardently debated. In 1772 Percival Potts introduced discission as a method of dealing with soft cataracts, and Saunders demonstrated its special value in the cataracts of children thirty years later. A new lease of life was given couching in 1785 when the maneuver was changed from depression to reclination. Argyll Robertson preferred reclination to extraction as the more successful procedure, but his contemporary, von Graefe, intensified interest in extraction by his stimulating contributions and secured its definitive acceptance. In Daviel's day, a cataract operation was placed in the successful listing if postoperative vision allowed walking without a guide. Hermann Knapp, in an analysis of cataract operations sixty years ago, considered a postoperative acuity of 20/200 or better a successful result. In 1000 intracapsular extractions reported in 1944, 85 per cent achieved a postoperative acuity of 20/30 or better, but our modern precautions have not eliminated all hazard—in 5 per cent vision was annihilated through various postoperative complications. Curiously, the increasing use of appositional sutures has favored a return to the technic of keratome incision enlarged by scissors as originally advocated by Daviel.

Reference

Lebensohn, J. E.: The bicentennial of cataract extraction. Am. J. Ophth., *30:* 922–923, 1947.

Biographical Note

Jacques Daviel (1696–1762) was born in La Barre, Normandy. Shortly after completing his medical studies at Hotel Dieu in Paris he volunteered for medical duty during the plague at Toulon and was cited for his ability. After two years of service he married the daughter of an army surgeon and resumed general practice in Marseilles, where he was soon appointed demonstrator in anatomy and surgery. For excellence in this post for over ten years he received Royal recognition. The dissecting room gave him a means of practicing the couching operation and his success at this procedure led him to limit his practice to ophthalmology. In 1746 he moved to Paris; in 1747 he successfully performed the first deliberate cataract extraction in history. By the end of 1756 Daviel had done 434 cataract extractions of which 384 were successful. Among his distinguished patients was King Ferdinand VII of Spain. In 1762 Daviel developed laryngeal paralysis, probably from carcinoma of the larynx, and went to Geneva, Switzerland, for his health where he died the same year. Daviel's grave is in the cemetery of the Grand Saxonix Church, two miles north of Geneva, and at this shrine an impressive memorial was placed in 1885.

Reference

Hildreth, H. R.: Daviel: modern surgeon. Am. J. Ophth., *36:* 1071–1074, 1953.

On the Corneal Suture in Cataract Extraction

E. KALT, M.D.

Physician to the National Eye Clinic of the Quinze-Vingts in Paris
ARCH. OPHTH., 1894, 23: 421–425*

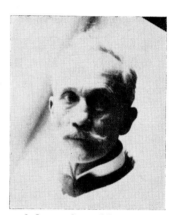

After the long discussions which have filled the scientific publications of the last twenty years, an agreement on the best method of operating for cataract seems to have have actually been reached. The great majority of operators have returned to the simple extraction, reserving the iridectomy for the cases complicated with adhesions or in which the iris refuses to take its normal position again. The partisans of the suppression of the iridectomy record from 8 to 12 per cent of iris prolapse. These and plastic iritis are dreaded as the chief complications now, the purulent inflammations having fortunately become very rare.

The mechanism of the prolapse of the iris is still partially unexplained. Prolapse has occurred in cases in which the coaptation of the wound was perfect and the patient quite manageable. We are not yet able to foresee it. It always is for us the most disagreeable surprise and a grave danger for the future of the eye.

If we suppose that the prolapse of the iris is due to the sudden escape of an inordinate quantity of aqueous humor stowed up behind the iris by a rupture of the wound still too feebly cicatrized, we may think of two, apparently opposed, preventive measures, *i.e.*, either to cause a delay of the complete closure of the wound and the refilling of the anterior chamber until the cicatrix has become solid enough, or to suture the lips of the wound in order to secure a firm closure.

The suture gives an immediate and sure result. Henry W. Williams, of Boston, published in 1867 encouraging results. He had to use chloroform and applied his suture after the extraction when every pressure

* Translated by H. Knapp from the (unpublished) French original.

on the eye may be dangerous. Suarez de Mendoza, of Angers, has recently recommended the systematic use of the suture and insisted on the important point that it should be applied before the opening of the anterior chamber and possibly through the superficial layers of the cornea and sclera. In his communication of 1892 he states to have used the suture thirty-eight times and to be very much satisfied with the results. He applies a single suture at the upper end of the vertical meridian. He begins with a shallow incision of the cornea, through the track of which the Graefe knife has to pass afterward, introduces the needle into the cornea two millimetres below his preliminary section, draws it out through the lower edge of the latter, reintroduces it through the upper edge, and brings it out 2 mm. above it. The middle portion of the thread forms a loop which is placed on the side. It is evident that a narrow knife could pass in the ordinary way through the cornea without cutting the thread. After the extraction the suture is tied. The wound is perfectly closed and the anterior chamber reestablished in two hours.

This is, in short, the procedure of Suarez. Without knowing it in its details I have, on my part, tried to suture the cornea quickly and safely.

I use very fine, short, sharp-pointed needles, and thin but strong silk threads. The needles when armed are sterilized in hot air and kept for use in a sterilized paper envelope. After cocainization and disinfection I pass the needle through the cornea, in the vertical meridian, about 1 mm. underneath the limbus; the point, without penetrating into the anterior chamber, emerges at the juncture of the opaque border, and the thread is drawn. Then the needle is introduced, about 1 mm. above its point of exit, into the episcleral tissue, as is done in the muscular advancement. So soon as I find that the point has penetrated into resistant tissue, I draw it out again, in order to involve as little of this tissue as possible. As it is impossible to draw the needle out at right angles about 2 mm. of conjunctiva are loaded on it, which is of no consequence. In drawing this thread I leave a loop, which is placed sideways toward the nose, and spread out carefully so as to avoid twisting.

The corneal section is made in the ordinary way, care being taken that the knife passes nicely through that portion of cornea which the suture has left free. Then I take off the speculum, and remove the cataract as usual. When the iris is well in position, an assistant holds the upper lid up, and I tie the thread.

It is to be borne in mind that I do not, like Suarez, make a superficial incision into the limbus corneae, in the depth of which lie the points of entrance and exit of the thread, for this makes the corneal section with the narrow knife very difficult without cutting the thread in so narrow a passage. The coaptation in my procedure seems to me quite sufficient. Furthermore, I am not afraid to draw the knot tightly at the risk of folding the cornea. This folding disappears in a day, and the corneal astigmatism is neither increased nor diminished.

The suture does not inconvenience the patient. Rarely I remove it before the tenth day, when it has become quite loose. With one stroke of the scissors I cut off the knots, and seize the thread with forceps.

Accidents to Guard Against.—Involuntary cutting of the thread with the Graefe knife. This is rare. Generally a new needle can be passed through the hole of the old.

When the suture is tied, we should draw on the superior, scleral end of the thread. The coaptation takes place by itself. The opposite would be dangerous.

I can affirm that the suture infects the cornea in no way. The slight opalescence left in its track disappears quickly.

Operative Results

I have practised systematically the corneal suture in 50 cases of simple extraction. In 45 the operation has been normal. The iris went back to its position, and the closure of the wound was perfect, without incarceration of the iris.

In 2 cases the reposition of the iris was laborious, and could not be maintained until the suture was tied anew. Nevertheless the result was excellent. Formerly I would have made an iridectomy.

In 1 case, a retrogressive cataract, prolapse of the vitreous ensued. When I had closed the suture, I was greatly surprised to see that the iris and vitreous had reduced themselves, and I have still been able to remove a few fragments of the lens.

In 2 cases of a normal operation I found, the next day, an angular incarceration of the iris. Thanks to the presence of the suture, the excision of the iris was very easy.

Thus, on the whole, there were 2 point-like hernias in 50 extractions, that is 4 per cent. I must say that without the suture I have never had less than 8 per cent of hernia in 180 extractions I make a year. This proportion has even been raised in some series to 10–12 per cent, for inexplicable reasons. These figures are not extraordinary; they are found in the statistics of excellent operators. Knapp, of New York, records 10 per cent of prolapse in a recent series of 600 extractions. The frequency of this deplorable complication explains why many operators still cling to the combined extraction. The corneal suture gives, I believe, a satisfactory solution of this prolapse question, which has become a real nightmare. It is to be hoped that neither the spirit of routine, nor the fear of making the operation two or three minutes longer will prevent the new procedure from spreading.

Comment: Methods directed toward an accurate closure of the cataract wound are of comparatively recent origin. Until thirty years ago only a few surgeons favored the use of sutures. Some attempted to improve the closure by leaving a bridge of unseparated conjunctiva beneath which the cataract was extracted. Elliot (1933) stated that a conjunctival bridge was a routine step in all his cataract surgery. Williams of Boston in 1865 used a perforating corneal suture after extraction of the lens but abandoned this for a conjunctival suture in 1869. Though in 1923 Lancaster rejected the suture, which he then considered prolonged the operation and added little to security, in 1931 he favored Verhoeff's modification of the Kalt suture. Kalt described the first preplaced corneoscleral suture in 1894 and in 1910 reported the outcome of over 2500 cataract extractions thus operated. The Kalt suture went vertically in the cornea and transversely in the sclera. Stevenson of Ohio in 1912 and Liegard of France in 1913 suggested that both sutures be horizontal, parallel and about 2 mm. apart. In 1922, Frisch of New Jersey advised placing a stop-knot at the corneal end of the Kalt suture so that drawing on the upper end of the suture would close the wound quickly at any time. With this modification, Frisch said, one is master of the situation even before tying the suture. After the intracapsular cataract operation attained general acceptance, corneoscleral suturing became mandatory, the Kalt-Liegard suture being usually favored. In 1891, Suarez de Mendoza had devised the method of making a preliminary groove in the cornea and inserting the ends of a double-armed suture in either lip prior to incision. Lindner in 1938 and McLean in 1940 modified the procedure by placing the groove at the corneoscleral junction instead of in the clear cornea and bringing the suture out through a previously dissected conjunctival flap. The Lindner-McLean preplaced nonperforating, appositional suture is now in established usage, and has changed the technique of cataract surgery since with these multiple, preplaced sutures it is far easier to use a keratome and scissors than the cataract knife. The Kalt needles have given place to swaged needles, an innovation originally introduced for intestinal surgery; and these needles have been made ultrasharp by a special process of reverse electrolysis to further facilitate work on the eye.

Reference

Roper, K. L.: Suturing in cataract surgery. Tr. Am. Ophth. Soc., *52:* 587–749, 1954.

Biographical Note

Jean Baptiste Eugène Kalt (1861–1941) was born in Alsace and educated in Nancy and Paris. His studies under Ranvier inspired an abiding interest in anatomy and pathology that was applied later to ophthalmic research. Eugène Kalt was trained in ophthalmology under Panas and became chief of the clinic. Among his numerous articles are contributions on tumors of the conjunctiva, dacryocystitis, congenital glaucoma and diseases of the retina. His last publication (1937) discussed the experimental production of retinitis pigmentosa by injections of sodium iodate. He was among the first to use contact glasses for keratoconus (1888) and he initiated the treatment of gonorrheal ophthalmia by profuse irrigation with a dilute solution of potassium permanganate (1892). He is particularly renowned, however, for his innovations in cataract surgery. He devised the corneo-scleral suture (1894), the bridle suture for the superior rectus muscle (1908), peripheral iridectomy with a fine hook, and the Kalt forceps for the removal of the anterior capsule of the lens (1909). He later used this forceps for intracapsular extraction. From 1892 to 1941 he was ophthalmologist to Hôpital des Quinze-Vingts where his operative dexterity attracted numerous students and visitors. He expired at the age of 80 on the day following a masterful surgical session. His celebrated son, Marcel Kalt, has proved a worthy successor to this post.

Reference

Kalt, Marcel: Personal communication.

Inflammations of the Eye Caused by Lenticular Material Dissolved in the Eye Lymph*

MANUEL STRAUB, M.D.

Amsterdam, Holland

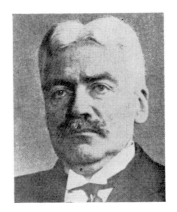

For several years there have been in the collection of my laboratory microscopic slides of eyes with an inflammation caused by resorption in the eye lymph of lenticular material which escaped through its capsule from a tear or by other means. I divide the great variety of material into the following groups:

I. Phacogenic inflammatory reactions following cataract operations and other perforating injuries of the lens.

II. Phacogenic inflammatory reactions after dislocation of the lens.

III. Phacogenic inflammatory reactions following spontaneous resorption of senile cataracts.

LaGrange and LaCoste agree that lenticular remains have less harmful effects in the infant than in the young adult and in the young adult less than in old age and that a large amount of lenticular remains is more harmful than a smaller amount. Observation has shown me that constitutional factors are of little importance. The lenticular remains itself give the impression of being harmful. Inflammation which we ascribe to lenticular remains show a completely different picture than the chronic inflammation caused by infection. Both types of reactions do not occur at the same time interval. Another argument for the influence of lens remains lies in the observation of cases in which the lens is completely removed. We all know how white and quiet the eyes remain when the lens is removed in its capsule. Most of the extracapsular operations leave posterior synechiae behind. Quivering of the iris then rarely occurs as we see after the intracapsular operation. The re-

* Excerpts from an unpublished English Translation by Volckerdt de Groot, M.D., of the Dutch monograph by Straub, published by J. H. de Bussy, Amsterdam, 1919.

tained lens material is the stimulus causing the posterior synechiae. Another reason why we accept the ability of lens material to cause inflammation are the cases of ruptured or perforated lenses which leave no doubt that the lens material is the irritating factor.

We performed an iridectomy in a case of chronic simple glaucoma which seemingly healed uneventfully, but after five months developed a chronic inflammation slowly increasing in severity. At operation a small incision was made in the lens capsule. The consequence of the wound revealed itself only slowly. Swelling of the cortical cataract first occurred. Then an increase in the size of the wound followed by the dissolving of lens fibers in the eye lymph produced inflammatory symptoms which betrayed this process. It is of great importance to determine this disease in time. A recognized case can be treated with lens extraction. This has already been done in our clinic three times. In this case the diagnosis could have been made by the increasing density of the cataract and the increasingly shallow anterior chamber. Further, the extent of the fibrin precipitate on the posterior corneal surface was conspicuous and likewise the bleb formation of the corneal epithelium. This is rarely seen in ordinary cases of iridocyclitis. I feel that the name of our disease process should not be iridocylitis. We deal with toxins that originate from an injured lens. The disease can, therefore, be called endophthalmitis phakogenetica.

The left eye of a 44-year-old woman was blind, painful and with a tension of two plus. Enucleation was performed. Histologic examination revealed a scar that perforated the entire cornea and because of its direction could not possibly be an operative scar. It corresponded in direction with an iris scar and a bundle of fibrous tissue strongly attached at the posterior pole of the lens where the capsule is torn open. Trauma in childhood had produced a non-progressive cataract. The lens was protected by fibrous tissue which preserved a useful eye for many years. The scar tissue, which extended from the ciliary processes to the posterior surface of the lens, contracted and caused a deep anterior chamber. With further traction on the lower lip of the capsule wound, the wound enlarged; the lens fibers swelled and the swollen mass was dumped into the vitreous. This case shows that whereas an anterior wound of the lens produces a cyclitis, a posterior one produces a hyalitis.

A combined cataract extraction was done on the right eye of a 62-year-old man with an uneventful post-operative course. Five months later, the left eye became painful and red, revealing mild corneal edema, keratic precipitates, hyperemia of iris and posterior synechiae. The eye quieted with treatment, but after four months the same condition recurred, responding again to therapy. But a third attack soon followed, accompanied by severe pain, high tension and shallow chamber, necessitating enucleation. Histologic examination revealed a tear in the capsule of the lens near its equator. Lens substance that entered the lymph stream by diffusion produced the endophthalmitis phacogenetica.

A few years later a similar case was treated by extracting the cataract from the inflamed eye. A 70-year-old woman was operated for left senile cataract with uneventful healing. Six months later she returned stating that the right eye became painful over the past few weeks. The cornea was edematous, and keratic precipitates and posterior synechiae were present. The eye was treated for two months but showed no response. Cataract extraction with peripheral iridectomy was then performed. The eye healed uneventfully. The keratic precipitates disappeared and the patient was discharged with a quiet eye. The diagnosis of endophthalmitis phacogenetica was made because of the intermittent course, the uncontrollable reaction, the haziness of the cornea and the numerous precipitates on the posterior corneal surface, and was confirmed by the operative result.

A 57-year-old woman suffered for many years a recurrent iritis in one eye, which eventuated in complete posterior synechiae, anterior lens opacities, phthisis bulbi and loss of light perception. Microscopic examination of the enucleated eye revealed signs of dissolved lens substance underneath the anterior capsular opacities. The iris angle was closed as in glaucoma. The eye showed a scattered infiltration of lymphocytes. This is a resorption-lymphocytosis and develops when only mildly irritating toxin is taken up in the eye tissues. The lymphocytes are found mainly in front of the posterior layers of iris tissue and if the process is of long duration in the anterior layers also, in the ciliary body and in the choroid at the ora serrata. The other part of the choroid shows scattered infiltrates such as is seen in sympathetic ophthalmia. These infiltrates result from the products of tissue decay that collect at these localities,—from dissolved substances that penetrate the intact lens capsule.

At the age of 46 a woman visited the clinic with a cataract in the left eye. At the age of 57 she returned complaining of severe pain in the eye of six weeks duration. Therapy proved ineffective and the eye was enucleated. Histologic examination disclosed atrophy of the cataractous lens and also of the iris and part of the pigment epithelium of the ciliary body. I consider the iris atrophy a result of the resorption of the lens substance. Lenticular opacification, maturity and hypermaturity preceded the iris atrophy. We know that lens toxins can cause an endophthalmitis producing exudates on the posterior corneal surface and that pigment granules are regularly carried away by the leucocytes of these iris exudates. A chronic process will, therefore, bleach the iris in the long run.

From where do the lymphocytes come? We must assume that they are drawn by different lure substances than the polymorphonuclear cells. We observe them regularly in chronically inflamed eyes, and consequently in those inflamed by lens substance. A gradual resorption does not necessarily cause an inflammation. However, when a weak spot or tear in the lens capsule develops and suddenly a large amount of lens toxin is thrown into the eye lymph, an inflammation will ensue. Secondary glaucoma may also result.

Comment: No proof of toxic substance in hypermature or degenerating lens material has yet been demonstrated. The tradition of toxicity arose from Straub's studies which had convinced him that such material called forth a secondary iridocyclitis of a special type that he called endophthalmitis phacogenetica. The evidence of toxicity was entirely clinical and circumstantial. After removing the cataract in a case that Straub would have diagnosed as phacotoxic uveitis, Maumenee in 1957 proved that the extracted lens was neither toxic nor irritating to normal animals or tissues and found that the concurrent uveitis was a typical hypersensitive reaction. Alan C. Woods studied the reports, histologic microphotographs and pathologic descriptions in Straub's monograph and perceived a striking similarity to Verhoeff's endophthalmitis phacoanaphylactica. Woods noted the characteristic mobilization of neutrophiles around the traumatized lens fibers, large mononuclear phagocytes and the monocellular infiltration of the iris and concluded that there could be little doubt that these cases were identical with endophthalmitis phacoanaphylactica. The latter entity was announced by Verhoeff and Lemoine in 1922. Straub was the first to present convincing histologic evidence of lens-induced uveitis and to differentiate non-granulomatous uveitis from that caused by infection. He also distinguished lens-induced uveitis from sympathetic ophthalmia and was the first to demonstrate that lens-induced uveitis could be cured by the extraction of the ipsolateral cataract. Observes Wood: "How unfortunate that the post-war chaos in Europe prevented the appreciation of Straub's contribution! Had it been realized in 1919 that lens-induced uveitis in the second eye was a clinical entity, was quite distinct from sympathetic ophthalmia, and that this form of uveitis could be completely cured by the simple procedure of extraction of the lens in the affected eye, how many eyes might have been saved!" Credit is due Woods for the rediscovery of Straub's contribution and for establishing its place as a classic of ophthalmic literature.

Reference

Woods, A. C.: Manuel Straub and the tradition of toxicity in len protein. Am. J. Ophth., *48:* 463–472, Oct., 1959.

Biographical Note

Manuel Straub (1859–1916) graduated in medicine from the University of Amsterdam in 1882. For a few years he was assistant in pathology under Prof. C. H. Kuhn, after which he served as military surgeon in the

Netherlands army where he attained the rank of major. He then studied ophthalmology at Utrecht under Donders and Snellen. His earliest ophthalmic contribution was on the lymph flow in the cornea. He became interested next in finding why clinical emmetropia was so extremely common. His studies led him to assume a regulatory process by which excess refractive power in one constituent of the eye was balanced by less refractive power in other elements. He conceived that this tendency toward an optimum equilibrium, which he termed "Emmetropization" in 1893, was due to the correlation of structural development with motor, sensory, psychic and nutritional factors. In 1895 he was appointed professor of ophthalmology at the University of Amsterdam, a post that he filled with distinction until his death at age 57. From 1895 to 1903 he also edited the Tijdschrift vor Geneskunde. Straub bubbled over with original ideas. His numerous publications covered every phase of ophthalmology and its inter-relations with physiology, pathology, bacteriology and biochemistry. His interest in refraction never ceased. In 1899 he emphasized the progressive increase of hyperopia in the elderly which he aptly labeled "senile hypermetropia"; and in 1909 he depicted the relative incidence of refractive errors at various ages. For some years before his demise he had been studying lens-induced uveitis. During his lingering final illness he called Zeeman and de Vries to his bedside and charged them with the task of compiling and publishing his notes and illustrative material. The monograph appeared in Dutch three years later. In 1958 de Groot made a complete English translation for Alan C. Woods which Dr. Woods very kindly let me read.

Reference

Zeeman, W. P. C.: Obituary. Klin. Monastsbl. f. Augeng., *57:* 129–134, 1916.

The Adjustment to Aphakia

ALAN C. WOODS, M.D.

Baltimore, Maryland

Am. J. Ophth., *35:* 118–122, January, 1952

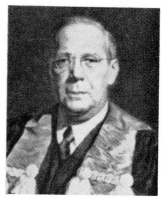

Patients with the best possible visual result from cataract extractions show a wide difference in their ability to adapt themselves to their aphakia. A few accept their correction with avidity and their happiness over their restored vision dwarfs any unpleasant symptoms they may experience. Probably a majority have various difficulties before they finally become reconciled to their new visual status. The second group comprises individuals with more acute visual needs, to whom the peculiarities and limitations of aphakic vision present a real rehabilitation problem.

Even when the second eye is operated on successfully and tests on the Howard-Dolman apparatus show accurate depth perception, the size difference of familiar objects introduces a spatial element of false orientation. There ensues an unpleasant period when tumblers are overturned, when, reaching for the salt, the unfortunate patient puts his fingers in the gravy-boat, flower vases are upset, ink is spilled, all exasperating to the patient and trying to the members of his household. It usually takes several weeks for the neophyte in aphakic vision to accustom himself to the magnified aspect of the outside world, forget his previous concepts of the size of objects, and overcome the false orientation.

The second, and fortunately transient, unpleasant phenomenon is spherical aberration. At first it appears almost impossible to live in a world in which all straight lines are transformed into curves. This difficulty is augmented when he discovers that the movements of his eyes suddenly cause the curved outside world to squirm like writhing snakes. Thus the newly elected aphakic regards a door through which for years he has been accustomed to pass and, to his amazement, he finds the jambs in each side curve in toward the middle and leave only an

188

aperture a few inches wide at the center. When mature thought persuades him that this is an optical illusion, he finds to his delight that as he approaches the opening, the curves recede gracefully and he finds unimpeded passage.

Similarly, when entering a high room with tall columns such as a hotel lobby or a railroad station, he finds the supporting columns bending and waving precariously. Gradually he learns the secret of persuading the outside world to abandon its sinuous behavior. The secret consists in holding his eyes motionless, his gaze fixed through the optical center of the correcting lens and to move his head slowly to look at any desired object not in his direct view. When this trick is mastered, the spherical aberration disappears.

The next step in the thorny pathway of the new aphakic is the coordination of manual movements with the new visual imagery. The most elementary tasks—sharpening a pencil, carving a fowl—are done with a sense of insecurity and clumsiness. There is nothing to do except to patiently repeat some manual task until confidence is again regained. For many, small jig-saw puzzles and the like are of decided value, teaching the individual how to handle objects and at the same time tickling his ego with a sense of accomplishment when the puzzle is solved.

Thus the newly created aphakic can be assured that his three most obvious troubles—false orientation, spherical aberration, and lack of coordination—can ultimately be overcome with time and practice. There remain two other difficulties which must be endured. These are the limitation of the visual field due to the ring scotoma and the continual necessary adjustment of the aphakic correction.

The magnified central visual field seen through the optical center of the glass overlaps and blots out a portion of the dimmer peripheral field and so produces a ring scotoma. At ordinary reading distance, the aphakic is unconscious of the scotoma. Beyond 20 feet the field is also sufficiently wide to permit driving a car and the scotoma presents no problem. For intermediary distances, especially between two and 10 feet, the presence of the ring scotoma imposes a handicap which cannot be overcome. In ordinary group conversation, faces pop in and out of the blind area with the annoying insolence of a jack-in-the-box. Going up and down stairs the aphakic must look at the steps to avoid falling and to learn when to stop ascent or descent. Crossing a street with a green light the unfortunate aphakic is at the mercy of any motorist who chooses to turn into his pathway.

The second difficulty is the annoyance of cataract glasses. The greater the base-curve of the correcting lens the larger the visual field, but the greater and more troublesome the spherical aberration. Within the average range, a —3.0 D spherical base curve affords the best compromise. For the bifocal addition, the flat top segment is vastly preferable to a rounded addition. The aphakic invariably prefers the upper portion of his add, avoiding use of the lower portion on account of prismatic deviation and peripheral spherical aberration. Since the aphakic uses only the optical center of his lens, any maladjustment introduces a prismatic error which greatly reduces visual efficiency. After the correcting prescription is filled, the patient must again be seen by the ophthalmologist to determine if the finished glasses give the maximum of vision, or if one lens must be set in or set out. His glasses rarely break but they constantly become bent out of adjustment. When this happens, his only resource is to have on hand spares and to seek the aid of a skillful optician.

Concerning the elderly individual without great visual requirements whose vision is reduced to the 20/70 or 20/100 level, is it proper to subject him to the visual and physical reorientation incidental to aphakia for the sake of the improved central visual acuity? It should be carefully considered on the basis of the individual's visual requirements and his physical and mental status before surgical interference is advised.

Comment: This classic editorial of Woods excited widespread attention, stimulated certain optical improvements in cataract spectacles and accelerated indirectly a more extensive use of contact lenses in aphakia. The article was republished repeatedly, the latest reprint being in the Brit. J. Ophth., *48:* 349–353, 1964. In a personal experiment R. C. Welch fitted his eyes with —14.0 D contact lenses and corrected the simulated aphakia with spectacle lenses, whereupon he marveled how the aphakic patient finally adjusted to the handicaps that a spectacle correction imposes (Brit. J. Ophth., *49:* 84–86, 1965). The aphakic correction with spectacles establishes in effect a Gallilean telescope with a magnification of nearly 30 per cent. Hence, as Boeder detailed, the patient is baffled by new size relationships and the disharmony between visual and tactile perception. He underestimates distances and sees straight lines curved as a result of an increase of magnification from the center to the margin of the lens. Because of apparent changing curvature when the eyes move, vertical lines appear to wave and may cause giddiness. The prismatic effect at the margin of the lens produces a "ring scotoma" that measures about 10° in a 44-mm. 12.0 D lens. When an object moves from the blind area into the field of view it seems to come from nowhere. Most of the unpleasant effects are avoided by using only the central portion of the cataract lens. In shifting fixation the patient learns to move his head slowly and so evades rotation of the eyes. A flat top bifocal is desirable as it provides a wide reading portion and minimizes the magnified jump. It should be fitted only slightly below the optical center of the principal lens. The proper inset of the segment can be calculated from the P.D., reading distance and power of principal lens in the horizontal meridian. For P.D. 60 mm.; reading distance, 14 inches; horizontal power, 10.0 D; the segment should be displaced 2.5 mm. For aphakic corrections aspheric plastic lenses offer a larger usable field, half of the weight of glass, less fogging and less internal reflections. The final prescription must be precise as plastic lenses cannot be resurfaced. Because of the electrostatic affinity of plastic for dust, a cleaning solution of the type used for contact lenses is advisable.

The aberrations inherent in a spectacle lens are practically eliminated by contact lenses since the contact lens moves with the eye and hence the visual axis passes through its center at all times. The improvement in visual comfort and cosmetic appearance has been a boon to the aphakic and the past 15 years have witnessed their steadily increasing use. Bifocals give the refractionist an opportunity to refine the contact lens correction. The magnification with the contact lens is about 7 per cent and can be reduced still further by fitting the contact lenses for near vision and correcting for distance with minus lenses. This arrangement also facilitates the insertion of contact lenses. For a patient with binocular aphakia, who wears contact lenses, spectacles should be prescribed fitted with one near vision lens and with the lower half of the frame of the other eye wire cut away so that the contact lens can be inserted. After this is done, the spectacles are removed and the other contact lens inserted with the vision of the corrected eye. Successful tolerance of contact lenses can be anticipated in two-thirds of aphakic eyes. Aphakics tend to wear their contact lenses overly prolonged and because of abnormal tolerance may be unaware of deleterious changes; hence they must be urged to have the condition of their eyes checked periodically.

References

Benton, C. D., Jr., and Welch, R. C.: *Spectacles for Aphakia*. Charles C Thomas, Publisher, Springfield, Illinois, 1966.
Boeder, P.: Spectacle correction of aphakia. Arch. Ophth., *68:* 870–874, 1962.
Symposium: contact lenses. Trans. Am. Acad. Ophth. & Otolaryng., *66:* 277–307, 1962.

Biographical Note

Alan Churchill Woods (1889–1963), the son of Hiram Woods who headed the department of ophthalmology at the University of Maryland, graduated from the Johns Hopkins Medical School in 1914. After a 2-year research fellowship at the University of Pennsylvania in the problems of allergy and immunity, he served in World War I under Sir William Lister under whose direction he did a vast amount of eye surgery. On his return he began work at the Eye Clinic of Johns Hopkins Hospital. In 1925 he became assistant director of the newly founded Wilmer Institute and on the retirement of Wilmer in 1934 succeeded him as director. He was a brilliant teacher and administrator, and inspired his staff which included Jonas Friedenwald, Frank Walsh and Louise Sloan. Among his many outstanding residents were McLean, William Hughes, Guyton, Becker, Iliff, McPherson, Sanders and Maumenee. The investigation of uveitis, begun during his research fellowship, was still his prime interest and during his career he contributed 160 articles and two books on the various facets of the subject. In 1946 he joined the full time staff of Johns Hopkins University and was promoted to full professor of ophthalmology. Upon his official retirement in 1955 he was succeeded in his post by Maumenee but he continued to

192

be active at his office in the Wilmer Institute until shortly before his death from coronary occlusion. In 1941, 22 years before his decease, his vision became affected by rapidly developing cataracts. Jack Guyton, who had just finished his residency, operated. The result was perfect, two round pupils and a corrected vision of 20/15 in each eye. He was elected to the presidency of the American Academy of Ophthalmology and Otolaryngology in 1947 and of the American Ophthalmological Society in 1956. Among his other honors were consulting editor and director of the *American Journal of Ophthalmology,* an LL.D., membership in the Ophthalmological Society of the United Kingdom and fellowship in the Royal College of Surgeons of Edinburgh, award of the Research Medal of the A. M. A. Section of Ophthalmology and the Howe Medal of the American Ophthalmological Society.

References

Randolph, M. E.: Alan Churchill Woods, M.D. Am. J. Ophth., *41:* 374–383, 1956.
Maumenee, A. E.: Obituary. Alan Churchill Woods, M.D. 1889–1963. Am. J. Ophth., *55:* 842–845, 1963.

Part Seven

Glaucoma

Glaucoma

WILLIAM MACKENZIE, M.D.

Glasgow, Scotland

EXCERPTS FROM CHAPTER XXIII OF *A Practical Treatise of the Diseases of the Eye,* 4TH EDITION, LONDON, 1854

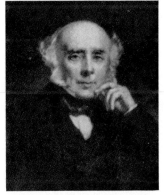

Brisseau appears to have been the first to announce to the profession the opinion that, while cataract was an opacity of the lens, glaucoma was a similar affection of the vitreous humor. Brisseau was not aware that the chief cause of the loss of sight in glaucoma resides neither in the lens, nor in the vitreous humor, but in the retina.

I have already had occasion to mention the occurrence of glaucoma in cases of arthritic iritis. The patient suddenly becoming blind, and the eye presenting a green reflection behind the pupil, the name *acute glaucoma* has been employed. The disease we now consider is, in contradistinction, designated as *chronic glaucoma*. It is of frequent occurrence, is in its early stages attended by no external signs of inflammation, and being slow in invading the perfection of vision, is apt to be confounded with cataract.

Glaucoma is a disease which does not occur except after middle age. It comprehends a series of morbid changes:

1st stage. The earliest appearance of glaucoma is a greenish hue, reflected from behind the pupil, and is not necessarily connected with any material deterioration of vision.

193

2nd stage. There is a sluggishness of the pupil, and more or less obscurity of vision. The eyeball is rather firmer than natural. This stage may last for five or six years, or more, vision declining by insensible degrees all the time, but without pain or external redness of the eye. Vision is thereby impeded nearly as in cataract; but there is little or no coagulation of the lenticular substance.

3rd stage. An abnormal hardness of the eye, with immobility and unequal dilatation of the pupil, a varicose state of the external, and probably of the internal, blood vessels, and a still more marked loss of sight, are signs of the third stage. In this stage the retina is compressed; the vitreous tissue is disorganized, and a superabundant watery secretion comes to occupy its place. For a time, the eye may continue sensible to objects placed to one side or other side of the patient, while in every other direction nothing is distinguished. At length, the retina becomes totally insensible.

4th stage. In the fourth stage, the lens appears augmented in thickness, and pressing forwards through the pupil, it at length touches the cornea. The iris is changed in color, its texture appears thinned, its fibrous structure is no longer discernible, and patches of it seem eroded. Varicose vessels are observed traversing its surface. Perception of external light is totally lost.

5th stage. In the fifth stage, the cornea, irritated by the projecting lens, appears hazy and rough; it inflames, and gives way by ulceration.

6th stage. The sixth stage presents the eye quiet and atrophied. This state may ensue even without bursting of the cornea; the inflammatory symptoms subsiding of themselves, and the contents of the eyeball undergoing absorption, so that it shrinks to less than its normal size; and, instead of the preternatural hardness which it formerly presented, becomes boggy, and sinks into the orbit.

These different stages of glaucoma run insensibly into each other. Although the disease is scarcely at any period of its course amenable to treatment, it is no uncommon thing for it to be spontaneously arrested in one or other of these stages. Sometimes amaurosis accompanies glaucoma from the very commencement. The anomalous appearances which we occasionally meet with in glaucoma are numerous. One of these implicates the epidermis of the cornea; its epithelium is separated from it by a fluid, and rises in the form of an irregular vesicle. The glaucomatous lens, viewed in its natural situation, seems of a greenish color. Taken out of the eye, all greenness is gone; the lens is of a deep amber color.

Diagnosis.—Attention to the following circumstances will enable the observer to discriminate between glaucoma and cataract:—

The eyeball, in cases of amaurosis combined with glaucoma, always feels firmer than natural; while in cataract, it presents its usual degree of resistance to the pressure of the finger. The crystalline should be examined catoptrically, according to the method of Purkinje. The observer and the patient should be placed in a room from which the daylight is entirely excluded. When a lighted candle is held before a healthy eye, at the distance of a few inches, three reflected images of it are seen. Of these, the anterior and posterior are erect, the middle one inverted. The anterior is formed by the cornea; the middle, by the posterior surface of the crystalline; the posterior, by its anterior surface. The focus of the inverted image is positive, and is situated within the crystalline. Cataract, even at an early stage, obliterates the inverted image, and renders the deep erect one very indistinct. Glaucoma, in all its stages, renders the deep erect one more evident than it is in the healthy eye. When the candle is held in the axis of the eye, the inverted image is indistinct in both diseases; but whenever it is moved to one side, it becomes distinct in glaucoma; whereas in cataract it is obliterated.

Prognosis.—When glaucoma has commenced in one eye, it generally extends also to the other. We often see the disease in different stages in the two eyes. Fully developed glaucoma is absolutely incurable.

Treatment.—Anti-neuralgic remedies, such as Fleming's tincture of aconite in doses of 3 or 4 minims, thrice a day, are of much use in alleviating the pain, which often attends the disease. As a superabundance of dissolved vitreous humor appears to form an essential part of the morbid changes, occasionally puncturing the sclerotica might prove serviceable, by taking off the pressure of the accumulated fluid on the retina. A transient amelioration of vision, as well as relief from pain, is sometimes the result of the operation, or even of that of puncturing the cornea, and evacuating the aqueous humor. It is necessary to be aware that a glaucomatous eye is always very susceptible of suffering inflammation and disorganization, even from the slightest operation which may be practiced upon it.

Comment: In his day William Mackenzie was the most distinguished ophthalmic surgeon in the United Kingdom. His textbook ran through four editions in English, and was translated into German, French and Italian. The original edition, published in 1830, was the first publication to emphasize that an elevated intraocular tension was the most important distinguishing character of glaucoma. Though Mackenzie did much to advance ophthalmic surgery, he opposed strongly von Graefe's operation of iridectomy for glaucoma. In 1958, when he was 67 years old, and von Graefe then was age 30, he wrote:

"Everyone who has practiced the operation of evacuating the aqueous humor in cases of acute internal inflammation of the eye knows that a single evacuation is often sufficient to check the inflammation and render it amenable to the remedies which it had before resisted. In abnormal hardness of the eyeball, Dr. Graefe first tried the local application of mydriatics but without effect. It is not easy to perceive on what grounds any effect in diminishing intraocular pressure could have been expected. The contrary was to have been feared, for mydriatics generally impair the sight still more in glaucoma. Iridectomy has been practiced frequently of late at the Moorfields Ophthalmic Hospital. In chronic glaucoma, not much is said in its favor, but the cases described as inflammatory glaucoma are sufficient to confirm Dr. Graefe's reports that good effects result from the operation in the latter disease. Notwithstanding this, the objection remains that the excision of a piece of iris is a proceeding unnecessarily super-added to a means long known as calculated to give relief, and to which alone the benefit obtained is to be attributed, viz. the removal of the tension by evacuation of the superabundant fluid within the eye. We have no doubt, however, that in a short time iridectomy as a means of treating glaucoma will be abandoned."

To this von Graefe courteously replied: "I should indeed have expected more moderation from the Nestor of English ophthalmology. I see, with regret, that Dr. Mackenzie maintains a procedure to be bereft of common sense which others name one of the most thanksworthy improvements in ophthalmological science, and this without having procured the slightest experience of his own on the subject. The future, which I look forward to with confidence, will decide who shall have to regret his too hasty expressions in this matter."

Mackenzie's unfortunate attitude is but another instance in which eminent authorities failed to estimate justly the work of younger men and to appreciate correctly the trends of progress. Wharton Jones dismissed the ophthalmoscope of Babbage as valueless four years before that of Helmholtz appeared. Dollard, who had achieved the first achromatic lens, said of Franklin's bifocals: "They can only serve particular cases, but are not for eyes in general." A British commission that investigated cocaine considered the drug inconsequential four years before Koller's discovery of local anesthesia.

References

Jones, T. W., and Mackenzie, W.: M. Times & Gaz., o.s., *37:* 342–345, 1858.
Graefe, A.: On iridectomy in . . . glaucoma. M. Times & Gaz., o.s., *37:* 447–448, 1858.

Biographical Note

William Mackenzie (1791–1868), the son of a muslin manufacturer, was born and educated in Glasgow. He graduated from the University of Glasgow with the intention of becoming a minister, but finally decided on a medical career and graduated from the Medical School of the University of Glasgow in 1815. After postgraduate study in London, Paris, Pavia and Vienna, he tried to establish himself in London in 1818. Not being successful, he returned to Glasgow the following year. In 1824 Mackenzie helped to found the Glasgow Eye Infirmary, which has been adorned for many years by his portrait painted by Macnee. In 1828 he was appointed lecturer in ophthalmology at the University of Glasgow, and in 1838 he received the distinction of being named Surgeon-Oculist to the Queen. His textbook, since its advent in 1830, was considered the ophthalmologist's bible for a quarter century. In 1843 Mackenzie was made an honorary fellow of the newly instituted Royal College of Surgeons of England. His extensive ophthalmologic library now belongs to the Faculty of Physicians and Surgeons at Glasgow, and his extraordinary collection of eye specimens is preserved in the medical school of St. Mungo's College. The ophthalmologists of Glasgow revere his memory through the William Mackenzie Lecture and Medal instituted in his honor.

Reference

Rainey, G.: Obituary. Glasgow M. J., *1:* 6–13, 1868.

Iridectomy in Glaucoma: A Study of the Glaucomatous Process

ALBRECHT VON GRAEFE

Berlin, Germany

ARCHIV FÜR OPHTHALMOLOGIE, 1857, *3:* 456–560*

The incurability of glaucoma seems to be due to the fact that ocular changes are consecutive and originate from an extraocular source. The whole question of glaucoma therapy took on a different aspect, however, when I realized that the blindness was to be attributed not to changes in the optic nerve, but to an increase in intraocular pressure. The increased pressure is the main cause of the damage, particularly of the excavation of the optic nerve. As a curative measure I propose that by some means or other a lowering of intraocular pressure be effected.

All efforts to produce a rapid outflow of fluid from the eye by general measures failed. Finally, I experimented with repeated paracentesis which gave such startling results at first that I published them without hesitation (Arch. f. Ophth., 1855, *1*). Visual acuity was improved by the outflow of the turbid aqueous and its replacement by transparent fluid. The paracentesis had the great advantage of proving that many symptoms of glaucoma, such as the corneal anesthesia, depended on the rise of pressure. As a result of the paracentesis, I could distinguish the ecchymotic changes in the fundus in the early stages of the disease, since the refractive media cleared immediately. Unfortunately, however, the beneficial results proved only temporary in the vast majority of cases. In the few eyes which were improved by the operation, visual acuity was not greatly reduced by the inflammatory exudation, in spite of all the initial symptoms of acute glaucoma. In the other cases after a period of improvement of days, weeks and even months, deterioration began, not, as a rule, in the form of a violent inflammation, but as chronic glaucoma. Even when the improvement lasted longer than three months, an unfavorable prognosis could be given because of the gradual constriction of the visual field. I tried to combat these relapses, at first, by methodical repetition of the para-

---

* Excerpted from a condensed translation by Francis Heed Adler, M.D. Arch. Ophth., 1929, *1:* 71–86

centesis, but each time the therapeutic effect became shorter in duration and finally the vision ceased to improve.

It was the use of iridectomy in ulcerations and infiltrations of the cornea which led me to the discovery of its pressure-reducing action. Operations for partial staphyloma of the cornea and staphyloma of the sclera usually consisted of an attempt, first, to remove the staphyloma, then to form a new pupil, if this was needed. When I reversed this order for another purpose, I noticed that after an iridectomy the ectatic part frequently receded to the normal level of the cornea, and that the second operation was unnecessary. In fact I saw cases in which repeated attempts to correct the staphyloma failed until an iridectomy was performed.

Fortified by these facts and hypotheses I felt justified in performing an iridectomy in glaucoma. I knew the favorable effect of the operation on the choroidal circulation. Everything seemed to promise that the operation might have a physiologic and a therapeutic effect in lowering pressure. The first attempts varied extremely, since I had no criteria for the choice of cases or for the details of the operation. I began to use this method in June, 1856, and from that time applied it in cases of acute glaucoma. The immediate effect appeared favorable, but recalling my disappointment with paracentesis, I was extremely mistrustful. A continuous improvement became apparent, however, as the observations were prolonged. The signs of glaucoma gradually disappeared. After observing a few of the patients for more than a year and many of them for more than nine months, I believe the operation of iridectomy to be a curative measure to combat glaucoma.

Iridectomy in the Prodromal Stages of Glaucoma

It is not often that patients seek medical assistance when prodromal symptoms of glaucoma appear in the first eye affected; these are either overlooked or regarded as of little importance. On the other hand, it often happens that after the vision in one eye has been lost from glaucoma, the patient is alarmed by prodromal symptoms in the other eye. The question then arises as to whether one should await the distinct outbreak of the disease in the other eye or should he interfere during the prodromal stage. I hesitated a long time before doing the latter, because vision was still good intermittently, and because I lacked complete confidence in the procedure. As I gradually became bolder, I began to operate in a few cases during the prodromal period, and was entirely satisfied with the results. Loss of vision did not occur in a single case following iridectomy. The ciliary pain and colored halos disappeared. The periodic clouding of the aqueous also vanished and did not return. The anterior chamber appeared deeper than before. I could not decide whether or not a slight decrease in presbyopia occurred. In three of these cases, clouding of the vision had occurred rather frequently for several months before the operation. For this reason the effect seemed to be permanent. Visual acuity is as little influenced as is the accommodation by the presence of a moderately broad coloboma. Moreover, the possible small changes in this respect, contrasted with the certainty of complete blindness, are not worthy of consideration.

There cannot be any disadvantage in temporizing and in using internal medication. Any operation, however safe, may harm the patient accidentally or as a result of his disobedience. I usually advise patients in whom one eye is blinded from glaucoma and the other eye is threatened to submit to an operation when the prodromal symptoms appear in the second eye, especially if diminution of vision occurs. One should not wait for a severe inflammatory attack. Even if an iridectomy affords complete relief from symptoms during the acute stage, the whole management of the patient at this time demands greater care and caution, and the operation itself is more painful. Massive retinal hemorrhages may occurr making the restoration of vision slower. Changes in the iris, fixed pupils and paralysis of accommodation usually continue. The prodromal stage may never pass into the acute form but may develop gradually into the chronic form through the continuous protraction of the exacerbations.

Even when the prodromal symptoms have lasted a long time, iridectomy gives the same result. In this connection, I might mention a patient whom I treated for two years. One eye had been blinded by glaucoma and the second was in the prodromal stage. The periodic obscuration of vision became more frequent and more intense and I knew of no means to check the glaucomatous process. I gave, therefore, the most pessimistic prognosis and sent the patient home. About nine months ago one of my assistants, Dr. Alfred Graefe, performed an iridectomy on this patient, with splendid results. The reduction in visual acuity in the meantime, however, had become severe.

Iridectomy in the Acute Period of Inflammatory Glaucoma

My experiences are far more numerous in cases during the acute period of inflammatory glaucoma than in those during the prodromal stage. I operated more than twenty eyes shortly after the outbreak of the first marked inflammation which, in a few cases, was so severe that an operation seemed disastrous from the start.

I sought, at first, to alleviate the symptoms by antiphlogistics, opiates and similar treatment. I became convinced, however, that immediate iridectomy was necessary. Under these conditions every delay causes increased damage, and the surest help for the inflammation lies in the operation itself. After the operation not only did the symptoms improve without other means of treatment, but a rapid clearing of the refractive media occurred in every case. Seven days after the operation, the eye-ground could be seen clearly with the ophthalmoscope. I thus ascertained the following facts about the process which later were of considerable aid:

1. The optic nerve is entirely normal after the first attack. Cupping or displacement of the vessels is not present, provided that chronic glaucoma has not preceded the attack but that the disease has occurred in a normal eye or after an intermittent prodromal period.

2. The same condition exists in respect to the arterial pulse.

3. The punctate hemorrhages in the retina are present constantly, but, undoubtedly, most of these occur after the operation.

4. In a careful observation of the equatorial region frequent choroidal hemorrhages are seen. These disappear quickly, however. It is not yet clear whether their inconstancy is not due entirely to the time of observation, since I have discovered them several times prior to operation.

Visual acuity as a rule improves immediately after the operation. This seems to depend, as in the case of paracentesis, on the outflow of the turbid aqueous. The degree of improvement, however, is not considerable when compared with the subsequent improvement, which may be explained partially as the clearing of the ocular media. In my opinion, however, this improvement results more from the resumption of the retinal functions which have been depressed by the intraocular pressure.

The condition of the iris varies according to the degree of involvement. I have never seen a completely movable, normal iris once marked inflammation has occurred. Partial mobility is found frequently, but in the majority of cases the pupil remains completely paretic although not as dilated as before. Occasionally the pupil is somewhat narrower than normal, with due allowance for the coloboma. The irregular form and position of the pupil seldom disappears even if posterior synechia are not present. This may be attributed to an irregular distribution of the paralysis of the ciliary nerves. Hence, it is a question whether the permanence of the pupillary damage is due to structural changes in the iris itself or to changes in the ciliary nerves. It is difficult to decide this, but I am rather inclined to the first opinion. The iris never regains its normal appearance in well marked cases. An ashy gray discoloration remains, as well as an indistinctness of the trabeculae, either in spots or in large areas, especially toward the periphery. This fact, which affords ample evidence of the disease, is important in the later recognition of the case. The tension of the globe returns entirely to normal; in fact, in some cases the eyes seem a trifle softer after operation than before.

In all the cases in which operation was performed within two weeks after the beginning of the inflammation, a complete restoration of vision occurred. The patients in several of these cases seemed desperate, having lost every trace of the perception of light. It is hardly necessary to add that I offered them little hope. I merely undertook the operation because of the violent ciliary pain. The result, however, was truly astounding. For the last half year I have predicted the complete return of function, provided that less than two weeks have elapsed since the inflammation and that some perception of light still exists. My early anxiety that the results might not be permanent gradually vanished. The visual field remained absolutely normal. Eccentric vision maintained its acuity once it had returned to the previous level. Not the slightest prodromal symptom recurred. The congestion of the subconjunctival vessels disappeared entirely; the anterior chamber became deeper and nothing betrayed an abnormal condition of the eye except the discoloration of the iris and the inactivity or paresis of the pupil. I cannot absolutely allay fear of a recurrence because of the short duration of my observations. It is certain, however, that a similar inhibition of the glaucomatous process has never occurred spontaneously or after any other form of treatment.

In spite of the surprising results of iridectomy shortly after the beginning of the inflammation, an exact analysis of the facts shows the correctness of the argument in favor of operating during the prodromal state. I would call special attention to the relative danger of the operation during the two periods. In the prodromal stage a chance accident seldom occurs even when the operation is not performed correctly. In the acute period, on the other hand, with every precaution, the result may be disappointing because of retinal hemorrhages and other adverse conditions which may occur in isolated cases in spite of the greatest care. This can be decided only after comprehensive statistics are gathered.

Observation of these patients showed that iridectomy does not influence the second eye. Frequently the process starts in the second eye after the first has completely recovered. It can be said with certainty that the glaucomatous inflammation of the second eye does not arise sympathetically from the disease of the first eye.

Iridectomy in the Later Periods of Acute Glaucoma

Although the curative value of iridectomy is most marked in cases of short duration, it loses none of its importance in disease of longer standing. My observations in this group are even more numerous than in the others. Because of variability of the results, however, their final evaluation has been more difficult, and a continuation of these studies is necessary. The following is only a preliminary report.

1. A lapse of weeks or even months after the first glaucomatous attack does not prevent complete restoration of sight; this depends entirely on the characteristics of the individual case. Occasionally the first inflammatory symptoms are intense, but the acuity, visual fields and optic papilla may remain normal for a long time in spite of iridoplegia and discoloration of the iris. These are the cases in which the actual beginning of the disease is not sharply defined from the prodromal period. In these cases iridectomy can effect a complete recovery many months after the outbreak. Even though the visual field and optic papilla are normal during the remissions, central vision may be considerably reduced. The cure seems to be just as permanent here as in the initial period. In malignant cases, as early as a few weeks after the first attack, conditions may be much more unfavorable for operating; in fact, there are fulminating cases in which vision is destroyed forever, so that after the first few weeks nothing is of avail.

2. The prognosis is different as soon as the visual field is constricted. A moderate concentric contraction is the most favorable. It occurs far less frequently, however, than a marked constriction coming in from one side; that latter affects the prognosis the more it approaches the midline. The condition of the papilla is equally important. When the papilla is but little cupped and, on the other hand, the field is decidedly cut down, there is naturally only slight improvement. This is particularly true of the visual acuity but also applies to changes in the field which occasionally may increase four-fold. The improvement usually continues. If, on the other hand, well marked cupping is associated with a high degree of contraction of the field, which is unfortunately the most frequent condition, a warning against too hasty an optimism is hardly necessary.

3. Tension of the globe, iridoplegia, corneal anesthesia and shallowing of the anterior chamber are favorable in that they prove the reduction in vision to be attributed partly to increased pressure, on which iridectomy has a beneficial action. This is also true of clouding of the aqueous and vitreous.

4. If the improvement in an advanced case of glaucoma is not permanent following iridectomy, the decrease in vision is not accompanied by symptoms of a fresh glaucomatous choroiditis. One should not speak, therefore, of a recrudescence of the original disease; the blindness must be caused by a continuation of the disease in the optic nerve. In a few cases which are exceptional, the subsequent deterioration occurs with symptoms of a rise of pressure.

5. In all cases of glaucomatous blindness an iridectomy has the advantage of alleviating the existing inflammation and the ciliary pain. The ophthalmologist who knows the torture which these blind eyes cause patients for years will greet the effect of iridectomy most heartily. Treatment with frequent blood-letting and narcotics is not necessary any longer.

Iridectomy and Chronic Glaucoma

Although it was on patients with chronic glaucoma that I first performed iridectomy, I yet cannot pass final judgment on this method of treatment in this group. Since the therapeutic value of the operation in any case exceeds that of all other remedies that have been tried, it is clearly necessary to continue to multiply the observations.

In general, a rather early cupping is unfavorable; hence, an extremely early diagnosis is of essential importance. This is not made as easily as in acute glaucoma, in which at the first inflammatory attack an iridoplegia can be discerned easily. Once cupping of the optic nerve occurs, it never disappears.

Iridectomy in Amaurosis with Cupping of the Optic Nerve

I have never observed any direct curative value of iridectomy in these cases. I have never seen improvement of visual acuity or widening of the visual fields beyond the limits of error in observation.

Concerning the operative procedure itself, I have little to say. A piece of iris is excised as in operations in which an artificial pupil is formed. The following points should be observed:

1. The wound must be as eccentric as possible so that the point of entrance is about one-half a line out in the sclera and the internal wound just at the limbus. In this way it is possible to draw out the iris up to the point of its ciliary insertion; this seems to be necessary for a good result. Any deviation of the internal wound from the limbus will diminish the size of the coloboma considerably.

2. Since the excised piece must be as large as possible, a broad, lance-shaped knife should be used, or the usual knife must be thrust in rather deeply. The operation differs, therefore, from that for the formation of an artificial pupil, in which one should excise only a medium-sized piece of iris for optical reasons. The more severe the symptoms and the higher the tension, the more iris would I advise being excised. There is little choice as to the site of the operation. I usually make my incision toward the nasal side; if the cosmetic effect is considered on account of the age of the patient, the incision can be made above this area, although I find that the colobomas made to the nasal side are scarcely noticeable in dark eyes. The excision above is rather difficult and demands a

greater rotation of the globe with the ophthalmostat, perhaps producing a greater inflammation.

3. The aqueous must be evacuated carefully, because too sudden a release of the pressure may cause numerous hemorrhages. In glaucoma, however, these massive hemorrhages tend to occur less frequently than in cases of iridochoroiditis with atrophy of the globe, probably because of the relatively greater pressure after the escape of the aqueous. On the other hand, from the very nature of the disease there is a disposition to rupture the blood vessels. Whether this is due to direct involvement of the wall of the vessel or to venous stasis, I cannot say. I have noted the presence of retinal hemorrhages many times. During the outflow of aqueous I usually exert slight pressure with the finger on the globe. A compression bandage is put on immediately after the operation, and loosened a few hours later. I have not found any other after-treatment necessary. Even when the operation is undertaken at the peak of the inflammation, the symptoms subside spontaneously. It may be necessary in exceptional conditions to apply some antiphlogistic remedy in order to hasten the subsidence of the inflammation. Naturally in these cases the eyes must be more protected from the light and the usual precautions more strictly observed than in the ordinary operation for an artificial pupil.

If the statements concerning the action of iridectomy are summed up, the following facts appear:

1. The surest results are obtained in those cases in which one eye is threatened after the other has became blind. In such cases it is the duty of the physician to refer the patient as soon as possible to an oculist for strict observation, and, vice versa, it is the duty of the oculist to warn the family physician to look for those symptoms which call for operative intervention.

2. Once the glaucomatous process has set in, the results are the more favorable and permanent the earlier the operation is performed. In the acute cases in which vision is lost almost immediately, iridectomy must be performed whenever possible in the first few days of the disease. This is of the utmost importance. Previously a glaucomatous eye was considered incurable the moment the diagnosis was made. It was comparatively unimportant, therefore, which type of medical treatment was used and whether this was instituted relatively early or late. A physician never had to reproach himself for delay in this respect. If I am not mistaken, conditions now are changed. An eye which has been blinded from acute glaucoma may as well excite suspicion of neglect as a badly set fracture, or atresia pupillae following simple iritis.

3. It has been shown that iridectomy is not suitable for all stages of the disease but that its action in a later stage, at least in some cases, is

extremely uncertain. It is sad to see the number of incurably blind persons who make long journeys because they think their disease is still curable.

I adopted this treatment with the idea of diminishing the intraocular pressure. Pursuit of this point of view seems to have obtained a result. At the same time, this is not a proof of the correctness of the explanation. It is possible that the effect of iridectomy is extremely complex. A decrease in the secreting surface of the iris might account for a reduction in the quantity of the fluid, but as yet information is lacking as to how much less aqueous is secreted in these cases and whether such a deficiency could explain such a striking change in intraocular pressure. The cooperative effect of the muscles of the iris with the tensor choroidea, which was pointed out in a recent theory of accommodation, might explain how the excision of a piece of iris would produce a diminution of intraocular pressure by a relaxation of this muscle. The persistence of accommodation after the coloboma has been made, however, does not support this view. Perhaps interference with the iris acts primarily on the choroidal circulation, the therapeutic pressure-reducing effect being only secondary. The presence of the hemorrhages proves that iridectomy in glaucoma is of considerable influence on the ocular circulation. The treatment, undoubtedly, will be still more efficacious when ophthalmologists are able to analyze more correctly all the foregoing points. It is conceivable that in selected cases the ordinary excision is not sufficient, but that removal of large pieces of iris will make the operation more successful. As already stated, the pieces of iris should be larger in proportion as the case is more severe.

The whole subject of glaucoma is open to the most varied investigations. After the marked change in our views on glaucoma produced by the first ophthalmoscopic examinations, I felt that further investigation was imperative. The difficulties which I encountered are apparent to any unprejudiced reader. I hope that I have assisted in solving some of these and that some one who is better equipped than I will soon bring this difficult task to a more happy conclusion.

Comment: Glaucoma was an incurable affection until von Graefe demonstrated the value of iridectomy. Acute glaucoma was originally confused with iritis. In 1813 Beer first recognized that certain cases, which he called arthritic iritis, had special characteristics; and in 1829 Sir William Lawrence identified the arthritic iritis of Beer as accute glaucoma, but the treatment of the new entity continued to be the same as that for iritis. The deleterious action of mydriatics, likewise discovered by von Graefe, was not noted till 1868. This observation led Laqueur to the thought that miotics should be beneficial and the consequent use of eserine, the first medical treatment of glaucoma of any value. Von Graefe attributed the curative effect of iridectomy to the reduction of the secreting surface of the iris, but this theory was discarded when the ciliary body was proved to be practically the sole source of intraocular fluid. The tension of the normal eye is not diminished by iridectomy. Not till 1876 was faulty excretion implicated; in that year Adolph Weber and Max Knies independently noted adhesions of the iris base to the cornea in eyes enucleated after congestive glaucoma. The validity of this view has been recently confirmed by tonography. In 1938 Otto Barkan proposed the separation of the primary glaucomas of the adult into two entities designated as narrow-angle (or angle closure) and open-angle (or trabecular). The mydriatic provocative tests give a positive result in narrow-angle glaucoma only. Doubtful cases of open-angle glaucoma are best diagnosed by combining tonography with the water-drinking test. If iridectomy is performed early enough in narrow-angle glaucoma, the filtration angle is permanently opened and the disease is actually cured. As the results of iridectomy in chronic glaucoma were frequently disappointing, De Wecker in 1867 proposed an operation to produce a filtering cicatrix. As the idea became accepted various procedures for this purpose were developed in rapid succession: cyclodialysis by Heine in 1905, iridosclerotomy by Lagrange in 1906, iridencleisis by Holth in 1907, and corneo-scleral trephination by Elliot in 1909.

Reference

Lebensohn, J. E.: Glaucoma simplex. Am. J. Ophth., 1955, *40:* 440–442.

Biographical Note

Albrecht von Graefe (1828–1870) was born in Berlin and graduated in medicine from the University of Berlin in 1847. He then visited Prague, where he was influenced by Arlt to specialize in ophthalmology. He continued postgraduate study in Paris under Sichel and Desmarres; in Vienna, under the Jaegers; and in London, under Critchett and Bowman. Both his father and his uncle had done work in ophthalmology and contributed original observations. His cousin and one-time associate, Alfred Graefe, two years his junior, became a celebrated ophthalmologist, co-editor of the Graefe-Saemisch Handbuch der gesamten Augenheilkunde, and was memorialized by the founding of the Graefe medal. Donders, while visiting the historically first World Fair, that at London in 1851, met Bowman and von Graefe; and forthwith the trio inaugurated a lifelong friendship. Von Graefe had started a successful practice in Berlin the year previously. He was one of the first to fully appreciate the newly invented ophthalmoscope, exclaiming: "Helmholtz has uns eine neue Welt erschlossen!" Von Graefe confirmed the discovery of the cupped disk in glaucoma by his favorite student, Adolph Weber (1855); described the ophthalmoscopic pictures of embolism of the central retinal artery (1859) and of choked disk (1860). In 1854 von Graefe established single-handedly the Archiv für Ophthalmologie, now the second oldest eye journal in continuous circulation, the oldest being the Annales d'Oculistique, founded in 1838. The first volume of von Graefe's Archiv contained 481 pages of which 384 pages were contributed by himself with discussions of keratoconus, ocular muscles, diphtheritic conjunctivitis and the arterial pulsation in glaucoma. In 1856, von Graefe introduced clinical perimetry and stressed the importance of visual fields in diagnosis, and in 1857 he announced the cure of acute glaucoma by iridectomy. He also noted the lid-lag in exophthalmic goiter (1864),

208

modified the cataract operation (1865), improved the operations for strabismus, made notable observations on sympathetic ophthalmia and reported the secondary glaucoma induced by rapid swelling of the crystalline lens (1869). His life was one of unhesitating sacrifice of self to ophthalmology, to teaching and to his patients in spite of continuous feeble health. In 1858 his recurrent hemoptysis and pleurisy became severe, and in 1870 he died of tuberculosis at age 42. How true that "we live in deeds, not hours"!

References

Ullman, E. V.: Albrecht von Graefe: The man in his time. Am. J. Ophth., 1954, *38:* 525–543, 695–711, 791–809.
Lebensohn, J. E.: Anno mirabile, 1850. Am. J. Ophth., 1950, *33:* 1160–1162.
Lebensohn, J. E.: German ophthalmology. Am. J. Ophth., 1954, *37:* 124–126.

A New Therapeutic Indication for Physostigmine

LUDWIG LAQUEUR

Strassburg, Germany

ZENTRALBL. MED. WISSENSCH. *14:* 421–422, 1876*

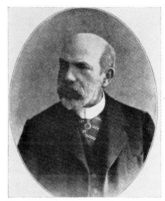

The experience of many observers that instillation of atropine precipitated acute glaucoma in predisposed eyes suggested this investigation as to whether the action of the alkaloid of the Calabar bean in regard to elevated intraocular tension was the reverse of atropine in this respect also. Aqueous solutions of neutral sulfate of eserine were prepared in concentrations of 0.3 and 0.5 percent, and three to four drops thereof were instilled at 20 minute intervals. The remedy was well tolerated and was continued for three weeks without any adverse reaction.

The study included five case of glaucoma simplex and one of secondary glaucoma due to subluxation of the lens. A definite drop of the elevated tension was soon noted, followed by a further and progressive diminution of tension and a considerable improvement of visual acuity as the treatment was continued in the next eight to ten days. In the patient with subluxation of the lens, the tension dropped from over T + 2 to normal, and has been maintained so since.

Though the permanency of the results has yet to be assured, it does seem that the effect of eserine in reducing tension continues much longer than the effect on the pupil and accommodation. In non-glaucomatous human eyes and normal rabbit eyes the repeated instillation of eserine causes no change apparently in the intraocular tension. The tension-reducing action of physostigmine in glaucoma can be explained by the stimulation of the smooth musculature of the choroidal vessels.

Regular and continued instillation of physostigmine would appear

---

* Translated by J. E. Lebensohn, M.D., Chicago.

indicated: (1) in all cases of glaucoma simplex, particularly if no abnormality of iris or anterior chamber is evident, as iridectomy in this group is almost always valueless; (2) in all cases of glaucoma in which a previous iridectomy has not been entirely successful; (3) in cases of secondary glaucoma in which the iris is not involved in either anterior or posterior synechiae.

The remedy has been tried without success in one case of hemorrhagic glaucoma.

Comment: The earliest studies on eserine emanated from Edinburgh and were inspired by a talk given before the local Ethnological Society by Dr. William Freeman Daniell, who described the use of the ordeal bean of Calabar in trials for witchcraft by the natives of Nigeria. Professor Balfour at the University of Edinburgh identified the woody vine from which the Calabar beans dropped into the adjacent river as a member of the pea family and christened it *Physostigma venenosum.* In 1855, his colleague, Professor Christison, tested the Calabar bean on animals and on himself. After swallowing one fourth of a bean he became extremely ill and weak, though vomiting was induced after 20 min. At his suggestion, Thomas R. Fraser, then 21 years of age, launched a thorough study of the pharmacology of the Calabar bean. Fraser noted that a small quantity of the extract applied to the conjunctiva caused extreme pupillary contraction in both rabbits and man. Aware that no substance previously known had such action, he disclosed his discovery to Argyll Robertson, who confirmed Fraser's observations on his own eyes. Robertson's article in March, 1863, preceded by a few months Fraser's detailed publication and was the initial announcement of the first known miotic. Robertson correctly concluded that the extract was a stimulant to the ciliary nerves, since pupillary contraction due to lesions of the sympathetic is not accompanied by spasm of the accommodation. The active alkaloid was isolated the following year. A year after Laqueur noted the tension-reducing action of eserine in glaucoma, Adolph Weber introduced pilocarpine, an alkaloid derived from a member of the rue family. Eserine is the first drug in which the mechanism was explained in terms of inhibition of a specific enzyme. Sir Henry Dale, in 1926, showed that eserine, because of a structural similarity to acetylcholine, unites with acetylcholine-esterase and thus protects acetylcholine from hydrolysis. His elucidation stimulated the production of synthetic miotics: neostigmine, 1929; methacholine, 1931; carbachol, 1932; isofluorate, 1946; demacarium bromide, 1959; and echothiophate, 1959. Acetylcholine-esterase accomplishes its result in about 30 μsec. In the hydrolysis of acetylcholine, an acetylated enzyme is first formed and choline eliminated; the acetylated enzyme then reacts with water to form acetate and restored enzyme. The organophosphorus compounds are irreversible inhibitors since after their use a phosphorylated enzyme is formed which does not react with water to form restored enzyme. The irreversibly inhibited enzyme can be reactivated by displacing the phosphoryl group by pyridine-2-aldoxime methiodide (PAM), a product synthesized for this purpose in 1955.

References

Rodin, F. H.: Eserine: its history in the practice of ophthalmology. Am. J. Ophth., *30:* 19–28, 1947.

Lebensohn, J. E.: The first miotic. Am. J. Ophth., *55:* 657–659, 1963.

Biographical Note

Ludwig Laqueur (1839–1909) was born in Silesia and began his medical studies at Breslau, but finished in Berlin, where he received his M.D. degree in 1860. He then trained in ophthalmology by working as an assistant successively to von Graefe and Liebreich. Deciding to practice in France, he obtained an M.D. degree in Paris in 1869, his doctoral thesis being on sympathetic ophthalmia. For the next three years Laqueur practiced ophthalmology at Lyon and lectured at the Ecole Préparatoire de Médecine. In the meantime Germany annexed Alsace and Laqueur was invited to Strasbourg as extraordinary professor of ophthalmology because of his recognized ability and his proficiency in the languages of the bilingual city. Laqueur was appointed five years later to the chair of ophthalmology at Strasbourg, which he occupied for the next 30 years.

Laqueur was born in the same year as Javal and like Javal was of Jewish origin and became afflicted with glaucoma. In 1874, at the age 35, he suffered his first attack of dimness and halos after performing an arduous plastic operation. He tried eserine on himself in 1876, and the remedy never failed to abort an attack though it did not prevent recurrences. A comprehensive article followed his preliminary report on the tension-reducing efficiency of eserine in glaucoma (Ein Beitrag zur Therapie des Glaucoms. Arch. Ophth., *23:* (part 3), 149–176, 1877), in which he concluded that eserine was a useful adjunct in glaucoma but did not supplant iridectomy. Strong opposition to the use of eserine ensued, but Laqueur maintained his stand firmly as he knew first-hand the value of the drug, though his affliction was only revealed after his death. In 1902 he wrote a secret account of his experience with glaucoma which was published two months after his death.

Before the advent of glaucoma Laqueur observed that he was emmetropic, with 20/20 visual acuity in each eye, had congenital red-green color deficiency, and suffered from photophobia and a recurrent blepharo-conjunctivitis that was relieved by applications of silver nitrate. His glaucoma was manifested by recurring attacks of dim vision and halos, 8° to 9° in diameter, in one or the other eye. He never had pain, great congestion or loss of visual field. His case would be diagnosed now as chronic non-congestive angle-closure glaucoma. In 1880 he consulted Johann Friedrich Horner of Zurich, who performed an iridectomy on his right eye without any anesthesia. The keratome incision caused an intense burning sensation but no particular pain. Healing was uncomplicated. A week later, on Horner's advice, an iridectomy was done on the left eye. For the remaining 29 years of his life Laqueur retained a corrected acuity of 20/25 to 20/30. Though his vision was saved, his personality was strangely affected. Afraid that his iris colobomata would be noticed, he became a recluse, wore dark glasses outdoors, and seldom attended medical meetings. Laqueur was a cultured man of much charm and a popular teacher. His parental grandmother was blind in the last 30 years of life from bilateral glaucoma.

References

Laqueur, L.: Geschichte meiner Glaucomerkrankung. Klin. Monatsbl. Augenh., *47:* 639–646, (June) 1909. English translation, Jackson, E.: Am. J. Ophth., *12:* 984–989, (Dec.) 1929.
Landolt, H.: Obituary. Klin. Monatsbl. Augenh., *47:* 536–539, 1909.
Bett, W. R.: Ludwig Laqueur. Arch. Ophth., *22:* 316–317, (Aug.) 1939.

Tonometry, With a Description of a New Tonometer

H. SCHIØTZ, M.D.

Christiania, Norway

ARCHIV FÜR AUGENHEILKUNDE, 1905, *52*: 401; 1909, *62*: 317*

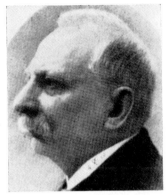

A number of instruments have been suggested to measure the intraocular pressure, but not one has, as yet, been generally used. The construction of the various instruments is given in the Graefe-Saemisch Handbuch, Vol. IV, page 206, with bibliography. The latest and best are those of Fick, Koster, and Maklakow.

There are two kinds of tonometers: first, those which which produce an impression in the capsule of the eyeball, of a constant depth, where the force necessary to accomplish this varies according to the degree of the intraocular pressure; and apparatuses with constant force, where the depth of the impression varies. A distinciton between tonometers of applanation and tonometers of impression, is not quite correct. Every applanation tonometer, with a pressure surface which is not too large, becomes, with increasing pressure, an impression tonometer. Moreover, there is no difference in the method of action.

It has seemed to me a great want that we did not possess a reliable instrument by which the intraocular pressure could be easily determined and translated into numerical values. I have been working for a long time upon this problem, and with the following results: At first I constructed an apparatus which produced a constant impression where a small mercury manometer permitted the reading of the recorded force. Finally, I used a tonometer with constant force and varying impressions. In other words, a combination of both systems. This apparatus is simple in construction and in manipulation. It will be seen that the long rod, *a*, is situated in a sheath in which it glides easily. It is 3 mm. in

* Abridged translation by Arnold Knapp, M.D., New York, Arch. Ophth., 1911, *40:* 518–525.

diameter. Its lowest extremity, which is to rest upon the cornea, is concave. The upper end is pointed and receives the weight, *1*. The sheath, *b*, has at its lower end a foot-plate, 9 mm. in diameter, with a concave lower surface, of a radius of curvature of 155 mm. During use, the pointed extremity of this rod is in contact with the short arm of a lever which rests upon it by its weight. Every movement of the rod causes a variation in the position of the long arm of the lever. At the extremity of the long arm of the lever there is a millimetre scale, by which the degree of the excursion can readily be read. About the sheath, *b*, there is a collar, *c*, supported by two arms. This collar is in contact with the sheath by means of very small rolling wheels. When the apparatus is to be used, it is most convenient to have the patient lie on a bench, with the head held back so that the eyes are directed upward. It is also possible to have the patient sit in a chair, with the head drawn back, though I do not think the determination is as accurate as in the previous position. The eye is anesthetized with a 2% solution of Holocaine. I have used this anaesthetic because it does not dilate the pupil. In eyes with increased pressure, after the testing of the tension, I employ pilocarpine. The patient is asked to look straight upwards; with the fingers of one hand the eyelids are carefully separated without pressing upon the eye, and with the other hand the apparatus is placed directly upon the cornea. The apparatus is supported by the collar, *c*, and then rests with its own weight upon the eye. The reading of the long arm in the millimetre scale can then be taken. Three measurements should be made, and the average determined. By means of a diagram it is easy to determine how many millimetres of mercury pressure corresponds to the reading in the milimetre scale. It is necessary to examine with weights of different weight. It is evident that in eyes with high intraocular tension, there is no reading when the weight is used which is sufficient in the measurement of a normal eye. The apparatus, therefore, is supplied with four different weights which, with the rod and the lever, together represent the weights, 5½ g., 7½ g., 10 g., and 15 g. When no weight is used, the rod and the lever represent a weight of 4 g., which can be used in very soft eyes.

The curves which were determined by measurements made by the open eye—that is, one directly communicating with a manometer—were supposed to be applicable for the estimation of the pressure in the closed living eye. This, however, has proved to be incorrect, because I at first assumed that the weight of the tonometer itself was of no particular importance. Later experiments have shown me that the weight of the tonometer influences, to a high degree, the intraocular pressure in the closed eye. The curves of the closed eye run differently, and are lower than those of the open eye. This, however, has very little practical significance. A variation of the lever from 6 to 3 mm., with the weight, 5½ g., still remains the normal variance of the normal intraocular pressure. This, however, does not correspond, as was previously assumed, to a mercury pressure of 24 to 31 mm., but a pressure of 15.5 to 25 mm. My attention to the great difference between the pressure of the open and the closed eye was first attracted after the using of a small apparatus which I have constructed to verify the tonometer. This consists of a small metallic cylinder, about 14 mm. in diameter, whose one extremity is closed by a thin piece of rubber. The other is connected with a manometer by a tube, and by means of a cock is opened and closed. The piece of rubber represents the cornea.

The almost daily use of my tonometer, during the past two years, has shown it to be practical and reliable. An experience which we soon make is, that the finger is not reliable in determining the intraocular tension. I have made a number of measurements after using mydriatics and miotics. The solutions were salicylate of eserine ½%, hydrochlorate of pilocarpine 2%, chlorate of morphine 3%, sulphate of atropine 2%, cocaine hydrochlorate 3%. The eye was first measured after Holocaine anaesthesia, then the medicament was instilled twice with an interval of fifteen minutes, and then the measurement was taken three-quarters of an hour and one and three-quarters hours later.

The miotics, eserine and pilocarpine, exert a powerful pressure-reducing action upon the normal eye; 2% of pilocarpine rather more than ½% eserine. It has generally been taken for granted that the action is the result of the miosis, but we observed a very marked reduction in tension in an eye with congenital aniridia, and in eyes in which an iridectomy has been performed the action is distinct.

Morphine, which is often used in combination with pilocarpine or eserine, has a distinct though transient pressure-reducing action, and is probably of no value in the treatment of glaucoma. The miosis is inconstant and not pronounced.

Atropine, in the normal eye, does not seem to have any particular effect upon the intraocular tension. This agrees with our daily experience. It is possible that there may be an unimportant and very transient increase in tension. In eyes, however, which are predisposed to increased tension, or where the pressure with the tonometer seems to be somewhat elevated, a drop of atropine always produces a decided increased tension. In a patient with pronounced glaucoma in the right eye, while the left eye had only a slight increase of tension, 27 mm. Hg (mercury), atropine was accidentally instilled in the left eye. In the course of the next hour the pressure rose to 41 mm. Czermack's explanation, that the increase of pressure after atropine is the result of the increased volume of the iris in its periphery by dilatation of the pupil, seems to me very plausible. It is conceivable that the thickening of the iris-periphery, to a certain extent, may impede the access to Fontana's spaces, and that thus the escape of fluid can be retarded which, in an eye predisposed to it, may be followed by increased tension. It cannot be assumed that the interference with the escape of fluids in glaucoma is produced by an occlusion of Fontana's spaces. In those cases with increased tension, with a normal or even deepened anterior chamber, as in buphthalmus, or not infrequently in serous iritis, we can assume that the obstruction to the intraocular circulation is caused by an occlusion of Fontana's spaces or of the canal of Schlemm. On the other hand, in those cases—which are, or course, the more frequent— where the anterior chamber is unusually shallow, the obstruction to the intraocular circulation must be sought for behind the lenticular system. The obstruction of fluids in the vitreous chamber has pushed the lens and the iris forward.

Cocaine does not seem to have any particular action on intraocular pressure, though experience has shown us that cocaine, just as atropine, from its mydriatic effect, can produce distinct increased tension in eyes which are predisposed. A case of this kind was observed in my clinic. To use the tonometer, cocaine was instilled in an eye. Immediately the pressure rose, and this was only controlled after the energetic instillation of eserine and pilocarpine.

If we measure the normal eye repeatedly with increasing weights, we sometimes observe variations in the reading, and if the weight 5½ g. is then used, a different reading is recorded than was used at the first measurement. This is probably the result of the escape of a certain amount of fluid from the eye from pressure.

I have made a number of measurements at different times of the day, but have not found that in normal eyes there is any particular variation in the tension. In a young girl, with pigmentary retinitis, the pressure in the evening seemed to be somewhat lower than in the morning. In pathological eyes it is astonishing how quickly and how marked variations in pressure may show themselves, especially in glaucomatous eyes. In the so-called prodromal attacks, the pressure may rapidly rise to 50 or 60 mm. A young man whose right eye presented a sclero-kerato-iritis, with opacities of the cornea and posterior synechia, after a number of prodromal attacks, the eye became permanently hard. After an iridectomy the pressure became normal for some time. A few weeks later the eye seemed to be very soft. The tonometer gave, with a weight 5½ g., a reading of 17 mm., which corresponded to an intraocular pressure of only 3 mm. Hg. On the following day, the pressure had risen to 40 mm. He told us that frequently in the mornings the eye was very soft and towards evening it would become harder again.

It is, perhaps, possible that the rapidity of the increased tension is a determining factor of the development of congestive glaucoma. The height of the pressure is not necessarily of importance. In congestive glaucoma I have not found very high pressure, frequently 60 to 70 mm. Hg. In glaucoma simplex, however, a pressure of 100 mm. Hg and even more, is frequently found. If the increase of pressure is gradually developed, the circulation becomes adapted to the variations of pressure. It is stated that a detachment of the retina is always associated with diminished tension. It has always seemed to me that this was erroneous. In the spontaneous retinal detachments in apparently normal eyes, I have found the pressure to be within the limits of the normal; thus, with a weight of $5\frac{1}{2}$ g., the reading would be 3 to 6 to 7 mm. In old detachments diminished tension is often present, especially in secondary detachments after irido-cyclitis.

The most marked hypotony which I have observed in a living eye occurred in an eye with chronic irido-cyclitis, which during the examination remained free from irritation, and with a vision of fingers in $\frac{1}{2}$ metre; projection was fairly good. With a weight of $5\frac{1}{2}$ g., the index on tonometer recorded 24 mm.—in other words, an intraocular pressure equal to 0. On palpating with the fingers nothing of the eye could be appreciated.

It is stated that increase of tension is of differential diagnostic importance in making a diagnosis of a retinal detachment and of a tumor. I have taken the tension in 3 cases in which the tumor was small. It is, of course, in the small tumors that the diagnosis is the most important. In two of these I found an unusually reduced pressure, namely, 11.5 mm. in one, and 19 mm. in the other.

Measurements before and after enucleation in a glaucomatous eye, with a very high pressure, 122 mm. Hg, showed, after enucleation, a pressure of 72 mm. Hg. In a normal eye, with 19 mm. Hg, pressure, after enucleation the pressure was equal to nothing.

Among a number of post-mortem measurements, one gave an excursion of 20 mm. Hg, with a weight of $5\frac{1}{2}$ g., showing that the intraocular tension was equal to nothing.

I should like to urge the colleagues who are using my tonometer to be very careful to cleanse the instrument thoroughly after its use. The rod is to be taken out and together with the foot-plate carefully washed. It is not infrequent that an instrument is returned to the maker, and a thorough cleaning is all that is necessary. It is well to use in cleaning some fluid which is indifferent to the eye, like water or boric acid. I should like to warn against the use of alcohol or ether. Some may remain in the cylinder and drop into the eye.

Comment: Of about 50 instruments devised for tonometry, the simply constructed and easily used Schiøtz design has achieved the greatest popularity. While Schiøtz was living, the tonometers manufactured by his instrument maker carried a certificate that they were replicas in construction and performance of the reference standard. As time passed and the manufacture of "Schiøtz tonometers" spread to other countries, the reproduction of the original design became increasingly faulty and instruments produced by different reputable manufacturers gave widely divergent readings on the same eye. This lamentable situation was ended in America through the continued efforts of the Committee on Standardization of Tonometers established by the American Academy of Ophthalmology and Otolaryngology in 1942. Testing stations for the rehabilitation and recalibration of aberrant tonometers were instituted in New York, Chicago, San Francisco, and Sao Paulo, Brazil, by individual committee members. Of more than 1500 tonometers checked, over 80 per cent were found grossly divergent from the official Schiøtz pattern. At the testing stations 28 measurements were made, of which 14 were found to affect the tonometer reading. The most critical items were the weight of the plunger assembly, the diameter of the plunger base and the plunger edge profile.

All reputable American manufacturers of tonometers now adhere to the specifications of the Committee and submit their instruments for certification to an impartial agency, the Electrical Testing Laboratories of New York City. Their certificate shows the identifying serial numbers of both the instrument and the plunger. From 1946 to 1951 nearly 4000 tonometers have been certified. With present tolerances the standard deviation for a single tonometer reading with a randomly selected tonometer is within the clinical error of measurement. Interconvertible readings with different certified tonometers is a valuable aid in consultation and institutional work. Though no one is compelled to submit his product for certification nor is forbidden to make uncertified instruments, the educational policy of the Committee has been so effective that ophthalmologists in increasing numbers are insisting on certified tonometers.

Reference

Standardization of Tonometers. Decennial Report. Am. Acad. Ophth. & Otolaryng., 1954.

Biographical Note

Hjalmar August Schiøtz (1850–1927) was born in Stavanger, Norway, graduated as bachelor of medicine in 1877, interned at the University Clinic at Oslo, after which he went to Vienna for postgraduate study under Arlt and Fuchs. He then worked with Javal for 15 months in the Laboratory of Physiologic Optics at the Sorbonne. Javal referred to the period of this association as "the best days of my life." The Javal-Schiøtz ophthalmometer, a product of their collaboration, was first exhibited at the Milan Congress in 1880.

Schiøtz returned to Norway in 1881 to become clinical chief of the ophthalmic service at the Royal Hospital in Oslo. In 1883 he secured his doctorate with a thesis "On some optical corneal characteristics." He was appointed professor of ophthalmology in 1901, the first in Norway, as the University had included ophthalmology previously as a service of surgery.

The tonometer, on which he had worked 3 years, was demonstrated first before the Norwegian Medical Society on May 12, 1905. Between then and 1927 he contributed 11 articles on tonometry. His calibrations, which continued for over 2 decades, are models of scientific care. After his first calibrations in 1905, he reported a revision in 1908, and a final revision in 1924, in which he proposed a set of three curves for eyes of average, low and high ocular rigidity. In 1927 he introduced a tonometer with a convex plunger, the Schiøtz X-tonometer, adaptable to all tensions without requiring accessory weights. Schiøtz also invented a self-registering perimeter, a lantern for testing color vision and an ophthalmoscope of his own design.

Reference

Lebensohn, J. E.: Professor Hjalmar August Schiøtz (A centennial tribute). Am. J. Ophth., *33:* 301–303, 1950.

Iridencleisis Cum Iridotomia Meridionali

S. HOLTH, M.D.

Oslo, Norway

EXCERPTED FROM ARCH. OPHTH., *4:* 803–816, 1930; "TECHNIC" FROM BRIT. J. OPHTH., *5:* 544–551, 1921

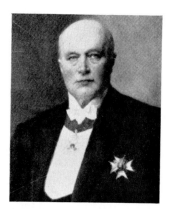

Among 640 operations for primary chronic glaucoma carried out in my private practice from 1904 to 1929, 223 were iridencleisis, 268 punch forceps sclerectomies and 149 Elliot trephinings. I have abandoned the methods of anterior sclerectomies. All gave an immediate fall of tension. After several years, however, the defect in the sclera may be completely obliterated by impermeable scar tissue. The tension is then often raised again. After my iridencleisis the condition is reversed. In only 50 percent does the tension become at once normal. In 35 percent one must use miotics for a fortnight to half a year. In both of these instances the resulting "filtering scar" will nearly always last for a lifetime. In the remaining 15 percent a continued use of miotics will keep the tension normal in most cases.

After iridencleisis I have never observed any late infection. In a patient with dipsomania a superficial infection was seen nine years after operation, but disappeared in a few days with the instillation of silver nitrate (0.5 percent) once a day. Dr. Enroth has shown that cataract may occur relatively early after Elliot's operation. I have never observed this result following iridencleisis. I was able to show post mortem that a subconjunctival iris fistula was the cause of the "filtering scars" obtained and thus of the normal tension and the good functional result.

Technic

A. *Iridencleisis simplex* is used in cases in which an iridectomy has been previously performed. The periphery of the iris at one border of the coloboma is drawn a little into the subconjunctival wound at one angle of the incision.

B. Iridencleisis cum iridotomia meridionale. A subconjunctival incision is made in the upper vertical meridian. The iris is drawn out so that the upper border of the pupil appears outside the limbal incision. The meridional iridotomy is performed with De Wecker's iris scissors, both blades of which have blunt ends. The lower blade is passed under the margin of the pupil as far back as the periphery of the prolapsed iris, which is released from the grasp of the forceps and the incision then made by closing the scissors. By this means scraping of the pigment epithelium from the back side of the iris is avoided. The sphincter corners slide back into the anterior chamber, so that the periphery of the iris only remains in and a little outside the limbal incision. I have rarely been obliged to cut away any of the prolapsed iris tissue. The cut in the sphincter causes the pupil, after re-establishment of the anterior chamber, to be considerably enlarged, and nearly central.

If the patient be a squeezer a transitory paralysis of the m. orbicularis after van Lint (1914) should be made. If the patient constantly turns the eye up, a transitory paralysis of the m. rectus superior may be made (Rochat, 1920).

In primary acute glaucoma I prefer the classical iridectomy; only when this operation fails and is not influenced by miotics, I perform iridencleisis. In cases of chronic glaucoma with some acute phenomena, *e.g.* redness of the conjunctive, hazy cornea and rainbows around the light, I have repeatedly had better results with iridencleisis than with iridectomy. In secondary glaucoma, iridectomy and medicamentous treatment are better.

Comment: Holth elaborated his ideas on iridencleisis in more than 10 papers published in Scandinavian, French, German, English and American journals and in talks before the 1909 International Congress of Ophthalmology, the Oxford Ophthalmological Congress, and the Heidelberg Society. During the first 30 of the 60 years that have elapsed since his initial paper in 1906, numerous ophthalmologists could not overcome a prejudice against this technic because of the dire consequences of accidental iris prolapse, but since then the popularity of iridencleisis has steadily increased, finally to become one of the most favored filtration procedures. In iridencleisis the cut pupillary margins lie everted in the subconjunctival space. The ocular irritability that so often follows accidental iris prolapse does not occur, since traction upon the iris is prevented by the meridional cut through the sphincter. The collagen-dissolving property of the draining aqueous converts the subconjunctival channel into a permanent filtering funnel in about 3 months. Atropine is instilled at the close of operation but not subsequently; as soon as the anterior chamber is reformed miotics are started, and light massage through the closed lids is performed for 2 min.

222

daily for 1 week in the same manner in which the eyeball is palpated in estimating ocular tension. The *ab externo* incision was introduced by Lundsgaard in 1928 and later popularized by Verhoeff and the Weekers (1948). In reference to this, Swan points out that the demarcation between the sclera and the posterior border of the limbus is clearly evident when the conjunctiva with the forward extension of Tenon's capsule is reflected, and that an incision here, slanted forward a few degrees, enters the anterior chamber safely, 1 mm. from the apex of the chamber angle in front of Schlemm's canal and behind Schwalbe's line. The iris usually prolapses spontaneously or with slight pressure on the cornea; if not, mild suction applied to the wound edge, as suggested independently by Christensen and Corboy, is effective. If the incision overlies the ciliary body because of the altered anatomy that occurs in glaucoma, del Barrio's technic of "internal iridencleisis" (1935) is indicated. The anterior chamber is entered by a cyclodialysis spatula; a dull hook then grasps the sphincter, which is carefully pulled out with the hook tilted sideways against the sclera, and sphincter iridotomy is performed. Other variations of technic are also used. A more cosmetically attractive pupil results, with an equally effective operation, if only the nasal pillar is incarcerated and the temporal pillar is replaced. Gjessing (1922), after grasping the sphincter, made parallel meridional incisions on either side of the closed forceps, and incarcerated only the tongue thus formed. Iridencleisis is not feasible if the iris is atrophic or bound by synechiae, but in the former case Swett's operation (1931) can be substituted. He made a moderate iridectomy through a keratome incision, floated the section pigment side up in physiologic saline, and with a repositor inserted it partly in the anterior chamber, to be gripped by the keratome incision. The present commentator can vouch for its efficiency. Iridencleisis is simpler, less harmful to the lens and less subject to late infections than are other fistulizing procedures. The operation is contraindicated in chronic inflammatory glaucoma because iridocyclitis may follow it.

References

Spaeth, E. B.: Principles and Practice of Ophthalmic Surgery, Ed. 4. Philadelphia, Lea & Febiger, 1948, pp. 833–841.
Weekers, L. and R.: Technique of iridencleisis. Brit. J. Ophth. *32:* 904–910, 1948.

Biographical Note

Søren Holth (1863–1937) was born in Naes, Norway, and received his certificate of medical qualification in 1891. While practicing ophthalmology in Drammen for 4 years, he collected data for his medical doctorate. He received it in 1896 for a thesis entitled "The indirect fixation blindness of the eye." Before moving to Oslo, Holth spent 1 year in study with Hirschberg in Berlin, with Tscherning in Paris, and with Vincentiis in Naples. For the following 6 years he was first assistant to Prof. Schiøtz; when the latter resigned, the chair was offered to Holth, who declined acceptance because of defective hearing due to otosclerosis. His chief interest was glaucoma and his great achievement was the operation of iridencleisis, about which he lectured in Stockholm, Oxford, Naples, Helsinki, and Budapest. His phenomenal industry is attested to by 110 scientific papers.

He was never afraid to try something new and once performed a reclination of a cataract on a lioness with good results. Profound deafness forced him to retire from active practice in 1935 and 2 years later he died suddenly of apoplexy.

Reference

Gjessing, H. G.: Obituary. Arch. Ophth., *18:* 1022–1023, 1937.

Sclero-corneal Trephining in the Operative Treatment of Glaucoma

ROBERT HENRY ELLIOT, M.D.

Madras, India

EXCERPTS FROM CHAPTER V, *The Technique of the Operation,*
PUBLISHED BY GEORGE PULMAN & SONS, LONDON, 1913

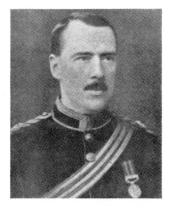

1. In which quadrant of the eye should trephining be performed?—Under most circumstances the upper is the quadrant of choice, for (1) the wound is then less exposed to infection; (2) the iridectomy lies under cover of the lid; (3) the conjunctival flap rarely requires a stitch when made above; and (4) the measurement from the angle of the anterior chamber to the limbus is greater in the vertical than in the horizontal meridian, and greater above than below the cornea. The consequent advancement of the limbus in this direction gives the operator a proportionate increase in the room available for the implantation of the trephine without risk of doing damage to the ciliary body.

An upward flap rarely required a stitch in India. If the flap is made in any other direction it is better to stitch it in every case as the lid movements will otherwise shift it from its proper position. The author's experience has shown that it is advisable to stitch the flap more often in Western than in Eastern practice.

2. The nature of the flap, and the method of making it.—Our decision has been the large flap for the following reasons: (1) it is a greater safeguard against infection of the eye; (2) we do not meet with any astigmatism in consequence of it; and (3) large flaps mean free and easy filtration. If one makes a flap of little length and if the line of union then cicatrises, it is obvious that the area left for filtration is very limited. The incision we now employ runs concentric with the limbus and ends opposite the highest point of the cornea, about 8 mm. from its inner and outer sides. Even if the line of incision cicatrises, filtering fluid can still find a free exit into the subconjunctival space outside the incision limits.

We may divide the fashioning of the flap into the following stages:—

(i) The incision.—The conjunctiva should be seized as high up as possible; one free horizontal cut, followed by a couple of snips at each side, will outline the flap.

(ii) The dissection of the flap.—We should carry our dissection down to the limbus over the central area only. As we approach the limbus we should work down to the sclera, and should expose the latter bare in the last few millimeters of the wound. The breadth of the dissection should contract as we approach the cornea, so that when we reach the latter we only expose just such a breadth as we mean to split and very little more. Our next landmark is the limbus, and we must clearly define this. The area over which we are about to apply the trephine must be carefully cleared of all tags of loose tissue. There is a little knack in getting the sclera clear; this consists in closing the blades of a sharp-pointed scissors and making a number of scraping movements from the center out to each side close above the cornea.

(iii) The splitting of the cornea.—The conjunctival flap should be drawn gently downwards by traction. At the same time the cornea is split with the scissors points; or if preferred a special wedge-shaped splitter as devised by McReynolds. The most important point is to work just behind the line of reflection of the flap; a number of short purposive lateral strokes speedily effect our purpose. The instrument is inclined at an acute angle to the cornea. As the dissection proceeds the so-called "dark crescent" of cornea can be seen clearly. If one sees the line of flap no longer curved at the corneal margin but crossing it in a straight line, we may rest assured that the cornea has been split. The split area has a smooth appearance, indicating that we have dissected up along a plane of cleavage. Experience has shown that one can safely split the cornea a little over 1 mm. and that such an area puts us in a secure position so far as the danger of trouble from the ciliary body is concerned.

3. *The application of the trephine.*—We place our trephine hole as far forward as possible. A failure to observe this rule (1) makes a clean entry into the anterior chamber uncertain; (2) complicates the free tapping of the aqueous fluid; (3) leads later to an interference with filtration due to uveal tissue blocking the trephine hole; and (4) exposes the eye to vitreous escape. The trephine is slid from the scleral side into place on the prepared sclero-corneal surface so that its edge will just clear the flap. Keeping the edge to one spot becomes quite easy if a sharp instrument be used. Assistance may be obtained by seiz-

ing the trephine blade low down, close to the eye, in the grasp of a conjunctival forceps and thus steadying the cutting edge. Various instrument-makers have supplied a handle to steady the trephine. Our preference is still for the forceps grip if any steadying is needed. It is necessary (1) to work in a good light; (2) to keep the area of operation clear of blood; (3) to make sure of cutting a definite groove before raising the trephine to see what has been done; and (4) to steady the trephine blade and keep it to one spot. Once a definite groove has been started, the trephine blade finds its way into it again; from this stage onwards the operator must raise his blade frequently to see how deeply he has cut. Place the index finger on top of the trephine and keep it there throughout the cutting, working the instrument with the thumb and middle finger. The heavier handle (9.7 gm.) has simplified the technique. No pressure need be used, as the instrument works by its own weight.

In the neighborhood of the limbus the cornea is thicker than the sclera. If we hold our blade perpendicular to the surface, we penetrate the coat first on its scleral edge. To make the blade cut through first on its corneal edge, we must slope the upper end of the instrument a little towards the patient's feet. As soon as the trephine has cut its way through, the disc, hinged on the scleral side, will be pushed outwards by a bead of iris tissue. This perhaps occurs with great regularity. It is, however, dependent on two factors, (1) the presence of a moderately contracted pupil, and (2) the use of a sharp trephine.

Of importance is the size of trephine. Our preference is in favor of a 2-mm. instrument. If we wish, we can cut off any desired portion of the disc, thus removing a third, a half, or more at will. We determine how much of the disc to remove and cut it off at right angles to the surface, thus leaving the posterior edge of the fistula as steep as its anterior edge. It is necessary to draw the hinge well away from the eye, and to cut with the plane of the scissors blades at a tangent to the eye, and as close to it as possible.

4. The iridectomy: its nature and the method of performing.—An iridectomy should be made in every trephine operation, simply to avoid the risk of iridic tissue becoming impacted in the trephine aperture. The iris bulges into the hole as soon as we withdraw the instrument. The most peripheral part is the first to pass into the hole. The appearance of the white disc, pushed upwards by the black bead of iris, is characteristic. It is easy to include both disc and iris in one grip of the forceps and to divide both together with a single snip of the scissors points. The resulting coloboma will be peripheral unless we drag on the iris. It is essential to put no traction on the iris and to carry the scissors-points right down into the wound. What are we to do if the iris reenters the chamber before we can perform an iridectomy, or if it never prolapses? If the iris fails to present, it is better to leave it alone. Experience shows that the use of a miotic makes the risk of a secondary prolapse comparatively small.

5. *The toilette of the wound.*—The iris should be thoroughly replaced. We use the irrigator, and placing the nozzle at the entrance of the trephine hole, we direct a stream of saline solution into the chamber; this quickly washes the iris back into place. The presence of a round central pupil affords proof that the iris has been thoroughly replaced. We next replace the conjunctival flap in good position, and stroke it well into place with the aid of some rounded blunt instrument. Both eyes are then closed with aseptic pads and a bandage.

6. *Instillation of drops.*—Our rule is to avoid all instillations immediately after operation. On the third day, provided the tension is down, we drop in a solution of 1-percent atropine. We find in congestive cases a strong tendency to the formation of posterior synechiae; the quiet iritis which leads to this exudation must be constantly guarded against.

In conclusion, the operation is *simple* sclero-corneal trephining. The motive is to reach, tap and sub-conjunctivally drain the anterior chamber, with a minimum of injury to the structures of the eyeball.

Comment: The trephination operation was introduced independently in 1909 by Fergus and Elliot. The procedure described by Fergus was actually a modification of Heine's cyclodialysis. A conjunctival flap was dissected down to the corneal margin and the sclera was trephined as near to the cornea as possible, after which an iris repositor was passed from the scleral opening into the anterior chamber. Elliot aimed to have the trephine cut its way consistently into the anterior chamber. To be sure of avoiding the ciliary body, he finally advanced the site of trephination to a sclero-corneal position. When Elliot addressed the American Academy of Ophthalmology and Otolaryngology in October 1913, he had performed more than 1000 trephine operations in all forms of glaucoma. The trephine procedure became rapidly the favored filtration operation. After World War II it was displaced in popularity by iridencleisis. Since Scheie introduced in 1956 peripheral iridectomy with scleral cautery, the "Scheie operation" is now being used extensively in America instead of iridencleisis. Scheie, however, is enthusiastic about the results of trephination in eyes with non-inflammatory chronic simple glaucoma in which the angles are wide open. He does not split the cornea but makes the trephine opening adjacent to the limbal insertion of Tenon's capsule, as in Elliot's initial report (Ophthalmoscope 7: 804–806, 1909). In such eyes the angle wall lies 1.5 to 2.0 mm. behind clear cornea and post-operative gonioscopy reveals the trephine opening to be in the trabecular area between Schwalbe's line and the scleral spur. His flap includes both conjunctiva and Tenon's capsule. The filtering cicatrix that results is thicker, less vesicular, and has no tendency to dissect downward into the cornea, as compared to the corneal-splitting method. Scheie uses a 1.5-mm. trephine tilted slightly forward so that the corneal side of the blade first enters the angle. As the iris pushes into the trephine opening, a small peripheral iridectomy is done before cutting off the scleral button. The flap is then secured to its original position by a continuous suture with each bite locked. In Scheie's experience the ocular tension of his glaucoma cases was adequately controlled by this trephine operation in 97 percent, by the Scheie operation in 86 percent and by iridencleisis in 85 percent, while hypotony after these procedures was respectively: 30 percent, 12 percent and 3.5 percent. In none of his cases did any impairment of vision result from the hypotony, though a more rapid incidence of nuclear sclerosis and other cataractous changes was anticipated. Filtering operations are indicated in chronic simple glaucoma only after failure of an adequate medical regime. The ophthalmic surgeon must not procrastinate then, since the less the eyes are damaged by advanced glaucoma the better the prognosis for surgical intervention.

Reference

H. G. Scheie: Filtering operations for glaucoma: a comparative study. Am. J. Ophth., *53:* 571–590, 1962.

Biographical Note

Robert Henry Elliot (1866–1936) was born in India, the son of an army colonel. He studied medicine in London at St. Bartholomew's Hospital, graduating in 1890, then continued his studies at Edinburgh for the degree of D.Sc., after which he entered the Indian Medical Service. The work in India gave him a wide experience in ophthalmic surgery. His intellectual brilliance and operative skill led to his appointment as superintendent of the Government Hospital, Madras. During this period (1904–1914) he was also professor of ophthalmology at the Madras Medical College. His preliminary work on sclero-corneal trephining for glaucoma, announced in 1909, was later extended to a definitive monograph, of which the first edition appeared in 1913 and a second revised edition in 1914. Equally famous is his Treatise on Glaucoma, published in 1918 and revised in 1922. In recognition of his contribution to the surgical management of glaucoma he was invited to speak in America in 1913 and received honorary membership in the American Academy of Ophthalmology and Otolaryngology and in various regional and local societies. After Elliot left Madras for London, he rapidly acquired a large practice and numerous honors. He was made chairman of the Naval and Military Committee of the British Medical Association (1917–1922) and gave the Hunterian Lecture for 1917 before the Royal College of Surgeons, his subject being the Indian operation of couching for cataract. He was appointed consulting surgeon to the London Hospital for Tropical Diseases, and ophthalmic surgeon to the Prince of Wales Hospital. Drawing from his vivid experiences in India, he contributed a text on *Tropical Ophthalmology* and in 1934, just 2 years before his death, published a remarkable book, *Myth of the Mystic East,* exposing the magic of the fakirs.

References

Keyser, G. W. R.: Sclero-corneal Trephining in Glaucoma. Grøndahl & Sons, Oslo, 1960.
Jackson, E.: Obituary. Am. J. Ophth. *20:* 203–205, 1937.

Clinical and Experimental Researches on Intraocular Drainage

M. J. SCHOENBERG, M.D.

New York, N. Y.

ARCH. OF OPHTH., 1913, *42*: 117–135

I. Introduction

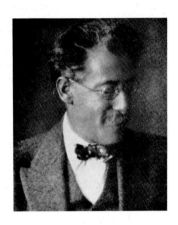

The advantage of the measurement of intraocular pressure by means of the Schiötz tonometer consists in its applicability to clinical work. One is thus enabled to get data more accurate and reliable than have been obtained in the laboratory, where the measurement is made on animals by connecting with a manometer a canula or hypodermic needle introduced into the anterior or posterior chamber of the eye.

The introduction of a cannula into the eye means a severe trauma to this most delicate organ. Such a trauma, I believe, must disturb at least for a certain length of time, the entire mechanism of circulation of intraocular fluids. Even the mere application of the tonometer on the eye, doubtless, produces a certain amount of traumatism, but this is inconsequent compared with that due to entering the eyeball with a cannula or a needle.

Since Prof. Schiötz's second article on tonometry a number of very valuable contributions discussing various questions in connection with the intraocular pressure has appeared. Some of the questions, as stated above, have been partly cleared up, but many have been left untouched. One of these is the following: What is the normal rate of drainage of intraocular fluids in animal and human eyes, and how is this rate of drainage affected in glaucomatous eyes?

All who have had experience with the tonometer have observed that when this instrument is continuously applied on the eye for a certain length of time, or at very short intervals, it registers a gradually decreasing intraocular pressure—*i.e.*, the eye becomes gradually softer. The rational explanation of this phenomenon is that the weight of the tonometer expresses a certain amount of fluid from the eye, thereby reducing its hardness. It is interesting to note that this fact has not been utilized in studying the drainage system of the normal and glaucomatous eyes. If by applying a weight on the eyeball, it is possible to express from this organ a certain amount of fluid, it is evident that there are channels in the eye through which this fluid is expressed.

It is almost universally admitted that the intraocular fluids are constantly renovated by a continuous slow flow of liquid which enters the eyeball and also by a continuous, just as slow exit of liquid. From the time of the researches of Leber and his pupils down to the latest work on this subject by Wessely, it is practically admitted by all ophthalmologists that normally fluid drains from the eyeball at the same rate at which it flows into the eye, that the "intraocular pressure is obviously a function of the volume of the contents of the globe and that the variations in internal pressure must be due to changes in the amount of fluid (blood and lymph)."

In eyes in which the draining function is more or less interefered with, there is a loss of balance between the two main factors (in- and outflow) regulating the intraocular pressure. The ocular fluid cannot leave the eye at the same rate as it does normally and the fluid contents of the eyeball will have a tendency to increase in amount, consequently the intraocular pressure will increase also. Supposing that a weight would be constantly applied on an eye with its drainage system in good order, that weight will gradually express from that eye a certain amount of fluid in a certain number of seconds. If the same weight is applied on an eye with its draining system partially obstructed (simple glaucoma), it will take a longer time to express the same amount of fluid. Finally, if the same weight is applied on an eye with its drainage entirely obstructed (absolute glaucoma), no matter how long we wait no fluid is expressed from that eye. Imagining that instead of the weight we use the tonometer, we readily see how we can judge at the same time the amount of fluid expressed from the eye by reading off the tonometric scale the degree of decrease of intraocular pressure when the tonometer is applied steadily for a certain time. In a normal eye the tonometer shows that the intraocular pressure is gradually decreasing at an average which we call normal; in an eye with an impaired drainage the weight of the tonometer still expresses fluid but at a much slower rate, and in an eye with absolute glaucoma the weight of the tonometer produces no decrease of the intraocular pressure.

From the above, it is seen that the tonometer may be utilized for the accurate measurement, not only of the intraocular pressure, but also of the index of ocular drainage.

The index of ocular drainage may be defined, in general terms, as the rate or rapidity with which the ocular fluid may be expressed by the weight of the tonometer applied on the eye.

Since I began to measure the ocular drainage in animal and human eyes, I have become convinced that the mere measurement of intraocular pressure, while very helpful in the diagnosis of certain cases of glaucoma, is a procedure which may be incomplete and misleading unless the index of ocular drainage is measured at the same time. It is misleading in those cases which have only occasionally a high intraocular pressure. If the tonometer happens to be applied during one of the intervals when the intraocular pressure is not above the normal limit, we may be induced to believe that the eye is normal. In fact, clinicians no longer rely upon a single examination. In suspicious cases, they have the intraocular pressure measured repeatedly. It is not improbable that in some cases the examinations should be made during the intervals when the intraocular pressure is not high. In such cases, the mere taking of the intraocular pressure with the tonometer is a crude and incomplete procedure.

The mere satisfaction of proving that the intraocular pressure of an eye is below 27 mm. Hg., *i.e.*, within normal limits, is sometimes deceiving and such an examination is incomplete. On the one hand, a low intraocular pressure does not exclude the presence of glaucoma, because the examination may happen to be made during an interval of nonirritability or because the original interocular pressure of the eye, when normal, was very much lower than the one now found. On the other hand, the measurement of the intraocular pressure is interesting only in so far as it reveals the condition of the safety devices which such an eye prossesses for keeping its draining system in good order. In other words, the measurement of the intraocular pressure alone throws some light upon the condition of the drainage system of the eye. This light is very dim, however, because the drainage capacity may be impaired to some degree and still the intraocular pressure may not exceed the normal limit. Therefore, a correct idea about the normal condition or about the state of impairment of the mechanism regulating the intraocular pressure, can be obtained only when we consider both the intraocular pressure and the index of drainage of the ocular fluids. The elucidation of this point is of great importance in the early diagnosis of glaucoma, when the various complaints of the patient are vague and indefinite and the information furnished by a most careful examination is very doubtful.

As to the method of examination for the index of ocular drainage, a correct technique is necessary and all possible precautions must be taken in order to avoid errors. The method which I have used in examining the rate of ocular drainage is as follows:

For rabbits, an assistant takes the rabbit on his lap and holding it stretched, fixes the head in such a manner that one eye is directed as nearly straight upward as possible. Another assistant, with a watch before him, records the initial intraocular pressure shown by the tonometer and the exact time in seconds at which the examination is begun. He then notes the number of seconds it takes the handle to move from the one division of the tonometric scale to the next one. The examination ends when the animal becomes restless or when the handle of the tonometer does not move while the instrument is applied for over 120 seconds. In human eyes the examination is made with the patient lying on a couch or a table.

II. Intraocular Drainage in Rabbits

It seems logical to expect that the same weight applied on the same eye will press out the same amount of fluid each time, in the same length of time. In reality it is not so, and the above tables, though very few, are suggestive with regard to the variability and relative instability of the draining mechanism of the eye.

From this apparent inconstancy of the index of drainage of intraocular fluid, one important observation may be made, namely: in all the eyes examined, drainage was present and fluid was expressed each time the tonometer was applied for a certain length of time.

It will be seen later that this is not so in glaucomatous eyes.

III. Measurements of Ocular Drainage in Human Eyes with Normal Intraocular Pressure

On account of the readiness with which patients with optic atrophy, submit themselves to repeated examinations, I have measured the intraocular pressure and the ocular drainage in three patients with optic atrophy. Their intraocular pressure does not seem to differ from that of perfectly normal eyes and the findings have given me valuable data with which to compare the tables furnished by numerous examinations of the intraocular pressure and of the index of ocular drainage in six glaucomatous patients.

From the tables of ocular drainage tests made on these three patients with optic atrophy (and with normal intraocular pressure) we see:

(1) That in these eyes, as in rabbit's eyes, the time required for a given amount of intraocular pressure to descend a certain number of millimeters of mercury is not the same in every patient.

(2) The same eye of the same patient does not exhibit the same index of drainage when examined at various intervals. In the first patient, the intraocular pressure went down from 13 to 11.5 in 62 seconds on

January 8th, in 65 seconds one week later, in 70 seconds five minutes later, etc.

IV. Measurement of Intraocular Pressure and Drainage in Glaucomatous Eyes

GROUP A. SIMPLE GLAUCOMA

Patient 4. The drainage system of the eyes of this patient seems to be in perfect order as long as a miotic is used and the pathological changes in the eye, wherever they may be, are very readily influenced by the use of pilocarpine. Parallel with the decrease of intraocular pressure we find an increase in the rapidity of ocular drainage. Ocular drainage suffers and grows less and less when the use of the miotic is stopped.

The readiness with which the ocular drainage is normalized and the intraocular pressure is reduced by the use of pilocarpine is strikingly indicative of the way these particular eyes will stand glaucoma. In this patient, neither the field, nor the acuity of vision has suffered during the year we have kept him under observation.

GROUP B. CASES WITH ABSOLUTE GLAUCOMA IN WHICH OCULAR DRAINAGE HAS BEEN MEASURED

In these four cases, contrary to what we have seen in patient 4, the use of miotics could not re-establish a normal ocular drainage.

GROUP C. MEASUREMENT OF OCULAR DRAINAGE IN PATIENTS WITH SUSPICIOUS GLAUCOMA

Patient 9. It is interesting to note that the right eye with the same intraocular pressure (18.5) on February 7th and March 22d, exhibited a normal capacity of drainage at the first examination and almost a complete stoppage during the second examination. The complaint of the patient of feeling an uneasiness in the right eye (the good eye) and the momentary impairment of the normal drainage are the only points leading us to suspect a prodromal stage of glaucoma in the good eye. Otherwise, neither the ophthalmoscope and field of vision nor the measurement of intraocular pressure would give us any help in the diagnosis.

Patient 10. In this case the question was whether the left eye is just starting on the same glaucomatous career as the other eye (with absolute glaucoma) did two or three years ago. Aside from the very indefinite complaint of the patient, that her vision is occasionally dim, we had no reason to think beginning of a glaucoma in the good eye. The acuity and field of vision, as far as could be determined in this patient, were normal and not receding during the ten months we have had her under observation. The pupil reacted well to light and accommodation and the fundus showed nothing abnormal. The i. o. pressure was always "within the normal limits" (16–26). The only disquieting phenomenon was the impairment of the ocular drainage on March 2, and April 10, 1912. I saw the patient again during Jan., 1913, suffering from an acute glaucoma of the left eye.

Patient 11. This patient is interesting on account of the difficulty experienced in deciding the presence or absence of glaucoma in the left eye. She gave a history suggestive of prodromal glaucoma: occasional pains in the left eye, dimness of vision, the seeing of various colors around the gas flame. The field of vision was about 20 degrees concentrically contracted in both eyes, but more limited nasally on the left eye. Both disks were deeply excavated (physiologic excavation?). On the other hand she was markedly neurasthenic and too much importance could not be attached to her complaints. Her vision was good and could be improved to 20/30 plus with glasses. The intraocular pressure was within the normal limits in both eyes. The opinions of two other ophthalmologists (A and B) of very wide experience was respectively, A: "No glaucoma"; B: "Glaucoma."

The careful study of the behavior of the intraocular pressure in the eyes of this patient and the repeated measurement of the ocular drainage, made the suspicion of prodromal glaucoma very plausible. The reasons are:

The intraocular pressure of the two eyes was always found to be different. Those who have made careful examinations of the intraocular pressure in a large number of cases have gained the knowledge that the intraocular pressure is usually the same in both eyes.

The mere fact that the intraocular pressure of an eye is within "normal" limits cannot be considered as conclusive, in my opinion, with regard to the quest on whether that amount of intraocular pressure is normal. This can be determined only by a comparison of the intraocular pressure and of the draining test of one eye with that of the other.

Patient 12. The miotic has reduced the intraocular pressure in the right eye from 60.5 to 27 and the patient assured me that in three years he has not seen as clearly as now. The ocular drainage however, was not so greatly influenced. In the left eye with the iridectomy, the miotic reduced the intraocular pressure and improved the rate of drainage. The right eye, as we see, responds readily to the miotics by a reduction of the intraocular pressure, but by no improvement of the drainage capacity.

Of the three groups of patients with glaucoma, the third one is the most interesting. The measurement of intraocular pressure and ocular drainage is important mostly for the establishment of a diagnosis in suspicious cases of glaucoma. In this group of cases in which the measurement of acuity and field of vision, as well as the ophthalmoscopic examination, could not advance the diagnosis even one step further, the method of measuring the rate of ocular drainage is perfectly welcome if it can help throw any light on the condition of these eyes. It is interesting to note that while the intraocular pressure in these eyes with suspicious glaucoma is within normal limits, the measurement of ocular drainage shows a reduced rate.

Summary

The degree of intraocular pressure depends in a great measure on the integrity of the draining system of the eye, and the examination of the rate of ocular drainage is of more importance than the simple measurement of the intraocular pressure. The rate of ocular drainage can be measured by the aid of the Schiötz tonometer in animal and human eyes with a certain amount of accuracy.

Normal eyes have an ocular pressure and a rate of ocular drainage varying within relatively wide limits; glaucomatous eyes have some impairment in the function of the draining system. It is safe to suppose that in incipient or prodromal glaucoma, the draining system may be undergoing slight alterations which, though too small to raise the intraocular pressure above the upper limit of the normal, yet sufficient to be discernible by the measurement of the rate of ocular drainage. There are patients with eyes in a condition of latent glaucoma in which the intraocular pressure is within normal limits—about 15 to 26 mm. Hg. The diagnosis in such cases can be cleared up to a certain extent by the measurement of the rate of ocular drainage.

Comment: Schiötz in 1908 observed that the tension became reduced when the tonometer set for some minutes on the cornea. In 1911, Polak-van Gelder discovered that, to produce the same fall of tension in this manner, glaucomatous eyes required a greater weight of the plunger assembly than normal eyes, and she suggested this finding as a diagnostic test. Since Schoenberg's paper, his simple method of assessing the drainage mechanism has been studied further. Wegner reported in 1925 that the Schiötz tonometer with the 5.5 gm. weight caused the tension of the normal eye to fall in five minutes to one-third to one-half its initial value; and that the relative drop in tension was constantly less in glaucomatous eyes. In 1953, Blaxter recorded the tension reading 15 seconds after the application of the tonometer as B, and four minutes later as C. The change in tension (B-C) divided by B was designated as the outflow fraction, and was over 30 percent in the normal eye. A lower percentage signifies a serious obstruction to outflow and, if the eye had been under miotic therapy, demonstrated the need of a filtering operation. In 1950 Grant utilized the electronic tonometer to determine the normal coefficient of aqueous outflow, after which he applied this method, named by him tonography, to glaucomatous eyes. No nonglaucomatous eye revealed an outflow coefficient of less than 0.14, the variation in normal eyes being 0.14 to 0.56. Methods that test the facility of aqueous outflow, tonography or the bulbar pressure test of Blaxter, provide an important advance in the early diagnosis of chronic open-angle glaucoma.

References

Blaxter, P. L.: Bulbar pressure test in glaucoma. Brit. J. Ophth., *37:* 641, 1953.
Kronfeld, P.: Tonography. A.M.A. Arch. Ophth., *48:* 393, 1952.

Biographical Note

Mark J. Schoenberg (1874–1945) was born in Rumania, graduated from the Bucharest University Medical School, and after 2 years of postgraduate study in Vienna and Germany, emigrated to New York City. In a relatively short time he became associated with Knapp Memorial Eye Hospital, the eye clinic at Mount Sinai Hospital and the eye staff of Columbia University Medical School. From 1912 he labored on the early detection of glaucoma; collaborated later with Loewenstein on pupillography applied to glaucoma and with Posner on the standardization of tonometers; and in 1935, with the cooperation of the National Society for the Prevention of Blindness, inaugurated glaucoma clinics in New York City. In 1914 he was awarded the Lucien Howe prize for his experimental studies on ocular anaphylaxis. In 1919 he reported the first case of bilateral retinoblastoma in which the nonenucleated eye was treated with radium and maintained useful vision during a 10-year period of observation. He observed Gonin's work at Lausanne and was the first to perform the Gonin operation for retinal detachment in the United States. He founded the New York Society for Clinical Ophthalmology and was its first president.

References

Esterman, B.: Obituary. Am. J. Ophth., *28:* 782, 1945.
Givner, I.: Obituary. Arch. Ophth., *33:* 322, 1945.

Part Seven

Conjunctiva and Uvea

The Bacillus of Acute Conjunctival Catarrh, or "Pink Eye"

JOHN E. WEEKS, M.D.

New York, New York

ARCH. OPHTH., *15:* 441–451, 1886

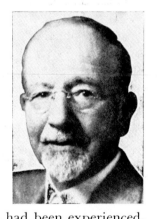

On the 21st of March, 1886 Dr. R. O. Born sent me a patient who was suffering from acute conjunctivitis, with the request that I should examine the rather profuse mucopurulent discharge microscopically. The patient, Anna F., age thirty, in good health, first noticed that her eyes were sore three days previous to her visit to me. A sensation as of a foreign body in the eye, burning and stiffness of the lids, followed by a mucopurulent discharge, preventing sleep, had been experienced.

St. Pr. The ocular and palpebral conjunctivae are greatly congested, lids slightly swollen, marked photophobia, profuse lachrymation and muco-purulent discharge. I made a cover-glass preparation (dry) of the secretion, stained it with gentian violet, and examined the specimen with a $\frac{1}{12}$ oil immersion. The examination disclosed large numbers of small well defined bacilli which were aggregated on and in the pus cells, and free in mucus. The patient complained of frontal headache, and had some coryza. By the use of constant cold applications for three or four days, and the use of mild astringents, the eyes recovered in two weeks from the beginning of the attack. There were two children in

238

the family, one of twenty months and one of four years, both of whom had sore eyes. The first had had conjunctivitis for two months. The palpebral conjunctiva was injected and was discharging muco-pus. The second was a case of six weeks' standing, and was in the same condition as the first. No corneal trouble was present in either case. The secretion from both cases contained many bacilli such as were found in the secretion from the mother's eyes. By keeping the eyes clean and the use of a zinc collyrium both children recovered in one week.

In frequent examinations of conjunctival secretions at the Ophthalmic and Aural Institute, for some months previous to the 29th of March, I had never met with this form of microbe. With a view to determining how frequently cases like the ones described occurred, I examined all secretions from cases of conjunctival diseases that came to the clinic after that time, but failed to find the bacillus again until May 21st, when Peter C., age twenty-three years, presented himself for treatment. On inquiry I found that his wife, three children, and a servant girl still had, or had recovered from, a similar form of conjunctivitis. They were attacked as follows:

Thos. C., two and a half years. Attacked May 4th. Muco-purulent discharge from both eyes; still persists.

Jos. C., fifteen months. Attacked May 7th. Muco-purulent discharge from both eyes; still persists.

Eliz. C., twenty-eight years. Attacked May 9th. Muco-purulent discharge from right eye only; recovered.

Katie O'C., servant. Attacked May 16th. Muco-purulent discharge from the right eye only; still persists.

Peter C. Attacked May 17. This case very closely resembles the first case reported. The eyes got well in five or six days by the use of cold and astringents. In three weeks he returned with a fresh attack fully as severe as the first, which readily responded to the same treatment. The bacilli were found, in quite large numbers, in the secretion from all of the last five cases.

A number of observations of the occurrence of the same disease in different members of the same family was perhaps sufficient evidence of the contagious nature of this form of conjunctivitis. I determined, however, to ascertain this point positively, by inoculating healthy conjunctivae with secretion from an affected eye. At first rabbits were used, but the inoculations failed to produce any inflammation of the conjunctivae. I then inoculated the healthy conjunctivae of six eyes in five men, who had previously lost their vision, by transferring a small amount of the secretion from the patient's eye to the eyes that were being experimented on. In five of the six eyes inoculated the same form of conjunctivitis was produced, the bacilli being found in secretions.

From March of this year up to the present time I have observed about one hundred cases of this disease. I find that it varies to a considerable extent in degree of severity; all the cases, however, resemble one another so closely in their clinical aspect that the diagnosis may be readily made without the aid of the microscope.

Cultivation

A mixture which contained only about 0.5% of agar was prepared. The bacillus developed rather feebly in this preparation in tubes. It would not grow on plates. Having found a medium on which the bacillus would develop, although feebly, my next endeavor was to make a pure culture. The bacillus in the tubes was contaminated with a club-shaped bacillus (or one which soon became clubbed), which developed as rapidly as the small bacillus, and repeated attempts to separate the two proved fruitless. It was easy enough to procure a pure culture of the clubbed bacillus as it grows quite readily on 1% agar. The 0.5% agar is the best medium that I have found on which to cultivate this bacillus; it leaves, however, much to be desired, which further experiments will probably satisfy. The method of inoculating tubes with the conjunctival secretion has been to thoroughly clean the conjunctival sac with clean water and cotton, direct the patient to keep the eyes closed, and after five or ten minutes to transfer a small portion of the newly formed secretion from the bottom of the lower conjunctival sac to the tube, using a previously heated platinum rod for the purpose. An even temperature from 34° to 37° C. is most favorable for the development of this microbe; it is also necessary to have abundant moisture. I have never succeeded in making a cultivation at the temperature of the room, nor on agar from which the water was in part removed. The bacillus varies considerably in length, being from 1 to 2 micro-millimeters long; in thickness it is always the same—namely, about 0.25 micro-millimeters. Compared with the tubercle bacillus it has about the same thickness, but is considerably shorter. In preparations from cultures on agar I have observed a number of bacilli joined, forming quite long threads (6 to 8 together), the division between individual bacilli being very indistinctly marked. There was no tendency to a double arrangement, as in bacillus subtilis or in Leber's bacillus of xerosis of the conjunctiva.

The bacillus under consideration stains readily with watery solutions of fuchsin, gentian violet, and methylene blue, taking the stain a little less deeply than do the cocci and bacilli ordinarily met with.

When the bacillus begins to degenerate it stains much less readily. It does not stain well with Bismarck brown, ammonium or picro-carmine, or with haematoxylin. Attempts at double staining have so far proven unsatisfactory. In staining sections of the conjuctiva, Gram's method with gentian violet has given the best results. I find nothing peculiar to this bacillus in the effect produced upon it by the various acids, alkalies, alcohol, chloroform, or ether. If colored with gentian violet or fuchsin the bacillus is quickly decolorized when treated with alcholol or a ten-per-cent solution of either nitric, acetic, hydrochloric, or sulphuric acid, taking the color again readily after the decolorizing reagent is removed by washing with water.

Inoculation Experiments

Not having succeeded in making perfectly pure cultures of the small bacillus, pure cultures of the clubbed bacillus were made and experiments conducted with this and the mixture.

Five inoculations of the human conjunctiva (to which I might add others) and two of rabbits are sufficient to prove the innocence of the clubbed bacillus in the production of acute conjunctivitis.

Experiments with the Mixture of the Small and Club-shaped Bacilli

Case 6. July 29th. M.I., six years. O. D. inoculated from a fifth generation.

July 31st. The ocular and palpebral conjunctivae of the inoculated eye are markedly congested, and are secreting a small amount of muco-pus; profuse lachrymation; no photophobia and but slight pain. Specimens from the secretion were examined with the microscope and were found to contain numerous bacilli exactly resembling the small bacilli in the culture tube. The left eye was perfectly normal.

Aug. 2d. The congestion of the ocular and palpebral conjunctivae of the right eye is very intense. Profuse discharge of muco-pus, which collects in the inner canthi, escaping at these points. Lachrymation, slight photophobia, some pain in the lids, and mild coryza. The left eye was becoming injected, probably having been inoculated with the discharge from the right eye.

Aug. 4th. Both eyes presented a typical picture of acute conjunctivitis, with intense congestion and slight swelling of the ocular and palpebral conjunctivae. Chemosis not prominent, with slight swelling of lids. The discharge has become thicker, and the accumulation of yellowish flakes at the inner canthi is marked. Continuous application of iced cloths was ordered.

Aug. 8th. The ocular conjunctiva is becoming white; the discharge still continues, but is less in quantity and thicker.

Aug. 10th. Still greater diminution in the congestion of the conjunctiva and in the amount of the discharge. A zinc collyrium, 1/3%, was ordered to be applied to the conjunctiva of the lids twice a day.

Aug. 16th. Ocular conjunctiva white. Palpebral still congested. Thick yellow masses of discharge appear at the inner canthi, an appearance quite characteristic of this form of disease. No photophobia, and but slight pain.

Aug. 30th. Still a very little of the yellowish discharge at the inner canthi. Conjunctiva almost normal.

Sept. 1st. Patient has entirely recovered.

Case 7. July 27th. S. D., seven years. O. D. inoculated with the mixture from a fourth generation. The disease ran a course identical with that in No. 5, except that on Aug. 8th some subconjunctival hemorrhages were present. The discharge ceased about the 28th of August.

Case 8. July 29th. A. S., six years. O. D. inoculated as in the two previous cases with the mixture of the fifth generation. The inoculated eye became injected on the second day, followed by the left two days later, with muco-purulent discharge, as in Cases 6 and 7. This case, however, recovered in three weeks from the time of the inoculation.

Case 9. July 29th. F. F., six years. This case was in every respect a repetition of Case 8; the inoculation having also been made from a fifth generation.

Case 10. Sept. 1st. M. T., thirteen years. The inoculation in this case was made from the eleventh generation of the same bacillus. The typical conjunctivitis appeared on the second day and ran a course as in Case 8, except that on the fifth day a very few marginal phlyctenulae appeared.

Case 11. Sept. 1st. J. A., ten years. O. D. inoculated from the eleventh generation. The typical conjunctivitis appeared, as in Case 8, running a similar but somewhat more protracted course.

Preparations of the secretions from all of the last six cases were made from time to time. The bacillus was present in all as long as the yellowish discharge persisted.

Sections of the conjunctiva from three of the cases, obtained by cutting out small portions from the bottom of the lower conjunctival sacs, some of which portions were hardened in Müller's fluid and others in alcohol, after which the sections were made by the use of the freezing method or by imbedding in celloidine. The sections were stained by Gram's method. The bacilli in rather scanty numbers were found in the anterior layers of the epithelium, either singly or in small colonies lying between the cells. Some leucocytes or pus cells found in the epithelial layer showed the bacilli apparently in the interior as well as on the surface of the cells.

No corneal complications occurred in any of the above cases. No corneal complications ever occur in this form of conjunctivitis, unless it is complicated by some intercurrent disease. In Case 9, a few phlyctenulae appeared on the fifth day. This I consider the development of a distinctly different disease, engrafted on the older conjunctivitis,—an accidental complication.

It will be noticed that in the last six cases described the inflammation in the inoculated eye (O. D. in all) appeared uniformly in about forty-eight hours from the time that the bacilli were introduced. In order to produce this effect there certainly must have been some causative agent in the cultures employed. Had it been a simple chemical irritant to the conjunctiva we would have expected to see an immediate inflammatory result. As it was, no redness of the conjunctiva, no sense of discomfort or any thing outside of the normal condition was experienced by the patient until thirty-six to forty-eight hours after the inoculation. A period of incubation was necessary to enable the bacilli to multiply sufficiently to produce an inflammatory condition of the mucous membrane.

The researches of numerous observers have demonstrated the fact that quite a large variety of microbes, cocci and bacilli, are present in secretions from the conjunctival sac. I have myself cultivated four forms of bacilli and five varieties of cocci from these secretions, not including the coccus of Neisser, nor the one recently described by Michel as the causative agent in trachoma. All which I have cultivated, except the very small bacillus described, grow on ordinary 1% agar, and do not (as has been determined by actual inoculation experiments, which my space here does not permit me to give in full) produce any inflammation when introduced into the conjunctival sac.

If additional proof of the contagious nature of this form of conjunctivitis was necessary, the auto-inoculation of the left eye in all of these cases—the appearance of the conjunctivitis in that eye on the fourth day—is conclusive. Cultivations of the small bacillus were made from the secretions from the inoculated eyes, which presented all the appearances of the original cultures.

In numerous examinations of secretion from the normal conjunctiva and from the conjunctiva in all its phases of disease, I have never met with this bacillus except in the form of acute conjunctivitis described. In this disease, of which as stated above I have observed many cases in the last six months, the bacillus is constant. The observations and experimental results given above, notwithstanding the defect in its cultivation, are, I believe, sufficient to establish the causative effect of the bacillus in this form of conjunctivitis. The difficulty in cultivating this pathogenic microbe on artificially prepared food is not unprecedented. Many, in fact the greater number of known pathogenic varieties, are cultivated with difficulty, and some are yet problematical in that respect.

This form of conjunctivitis is contagious and epidemic; it appears most plentifully in the spring and fall months, but isolated cases are found at all times of the year. From the peculiar congestion of the ocular conjunctiva it has become popularly known as "pink eye." Its epidemic character is well known. As before stated, corneal complications never occur in this form of conjunctivitis unless some other disease is engrafted upon it. The disease usually runs its course in from three weeks to two months, but may continue even longer if not treated. It may be much shortened by the use of constant cold applications during the acute stage, and the application of some mild astringents in the subacute and chronic stages.

So far as I am aware, no one has heretofore described a microbe as the cause of this form of acute conjunctivitis. Koch (Wiener med. Woch., 1883, p. 1550), while at Alexandria, Egypt, investigating the cholera epidemic, examined the secretion from fifty cases of conjunctivitis, which included two forms. One of the forms of conjunctivitis, which runs a very severe course, he asserts to be due to the presence of a bacterium, which closely resembles the gonococcus, and is probably identical with it. The other, a much less severe process, in which a constant condition was the presence of a very small bacillus in the pus corpuscles. The latter is probably the same form that I have described.

Comment: The organism causing acute epidemic conjunctivitis was originally observed as a contaminant of Egyptian trachoma, first by Julius Hirschberg and Krause in 1881, then by Koch in 1883. In recognition of this history, the most recent label for the germ is *Hemophilus aegyptius.* After Weeks had ascertained that the organism did not affect the cornea, he inoculated his own eyes, as well as those of six human volunteers. Morax, who among many others confirmed Weeks' discovery, felt strongly that Weeks awarded Koch undue credit, and that the eponym Koch-Weeks bacillus was unwarranted. He always called it the Weeks bacillus and it is still known in France by that name. Weeks, in pursuing his studies, clarified the clinical picture of acute epidemic conjunctivitis by a report of more than 100 cases, and in 1887 he successfully isolated the bacillus in pure culture. He found that the organism grows well only in media enriched by hemoglobin or yeast. The Weeks bacillus is morphologically similar to *H. influenza,* but the two organisms differ in pathogenicity, antigenicity and biochemistry. *H. aegyptius* is strictly an ocular path-

244

ogen. It is more easily found in scrapings than in smears. The germ is small, Gram-negative, hemophilic, and pleomorphic, especially in culture, appearing as very short rods or long filaments. It may be found free or intracellularly. In culture the colonies are tiny, glistening, translucent dewdrops emitting a pronounced sweet odor. The organism grows around a staphylococcus colony as an iridescent zone, and this aids identification. Acute epidemic conjunctivitis clinically resembles pneumococcic conjunctivitis. The bulbar conjunctiva has a cyanotic redness and under magnification petechial hemorrhages may be seen in the upper bulbar conjunctiva. The disease is highly contagious and school children should be kept at home for 1 week after all discharge has ceased. The organism is susceptible to the topical administration of streptomycin, tetracycline or sulfonamides, but is only slightly affected by penicillin. At office visits, resolution may be hastened by lightly painting the palpebral conjunctiva with 1 per cent silver nitrate.

References

Fedukowicz, H. B.: External Infections of the Eye, pp. 91–93. Meredith Publishing Co., New York, 1963.
Feldman, M.: The Koch-Weeks bacillus and John Weeks, M.D. Arch. Ophth., *70:* 430–432, Sept. 1963.

Biographical Note

John Elmer Weeks (1853–1949), who was born in Painesville, Ohio, worked as a painter of railroad cars until he accumulated sufficient funds to finance his medical education. After receiving his medical degree from the University of Michigan in 1881, he had a 1-year internship and a 2-year residency in general medicine. He then secured a 2-year residency under Dr. Hermann Knapp at the New York Ophthalmic Institute (1884–1886). In 1885, Knapp brought from Europe the equipment for a small bacteriological laboratory and soon started Weeks on the investigation of "pink eye," which culminated in the discovery of the causative organism. He served as chief of the clinic in the departments of ophthalmology successively at New York University (1886–1888) and the College of Physicians and Surgeons (1888–1890). While he was a staff surgeon at the New York Eye and Ear Infirmary (1890–1920), Weeks developed there a laboratory of pathology and bacteriology. He lectured on ophthalmology at New York University (1890–1900) and subsequently became professor and chairman of the department (1900–1921). During his 60 years in ophthalmology, Weeks contributed 125 publications, including "A treatise on diseases of the eye" (1910). He was chairman of the Section on Ophthalmology of the American Medical Association in 1905, president of the American Ophthalmological Society in 1921, and a member of the Ophthalmological Society of the United Kingdom and of the Royal Hungarian Medical Society. Weeks received the honorary degree of D.Sc. in 1934 from the University of Michigan, LL.D. from New York University and was made an honorary professor of ophthalmology of the University of Oregon. In 1921, he established a scholarship for research in ophthalmology at the University of Michigan. In 1925 he moved to Portland, Oregon and became deeply interested in the new University of Oregon Medical School. In 1939 he donated funds for its library and auditorium and in 1944 he assisted financially in the development of the department of ophthalmology. Finally, he established a laboratory for ophthalmic research and an ophthalmic museum, which have since been moved to larger quarters and named in his memory.

Reference

Knapp, A.: Obituary. Arch. Ophth., *41:* 752–754, 1949.

A Case of "Squirrel Plague" Conjunctivitis in Man (Bacillus Tularense Infection of the Eye)

DERRICK T. VAIL, SR., M.D.

Cincinnati, Ohio

OPHTH. REC., 1914, *23:* 487–497

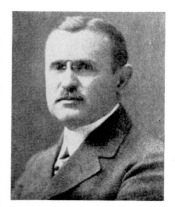

It is believed that this is the first report of infection of the human eye from the virus of a plague-like disease among certain rodents, notably the California ground squirrel, and now known as "Squirrel Plague."

The case which I bring to your attention in this report presented such unique, alarming and peculiar ocular symptoms that it was impossible from anything written in ophthalmic literature to render a clinical diagnosis.

Historical Data on California Squirrel Plague

The bubonic plague first appeared as an epidemic in the United States at San Francisco in 1900. The presumption was that plague-infected rats infesting incoming ships from the Orient found their way ashore and that they constituted the source of infection for the human cases through the fleas that they harbored.

The human epidemic was at first practically limited to the inhabitants of Chinatown, San Francisco. The United States officer in command of plague suppression was Surgeon Rupert Blue, the same who is in charge of the bubonic plague situation in New Orleans at this present writing (1914).

Blue first suspected in 1903 that the plague which was destroying ground squirrels in such great numbers, as was being reported from many parts of the country about San Francisco, was nothing other than bubonic plague. Soon, however, human cases of plague-like infection began to appear in country districts, in which no reasonable mode of conveyance other than through squirrels seemed plausible.

Take the case of Charles Bock, a country blacksmith, who came to

246

San Francisco (August, 1903) from a neighboring village, and died of plague. Surgeon Blue visited his town and learned that Bock had shot ground squirrels three or four days before his illness began. The following September (1903) another victim from another part of the country died from plague, a man who had been living in a railroad camp thirty miles from civilization, and it was learned that these rough laborers often killed and ate ground squirrels. In 1904 rural cases continued to be reported here and there, and Dr. Blue, who was keen on the suspicion that ground squirrels were furnishing the infection, conducted a series of experiments through the aid of Assistant Surgeon Donald Currie, bacteriologist for the plague laboratory, and proved that the ground squirrel was very susceptible to plague infection, both by inoculation and direct contact. Blue then (1904) sent a man to investigate the county of Contra Costa to ascertain the truth of the many reports that came through various sources that the squirrels were being exterminated by a plague. This agent reported that the farmers were everywhere rejoiced at the disappearance of the ground squirrel. He also learned that the squirrels had been suffering from an epizootic.

It was then learned by another investigator (Past Assistant Surgeon J. D. Long) that armies of ground squirrels were seen at different times between the years 1903 and 1905 to be migrating across the country. Farmers had endeavored to secure sick squirrels to carry home to spread the infection. They burrow the ground, feed on grain and multiply so rapidly that they had become a great pest. In fact, one man offered a bounty of $20.00 for a single sick squirrel.

After the earthquake of 1907 true bubonic plague cases appeared in alarming numbers in San Francisco. There were 156 cases with 78 deaths, and country cases continued to appear, so that Blue directed his men to trap and collect rodents from Contra Costa county that a thorough search for plague might be made. Four hundred and twenty-three ground squirrels were sent in and among them were found four genuine cases of glandular suppurations in sick squirrels.

In spite of this, many doubted that the disease in man was contracted from squirrels. Soon, however, a case appeared in Los Angeles, which proved the direct communicability of the infection from squirrel to man without the intervention of fleas or biting insects. A boy ten years old, living in Los Angeles, found a sick ground squirrel near his home. Being moved with compassion, and thinking he would take it home, nurse it and make a pet of it, he picked it up, but the animal bit him on the finger. On the fourth day after, he was taken very sick with fever, delirium, etc., and the glands of the axilla on that side became swollen and painful. The abscess in the armpit was aspirated, and G. W.

McCoy, who was studying the case, found by experiments on guinea pigs and rats that the organism was similar to *Bacillus pestis.* Suppurative glands appeared elsewhere, but the boy finally recovered. In view of the fact that Currie had demonstrated that the saliva from the mouth of an infected squirrel was laden with infection, due most likely to the influence of plague pneumonia that was demonstrated, it is beyond question that this boy was directly infected from the bite of the squirrel and not from flea bites.

It was then thought by many that squirrel-plague and bubonic plague were one and the same disease. This, however, proved untrue, for Past Assistant Surgeon George W. McCoy, of San Francisco, proved among other things that there was a distinct difference between true bubonic plague and squirrel-plague, the latter being less violent and the bacillus causing it being different from the true *Bacillus pestis,* although closely allied to it and that fatal squirrel-plague is not identical in its pathology with fatal bubonic plague.

Finally, in 1911, McCoy and Chapin identified the germ of squirrel-plague, grew it on egg-yolk culture, proved its entity, described it fully and named it *"Bacillus tularense"* after the county of Tulare, in California, in which the disease was first observed. They state "the essential pathological lesions (of fatal squirrel-plague infection in rodents) are many whitish or yellowish caseous granules in the spleen and liver." Caseous nodules also appear in the lymph glands.

Report of My Case of Squirrel-Plague Infection of the Human Eye

E.E., male, aged 28, referred to me on November 24, 1913, by Dr. Paul DeCourcy, of Cincinnati, on account of an acute and violent inflammation of his left eye.

Occupation: Meat cutter in restaurant.

Present Illness: Three days ago left eye became inflamed and swollen. Tried medicine prescribed by a druggist, but eye became rapidly worse. The lid margins were agglutinated of mornings. Notices a "sore lump" in front of the left ear. Eye discharges much watery secretion. Has no pain; vision unaffected.

External Inspection: Right eye, normal.

Left Eye: Marked redness and swelling of both eyelids. Intense chemosis is present. Eye discharges muco-watery secretion. Lashes are matted, tuft-like. General appearance of eye suggests gonorrhoeal ophthalmia. The pre-auricular gland on that side is swollen to the size of a small cherry and is tender to touch. Palpebral conjunctiva: On everting the eyelids, the seat of disease is revealed. The conjunctiva is riddled with about ten discrete deep, round, yellow necrotic ulcers, that run clear through the substantia propria of the conjunctiva quite to the tarsus. There are six such round ulcers over the upper tarsus and four at least over the lower tarsus. The ulcers appear punched out, but filled with golden yellow necrotic plugs. Sizes vary from 6.0 mm., the largest, which exists near the upper edge of the tarsus of the upper lid, to about 1.0 mm. The surrounding conjunctiva is deep red, very soggy and swollen, but does not bleed on being wiped with a wet cotton sponge. The necrotic plugs in the beds of the ulcers cannot be wiped away. The contrast between the deep red color of the conjunctiva and the brilliant golden color of the ulcers is as striking as a turkey-red calico dress with yellow "polka dots."

A smear was taken at once to search for the gonococcus, but none found. Diagnosis of Parinaud's conjunctivitis tentatively made.

November 25, next day. Eye looks worse, patient pale, temperature 100°, pre-auricular gland more swollen, the lymph glands of the anterior triangle of the neck and submaxillary region of that side are easily felt to be enlarged and are tender. Diagnosis of Parinaud's conjunctivitis withdrawn on account of the ulcers. Too acute for tuberculosis and certainly not chancre or syphillis.

November 28. Patient is losing weight rapidly, looks cachectic and sick, temperature 102°, glands of the left side face and neck are conspicuously large and now there is seen a discrete pustular eruption six or seven in number and 4 to 5 mm. in size, something like the pustules of varicella, located on the left temple and malar region. The appearance of the left eye is not improved; cornea, is, however, brilliant and vision unaffected. The left nostril discharges a watery muscus freely. The left turbinated bodies are swollen and red. On account of the nasal symptoms and the pustular eruption on the left malar, the diagnosis is changed to "Glanders or Farcy" and patient urged to go to the Cincinnati Hospital.

December 1. Patient did not go to the hospital. Wants to continue treatment at my office. A new symptom has developed since two days ago. Infection of the left lachrymal sac with every evidence of abscess formation. The ulcers of the conjunctiva remain about the same in appearance, but are slightly more numerous. They are not epithelial ulcers, such as we see in herpes, but perforate the conjunctiva quite to the tarsus. Evidently the solitary lymph nodes of the conjunctiva are the seat of the necrosis. His family physician, Dr. DeCourcy, finally persuaded him to apply to the Cincinnati Hospital for treatment. Dr. Robert Sattler was on duty at that time and we find the following clinical memoranda:

Right eye: Normal.

Left eye: Lids puffed and reddened. Swelling size of hazel nut at inner canthus (purulent dacryocystitis). Ocular conjunctiva much congested. On eversion of the lids the palpebral conjunctiva much thickened, roughened and reddened. Conjunctiva ulcers are present. Pressure on tear sac, which has consistency of well filled bladder, does not evacuate into the eye or nose. There are a half-dozen large pustules between the left eye and ear. The anterior auricular and anterior cervical glands and those about the angle of the jaw are enlarged. There are no glandular enlargements at the right side of the face.

December 9. Abscess of the tear sac incised, discharging yellow, creamy pus.

December 10. Drainage from the abscess has ceased. Conjunctiva ulcers gone. Ocular condition much improved, but the pre-auricular and other glands remain enlarged.

December 11. Patient discharged, improved. The temperature chart shows the typical rise and fall of a general septic infection, highest being 102.6°, evenings of December 4 and 5, but the morning temperature never below 100° until after December 5.

How could the infection of the California ground-squirrel-plague find its way into E.E.'s left eye in Cincinnati? This is a question that is hard to answer definitely. It has been proven by various students of the disease—Blue, McCoy, Chapin, Currie, Long, Wherry, and others —that all rodents are susceptible to infection by direct contact, squirrels and rabbits particularly so. Three facts are significant:

(1) Wherry says that "a year previously (to this case) we had heard from a hunter that wild rabbits were dying in large numbers across the Ohio River in Kentucky." Moreover, this man was infected during the hunting season when the market is open to the sale of rabbits, and I, myself (being a hunter), was interested in reading in a Cincinnati daily a note from rabbit hunters in the vicinity of Cincinnati, stating they were finding large numbers of dead rabbits in the fields, and the opinion that they were being exterminated by a plague of some sort.

(2) Health Officer Landis, of Cincinnati, learning the markets of the city were selling rotten rabbits, investigated and found large quantities of putrid rabbits on sale at five cents apiece. He rightly condemned all of them and reports that 36,420 pounds of decayed rabbits were seized and destroyed between November 1 and December 6, 1913. My patient was infected in the height of this season.

(3) My patient was by occupation a meat cutter in a cheap restaurant located in the tenement and slum district of the city close to the markets. The inference is fair that rabbits affected with caseous buboes came to his table for cutting, that he held the diseased meat in his left hand, cutting with the knife held in his right hand, and that he introduced the poison into his left eye from his left finger.

PROOF OF SQUIRREL-PLAGUE INFECTION IN THIS CASE BY PROF. WHERRY,
BACTERIOLOGIST, AND SENIOR STUDENT B. H. LAMB

"Guinea pig No. 1 received on December 4, 1913, an intraperitoneal injection of scrapings from a conjunctival ulcer from the patient's eye, suspended in normal sterile salt solution." Died December 10. Post mortem shows acute pneumonia; the spleen and liver are congested and enlarged and show numerous scattered foci of necrosis. No bacteria found on various smear preparations variously stained. Various culture media remained sterile as to aerobic and anaerobic bacilli for a month.

"The disease was kept going through a series of guinea pigs while isolation experiments were in progress"; nothing definite was found, but "after passing the virus through twenty-four animals, we became acquainted with the work of McCoy and Chapin and by using the coagulated egg-yolk on which they were able to grow *Bacillus tularense*, we isolated what we believed to be the same bacterium."

The Berkfeld filter prevented the germ from passing through, as proven by experiment injections on guinea pigs. The corroborates McCoy and Chapin's findings, "while guinea pig No. 20, used as a control, was injected subcutaneously with 2 cc. of the unfiltered extract. It died in three days with typical lesions and *Bacillus tularense* was isolated in an ovomucoid-yolk culture from an inguinal buvo."

The tests and measurements of the bacillus by Wherry tallied very closely to those of McCoy.

In carrying out their investigations to prove this case, Wherry and Lamb used "forty-nine guinea pigs, three Belgian hares, three white rats, three kittens and one pigeon." "The guinea pigs, as a rule, succumbed on the fourth or fifth day after cutaneous inoculation with spleen juice or when pricked in the eye with an infected needle" and again simply dipping a fine needle into the spleen of a dead animal or into a culture and pricking the ocular or palpebral conjunctiva of rabbits or guinea pigs results in the production of multiple areas of necrosis on the palpebral conjunctivae, just like those in the human case, and is followed by septicemia and death in a few days.

Wherry showed me the head and viscera of rabbit No. 1, which had been pricked in the conjunctiva, as above suggested. The eyelids were everted on toothpick stays and presented the same typical round necrotic ulcers my case had presented; moreover, the lymph glands in front of the rabbit's ear and down the side of its neck were greatly enlarged.

The white rats inoculated intraperitoneally died in two days or less. The kittens survived. An infected emulsion was dropped in the healthy eye of guinea pig No. 38. It died in four days' time. The conjunctiva presented the same round ulcers and the lymphatic glands of the neck were markedly involved.

Guinea pig No. 34 was fed on most of the spleen of a dead guinea pig. It died in three days' time.

From the evidence submitted, I think we may make the claim beyond doubt that the case of E.E. was one of squirrel-plague ophthalmia, and I believe the first case on record.

Comment: In 1912, G. W. McCoy of the U.S. Public Health Service announced the discovery of *Pasteurella tularense* and its agglutination by the serums of two laboratory co-workers who had contracted the disease while investigating a plague-like sickness of rodents. The oculoglandular form of tularemia with bacteriological confirmation was first reported by Derrick T. Vail, Sr., in 1914. The next two proved cases were also observed by Cincinnati ophthalmologists, Sattler (1915), Lamb (1917). After the detection of tularemia in the United States, the disease was noted successively in Japan (1925), Russia (1928), Norway (1929), Canada (1930), Sweden (1931), Austria (1935), Czechoslovakia and Turkey (1936). The conjunctiva is especially susceptible to the tularemia organism. Of 78 ocular infections reported in America by 1940, only 6 were accompanied by involvement of the hand although both were subjected at the same time to the same source of infection, tissue from rabbit, squirrel, ground hog, water rat, or crushed tick or fly. The incubation period, which averaged 3 days, varied in these cases from 1 to 14 days. Ulcers were located on the tarsal conjunctiva in 43 patients and on the bulbar conjunctiva in 8. Nonulcerating nodules were noted on the tarsal conjunctiva in 6 cases and on the bulbar conjunctiva in one. Unilateral enlargement of the preauricular lymph nodes occurred in 55 cases, of the submaxillary in 46, and of the cervical in 41. Suppuration of some of the lymph nodes occurred in 36 cases. Constitutional symptoms—fever and debility—are part of all forms of tularemia. Death occurred in 7 of the 78 oculoglandular cases, a mortality of 9 per cent. Attempts to identify the organism from smears of the conjunctival secretion are useless. The etiological diagnosis is made by agglutination tests which can be confirmed by culture on blood-dextrose-cystine agar. The antibiotic, tetracycline, is an effective remedy.

Reference

Francis, E.: Oculoglandular tularemia. Arch. Ophth., *28:* 711–741, 1942.

Biographical Note

Derrick Tilton Vail (1864–1930) was clinical professor of ophthalmology at the University of Cincinnati, and a founder member of the American Academy of Ophthalmology and Otolaryngology (of which he was president in 1908), the Oxford Ophthalmological Congress, the American College of Surgeons, the Gorgas Memorial Institute, and the Cincinnati Ophthalmology Club (of which he was president in 1919). In 1909 and again in 1924 he went to India, taking time out from his extensive practice, to study under Col. Henry Smith the latter's technique of intracapsular extraction of cataract. His subsequent writings, illustrated by many drawings of his own, testified to his enthusiastic advocacy of this method. He contributed to the *American Encyclopedia of Ophthalmology* the section on the pupil in health and disease and wrote for *Ball's Modern Ophthalmology* the chapter on the intracapsular operation for cataract.

Reference

Obituary. Am. J. Ophth., *14:* 70–71, 1931.

Irido-cyclitic Sympathica

ERNST FUCHS, M.D.

Vienna

Text-Book of Ophthalmology, 12th German Edition*

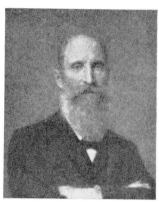

When an eye is affected with irido-cyclitis in consequence of an injury, either symptoms of irritation or else an actual inflammation my develop in the other eye.

Sympathetic irritation (irritatio sympathica) consists in photophobia, lacrimation, or actual pain. Sometimes also weakness of accommodation is present, so that when the patient tries to do fine work the vision gets indistinct and the work has to be given up. Such symptoms, however, are to be called by the name of sympathetic irritation only when objective signs of inflammation are absent, for when once these make their appearance, it is a question, not of sympathetic irritation, but of sympathetic inflammation. A characteristic sign, furthermore, of sympathetic irritation is that it disappears at once and forever when the primarily affected eye is removed.

Sympathetic inflammation (ophthalmia sympathica) consists in the development of an irido-cyclitis in the second eye. The eye primarily affected is called the "exciting eye," that which is affected secondarily the "sympathizing eye." Sympathetic inflammation develops sometimes in immediate conjunction with preceding symptoms of sympathetic irritation, sometimes without any intermediary symptoms at all and quite unforeseen.

The beginning is often insidious. In conjunction with an insignificant reddening of the eye, deposits—which are never wanting in the beginning of a sympathetic ophthalmia—appear upon the cornea. Then a few posterior synechiae and fine opacities in the vitreous develop, and the ophthalmoscope shows hyperaemia of the retina and optic nerve. In favorable cases the disease reaches no higher pitch and at length gets well, leaving either no trace of its presence or a few posterior synechiae.

* Translated by Alexander Duane, M. D., New York, N.Y., J. B. Lippincott Co., Philadelphia, 1923, pp. 682–685.

Unfortunately such mild cases are the exception. The rule is that the symptoms of inflammation slowly or quickly increase; more and more adhesions of the iris develop, and the visual power becomes more and more reduced. Hypopyon, however, ordinarily does not occur even when the inflammation is severe. Although sometimes intervals in the inflammation with some improvement in sight occur, yet these are not lasting, and finally, owing to the constantly recurring inflammation, there ensues in spite of all treatment the formation of a pupillary membrane and of an annular or total posterior synechia. Then, in consequence of the seclusion of the pupil, increase of tension may set in, but this is commonly not of long duration, since cyclitic membranes have also formed in the vitreous, and by their shrinkage the intra-ocular pressure is once more lowered and finally atrophy of the eyeball is produced. As a rule, therefore, the sympathizing eye is lost.

In view of the great gravity of sympathetic ophthalmia, it is important to know its early danger signs, *i.e.*, those that occur before the stage of actual exudation. According to Brownlie, these are a contraction of the visual field, a spindle-shaped enlargement (elongation of the vertical diameter) of the blind spot, congestion of the optic disc and retinal vessels, loss of visual acuity, paresis of accommodation, and changes in the blood count (marked increase in the large uninuclear leucocytes, some increase in the lymphocytes, decrease in the polymorphonuclear cells). According to Gifford, however, the blood changes, although well-marked in sympathetic ophthalmia, are not pathognomonic since they are found frequently in chronic uveitis and like conditions.

It is supposed that the sympathetic disease may appear not only in the form of an irido-cyclitis, but also under some other guise. The greatest variety of affections have been described as sympathetic. Among non-inflammatory affections, cases of paralysis of accommodation, of amblyopia, and of blepharospasm have been adduced as sympathetic; among inflammatory affections in the posterior division of the eye, neuritis, chorioiditis, and glaucoma; and in the anterior division of the eye, conjunctivitis and keratitis. However, the only conditions in which the connection has been surely proved are sympathetic neuritis and chorioiditis. The former occurs very rarely and gives a comparatively good prognosis. As regards the chorioiditis, this probably is present in all severe cases, of sympathetic irido-cyclitis, but cannot be diagnosticated, because the cloudiness of the media prevents ophthalmoscopic examination. Hence we get the ophthalmoscopic picture of chorioiditis only in those comparatively mild cases, in which the anterior segment of the uvea is affected but little or not at all; and such cases are rare. Sympathetic chorioiditis is marked by the presence of numerous small yellow patches which occupy especially the periphery of the fundus. In other cases observers have often gone too far in taking the sympathetic nature of the disease for granted. The fact that an eye has been destroyed through traumatism by no means justifies us in regarding, without further proof, any subsequent disease of the other eye as sympathetic. This assumption should be made only when such disease presents the characteristic clinical picture of sympathetic irido-cyclitis, or when, upon the enucleation of the eye first diseased, the symptoms in the second eye recede too rapidly to be accounted for upon any other assumption than that the affection of the second eye was caused by that of the first. The converse of this inference does not hold good—that is, the fact that enucleation of the first eye does not influence the course of the disease in the second is no argument against the sympathetic nature of the lesion; indeed, it is a well-established fact that when sympathetic ophthalmia has once broken out, enucleation of the eye first diseased is not generally able to cause much change.

The affection of the *exciting* eye, which gives rise to a sympathetic inflammation, is always an irido-cyclitis, and is, in fact, almost without exception, an irido-cyclitis traumatica, due to a penetrating injury. In this category, of course, are to be reckoned the operations that are attended with opening of the eyeball, in case they are followed by inflammation.

As a matter of prognosis and treatment, it is important to know that, in spite of there being a violent inflammation of the primarily diseased eye, sympathetic ophthalmia occurs very rarely in (1) suppuration of the cornea (in ulcus serpens, after acute blennorrhoea, etc.) and in its sequelae, phthisis corneae or staphyloma of the cornea, and in (2) panophthalmitis and the phthisis bulbi that follows it; and it never occurs in (3) absolute glaucoma.

The *point of time* at which the greatest danger of the transmission of the inflammation exists is when the irido-cyclitis in the injured eye is at its height. Hence sympathetic inflammation makes its appearance, in most cases, from four to eight weeks after the injury to the first eye has taken place. (It may occur as early as four days after the injury— Cahillous cited by DeLapersonne.) Later than this, when the traumatic irido-cyclitis has subsided and the eye has fallen a prey to atrophy, there need be generally no fear of sympathetic inflammation, so long as the atrophic eye is free from inflammation and is not painful, either spontaneously or to the touch. The danger for the other eye does not develop again until the atrophic eye becomes once more the seat of inflammation and of pain—an event which, to be sure, very frequently occurs. In this way an eye which has been carried for many years in an atrophic state without causing trouble may suddenly become the cause of a sympathetic inflammation. While, therefore, the minimum period for the development of sympathetic irido-cyclitis is but a few days, no limits can be set to the maximum period; sympathetic inflammation has been seen to appear forty years and more after the injury of the first eye. An eye which has been destroyed in consequence of injury is therefore a constant source of danger to the other eye.

To excite sympathetic inflammation it is not necessary for the injured eye to be perfectly blind. Cases occur in which the eye has retained a remnant of visual power after the injury and the irido-cyclitis following it, and has yet given rise to sympathetic inflammation. In that case it may happen that the sympathetically affected eye undergoes complete destruction, while the injured eye is still used to see with.

Can an irido-cyclitis of *non-traumatic origin* be transmitted to the other eye? We very often see irido-cyclitis develop spontaneously first in one eye, then in the other. But we must not therefore at once conclude that the inflammation has been transmitted from one eye to the other. It may be that we have to do with a deeply seated common cause, generally of constitutional nature, which makes itself felt first in one eye, then in the other. We should therefore regard an irido-cyclitis occurring in the fellow eye as sympathetic, only in case the inflammation in the first eye is certainly a purely local one and not dependent on constitutional causes. This is true of two varieties besides the traumatic, *i.e.,* of the irido-cyclitis which sometimes occurs after the perforation of a corneal ulcer, and of that which develops in eyes with an intra-ocular tumor. If the latter becomes necrotic, a violent inflammation of the inner coats of the eye results. In these two cases a genuine sympathetic inflammation of the second eye is observed, even though it is rare.

The way in which the inflammation is *transmitted* from one eye to the other is as yet unknown. Not every severe traumatic inflammation of the eye leads to sympathetic disease of the other; whether this develops or not depends upon two conditions:

1. Upon the character of the inflammation of the injured eye. To a certain extent this has been known for a long time; thus we are aware that in cases in which the injury produces ulcus serpens or panophthalmitis, sympathetic inflammation usually does not set in. To excite this an irido-cyclitis is required. But again it is not every traumatic irido-cyclitis, even when destructive, that causes sympathetic inflammation, but only an irido-cyclitis of a quite well defined sort, which is marked by a peculiar, very characteristic anatomical condition. Unfortunately, we have not as yet advanced so far as to be able to conclude from the clinical picture itself whether in a given case we are dealing with this particular sort of irido-cyclitis.

2. If now this particular kind of irido-cyclitis does really develop after

an injury, a possibility is then afforded that this inflammation may pass to the other eye, but such passage does not necessarily follow. For it to occur, a series of conditions must be involved, affecting the paths by which the passage takes place. What these conditions and indeed what the actual paths are we do not know. By some the transmission has been thought to take place by the ciliary nerves. But since the ciliary nerves of the two sides are nowhere in direct connection, the transmission in this case could be effected not by direct migration, but only in a reflex way. As a matter of fact it is scarcely to be doubted that sympathetic irritation is effected by way of the ciliary nerves. In fact even in slight changes occurring in one eye (for example, a foreign body in the cornea) we observe lacrimation and photophobia in the other. But that an actual inflammation with serious anatomical changes should develop in a reflex way is, in our present state of knowledge, inadmissible. Hence others, including Mackenzie, who first taught us to know sympathetic ophthalmia, have regarded the optic nerves as the medium by which bacteria or toxins are transmitted from one eye to the other. But this hypothesis is opposed by the fact that sympathetic ophthalmia does not actually begin in the optic nerve and when changes are found in the latter these decrease instead of increasing as we go backward. Furthermore, the optic nerve of the exciting eye may be completely divided and yet sympathetic ophthalmia may develop. Hence the view has prevailed that the transmission of bacteria or other agents exciting the inflammation takes place through the blood (Berlin). It has been suggested that bacteria by prolonged lodgement in the exciting eye may acquire a special affinity for the uvea so that when finally let loose in the circulation they start up a peculiar inflammation in the uvea of the other eye but affect no other organ (Gifford, O'Connor).

Another view is that sympathetic inflammation is an anaphylactic disease. In this view the transmission of bacteria or of disintegrated uveal tissue from the affected eye so sensitizes the other that the latter falls a prey to infection from other sources (especially to focal infection from the teeth, tonsils etc). There are a number of arguments in favor of this view, but it cannot yet be regarded as proved.

Investigation of this subject has been frustrated by the fact that we have been able in no way to demonstrate the presence of the bacteria that are supposed to excite the sympathetic inflammation. Furthermore we have had no opportunities for examining a sympathizing eye in the first stages of the disease, nor is experimentation on animals of any help to us either. Not only does sympathetic ophthalmia fail to occur spontaneously in animals, but the attempt to produce in animals an undoubted sympathetic inflammation experimentally has also failed of success.

Brownlie and others have pointed out the analogy that sympathetic ophthalmia shows in various ways to the protozoal diseases (syphilis, malaria, trypanosomiasis). This analogy is somewhat supported by the fact that salvarsan exerts a favorable effect on the disease.

Changes in Sympathetic Inflammation.—This infiltration has been especially studied in the exciting eye (that is the one which was injured and is the first affected). Here, in addition to the evidences of an ordinary plastic irido-cyclitis, such as cyclitic membranes with detachment of the retina, we find the uvea distended with densely crowded lymphocytes and plasma cells. In most cases there lie in the midst of this uniform infiltration focal collections of large (epithelioid) cells, which not infrequently have giant cells between them. Nodules are thus produced which often are like tuberculous nodules. This peculiar infiltration often is present in only a few spots, so that isolated nodules are seen here and there in the iris, ciliary body, or chorioid. In other cases the uvea is occupied by them either largerly or wholly and thus often becomes extremely thickened so as to fill, more or less completely, the interior of the eye. Sometimes the infiltration even makes its way into the sclera, which is permeated with scattered nodules, and in this way perforation of the sclera and extra-ocular proliferation may result.

Up to the present time it has not been possible to demonstrate the presence of bacteria in the nodules. Nevertheless there is scarcely a doubt but that here too we are dealing with an affection produced by bacteria, which, however, do not cause acute suppuration but, after the analogy of many other bacteria (for instance the tubercle bacilli), cause chronic proliferations. This inflammation has the property of being transmissible to the other eye. Of the sympathizing, that is the secondarily affected eyes, only a few have so far been got for examination, but then generally the same peculiar changes have been found.

Treatment.—If we wait to perform enucleation until the first signs of sympathetic disease show themselves, we are generally too late. Hence, to advise enucleation at the right moment is one of the most important tasks that the physician has to perform. To do this properly we must bear in mind the fact that the danger of sympathetic inflammation, is almost confined to the traumatic cases. If it is a case of recent inflammation, enucleation is indicated as soon as we see that blinding of the injured eye is inevitable. We recognize that this is the case by the increasing deficiency in the perception of light (this especially in the plastic cases; in purulent conditions, this not always an absolute guide). If the traumatic inflammation has already run its course, and a greater or less degree of atrophy of the eyeball has supervened, enucleation is still indicated if the eye is sensitive to pressure or if it gets inflamed often. It is only when the eyeball is entirely and permanently free from irritation that the demand for enucleation is not imperative. But the patient ought to be warned that he should report immediately for enucleation, if pain or inflammation happens to set in anew, and should be kept under periodic observation so that we can detect at once any evidences of inflammation or any of the danger signs of sympathetic disease.

When sympathetic ophthalmia has already broken out, the effect of enucleation is uncertain. In the lighter cases it appears to exert a favorable influence upon the course of the sympathetic inflammation; in severe cases, on the contrary, it is often of no avail.

Although enucleation generally affords a sure safeguard against sympathetic inflammation of the other eye, nevertheless a series of cases is known in which in spite of enucleation, inflammation has subsequently made its appearance. In every instance, it has set in within a short time—from a few days to a few weeks—after the enucleation. The longest interval so far observed is fifty-three days (in a case of Stephenson's cited by DeSchweinitz). Yet even when this does happen, enucleation does not fail to exert a favorable effect, since in the great majority of these cases the sympathetic inflammation runs an unusually favorable course, probably because the removal of the first eye prevents the constant emission from it of new impulses for the production of inflammation.

Operations in a case of sympathetic ophthalmia generally give a bad result, since they start up the inflammation again, so that the newly formed pupil is once more closed by fresh exudate. Hence operations are done only when it is absolutely requisite (e.g., when done on account of increase of tension); other operations, such as, for example, an iridectomy for optical purposes, are put off as long as possible, preferably for years.

Comment: In a histologic study of 200 eyes Fuchs was able by the pathologic evidence alone and without reference to the case history to separate accurately the 35 eyes which had excited sympathetic ophthalmia. Though an additional 16 eyes were found to have induced in a fellow healthy eye symptoms of photophobia, lacrimation, blepharospasm, pain, fatigue or paresis of accommodation, Fuchs proved that this syndrome of sympathetic irritation was simply reflex as the excised eyes showed none of the signs characteristic of sympathetic inflammation. His studies indicated no special age predilection, as he found that the incidence of sympathetic disease corresponded fairly well with the age distribution of the general population. Among the pathologic features of the disease Fuchs noted nodules of pigment cells undergoing depigmentation (Dalén-Fuchs nodules) which corresponded to the small drusen-like white spots seen ophthalmoscopically (Dalén's spots). The evidence suggests infection as the cause of sympathetic ophthalmia and a virus as the probable offending organism. Allergy to uveal pigment may be a factor in certain manifestations of the disease. The shorter the interval between injury and removal of the offending eye, the greater the prophylactic value of enucleation. Sympathetic involvement occurs most frequently between the 4th and 8th week after injury or operation. An attack is infrequent after 3 months and rare after 1 year. Once established the early administration of cortisone and ACTH is now considered the best available treatment. The use of antibiotics may be harmful as they kill the accessory flora and permit uninhibited multiplication of the virus of sympathetic ophthalmia.

References

Fuchs, E.: Ueber sympathisierende Entzündung nebst Bemerkungen über seröse traumatische Iritis. Arch. f. Ophth., *61:* 365–456, 1905.

Schreck, E.: Micro-organisms causing ophthalmia. Arch. Ophth., *46:* 489–500, 1951.

Biographical Note

Ernest Fuchs (1851–1930) was born in Kutzendorf, a village near Vienna where he received his medical education. After graduation he worked as Arlt's assistant for 6 years, and then assumed charge of the newly-formed department of ophthalmology at Liége. While there he submitted anonymously the prize-winning treatise on the prevention of blindness, surpassing Mules and Wilbrand, in a contest sponsored by the English Society for the Prevention of Blindness. In 1885 Fuchs succeeded Eduard Jaeger as director of the Second University Eye Clinic and became celebrated for his remarkable insight into the fundamental problems of ophthalmology. Salzmann, Meller, and Lindner were among his loyal assistants. The medical school, then at its zenith, included the Nobel Prize winners, Bárány, Landsteiner and Wagner-Jauregg. As pathologist Fuchs elucidated the processes of sympathetic ophthalmia, endophthalamitis septica, chalazion and pterygium; and as an astute clinician he isolated several new entities, such as epithelial dystrophy of the cornea, keratitis disciformis, superficial punctate keratitis, episcleritis periodica fugax and retinitis circinata. But his greatest gift to ophthalmology was his textbook. The admirable translations by Duane, begun with the second German edition of 1892, made the treatise a favorite among English-speaking nations. Fuchs was a masterful linguist and traveled extensively. In 1902 he delivered the Bowman Lecture at the Ophthalmological Society of the United Kingdom, and lectured in America in 1911, 1921 and 1929. Fuchs was the greatest ophthalmologist of his era, and his influence on ophthalmology is probably second only to Albrecht von Graefe.

Reference

Lebensohn, J. E.: Professor Ernst Fuchs. Am. J. Ophth., *34:* 772–774, 1951.

Part Nine

Ophthalmoscopic Detection

Lecture on Optic Neuritis from
Intracranial Disease

JOHN HUGHLINGS JACKSON, M.D.

London, England

EXCERPTED FROM MEDICAL TIMES AND GAZETTE *2:* 241, 341, 581, 1871

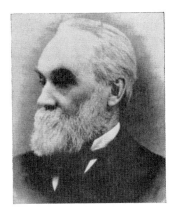

The physician is as much indebted to Helmholtz as the opthalmic surgeon is. You cannot investigate cases of cerebral disease methodically unless you use the ophthalmoscope. It is sometimes taken for granted that because sight fails from intracranial disease there will be no abnormal ophthalmoscopical appearances. One hears it said, "The changes are in the head, not in the eye." In very few cases of amaurosis there are no morbid ophthalmoscopical appearances.

I wish to speak of the commonest abnormal ophthalmoscopical appearances which occur in *medical* practice—of optic neuritis and its usual sequel, optic atrophy. Double optic neuritis does not point to the position of intracranial disease but is most important evidence as to its nature.

The Stages of Optic Neuritis

There are gradual changes from the beginning of the process through its ascent to a climax, and its descent to the permanent change—atrophy. We will make four stages. The following is an account of what is seen at different stages of a severe case. There may be retrocession from either the first or the second stage and not a progress to atrophy.

(*a*) *The onset.* The disc is redder, slightly swollen and therefore prominent. Its edge is indistinct, and the arteries are slightly obscured from the swelling. The veins are large, dark and tortuous. I confess that I often cannot tell whether there is optic neuritis or the swollen disc (Stauungspapille of Grafe). There is mostly no defect of sight in this stage.

(*b*) *Second stage.* The disc is quite lost in a patch, which is about two or three times the diameter of the normal disc. The arteries are not traceable, or only faintly here and there, in the patch, which is much raised above the neighboring fundus. The veins are very large and tortuous, and more or less obscured in the patch, and seem to knuckle over its edge. There are scattered blotches of effused blood on and beyond the patch, especially near its margin. There are often near the edge small shapeless white patches, sometimes edged with blood. Occasionally there are, especially near the macula, brilliant white spots. It is of importance to recognize that the appearances of this stage may clear away, the disc resuming a nearly healthy aspect.

(*c*) *Third stage.* The descent to atrophy begins. The blood has cleared away. We again see something like a disc, but there is much swelling and the edge merges into the fundus. We trace the arteries again, but they are still partly obscured, and the veins are tortuous.

(*d*) *Fourth Stage.* The stage of permanent atrophy. The disc is now white; its margin is distinct, but not so clearly defined as in health; and the vessels are traceable, the swelling having disappeared.

There are two kinds of optic atrophy. If we see an atrophic disc, we have to determine whether the atrophy really is consecutive or whether there has been slow atrophy from the first. The atrophy which begins by a noninflammatory process is the form of atrophy which occurs with locomotor ataxy. In the atrophy after optic neuritis the edge of the disc is not distinct; the whiteness is opaque; the lamina cribrosa is not well seen from remains of effusion; the arteries are thin, and the veins remain irregular; and we occasionally see very small whitish patches, extending over the boundary of the disc on to the neighboring fundus. Simple atrophy shows an atrophic, slightly excavated papilla of bluish gray color. The veins, although thinner than in the normal eye, are considerably larger than in other cases of atrophy.

There may be extensive changes, even of stage (b), when the patient does not know that there is anything the matter with his sight and when he can read the very smallest of our test types. In cases of cerebral disease you use the ophthalmoscope as a matter of course, just as you examine the urine as a matter of course. You must never omit to use this instrument when the patient has a severe headache.

It is a rare thing to see uniocular optic neuritis; but it unquestionably occurs. One eye may suffer more than the other, but nearly always both suffer somewhat; nearly always at the same time; and they are nearly always in the same stage.

Occasionally sight fails rapidly—in a day or two. If we use the ophthalmoscope, or if we use atropine, or adopt any new kind of treatment, the patient may blame us for his blindness if he saw well before such procedures. We must, then, when we discover neuritis, tell the patient that his eyes are really not good and that we are anxious about his sight.

The Nature of the Intracranial Disease Associated with Double Optic Neuritis

There is usually a gross change or "coarse" disease, in short a "lump of something"—an adventitious product. Double optic neuritis does not point to any particular kind of coarse disease but simply to coarse disease of some kind. That some "foreign bodies" are more likely to produce optic neuritis, I need not deny. Certain adventitious products affect particular localities. Abscess occurs in the mass of the cerebrum or cerebellum and blood clot in the motor tract. Blood clot is rarely associated with optic neuritis. If you find swelling of the discs, with or without hemorrhages, you may infer in the vast majority of cases that there is an adventitious product within the head. You usually have other evidence. There is severe pain in the head and perhaps urgent vomiting. In chronic cases you will scarcely ever be wrong; in acute cases there is more difficulty. In certain nervous affections optic neuritis scarcely ever occurs. I have never seen optic neuritis with hemiplegia from local softening, the result of embolism or thrombosis.

The coarse disease does not, as a rule, directly involve any part of the optic nervous system, there may be disease of the base of the skull which squeezes or involves the optic nerves, but double optic neuritis does not help you to that diagnosis unless other symptoms are present such as palsies of cranial nerves. Adventitious products rarely occur in the motor tract. A tumor does not cause amaurosis because it has destroyed so much of the hemisphere, but because it has led to secondary changes. Coarse disease in either cerebral hemisphere may lead to loss or defect of sight. Optic neuritis most frequently results from the presence of a foreign body in parts of the cerebral and cerebellar hemisphere, destruction of which parts may produce no symptoms at all.

The coarse disease may have led to pressure transmitted to the optic nerves and venous sinuses at the base. I do not think it owing to pressure on the optic nerves, because none of the other nerves at the base suffer; and if the optic nerve fibers were partly or wholly destroyed by squeezing I should rather expect slow atrophy than neuritis. Nor do I think impeded exit of blood is the cause, because the swelling of the discs subsides although the intracranial pressure goes on increasing. I confess that optic neuritis is a very great puzzle.

Comment: Early observers labelled all cases with acquired changes in the optic discs other than atrophy as "optic neuritis." In 1911 Paton and Holmes differentiated passive edema of the disc (papilledema) and inflammatory involvement (optic neuritis). "Papilledema," a term introduced by Parsons, is now used to cover both edema of the nervehead due to increased intracranial pressure and noninflammatory edema from other causes such as orbital tumor, reduction of intraocular pressure or blood dyscrasia; but the term "choked disc" is reserved for papilledema caused by increased intracranial pressure. The mechanism for the production of choked disc is definitely mechanical in origin. The discovery by Schwalbe in 1870 of a perineural space surrounding the optic nerves (the intervaginal space) that communicates with the subdural space about the brain suggested to Schmidt that pressure was transmitted to the fluid in the space of Schwalbe. Cushing and Bordley (1909) found that fluid under pressure in the subdural space produced engorgement of the retinal veins and that, when the fluid pressure approximated the arterial pressure, high-grade choked discs developed. Lauber and Sobanski pointed out that when the pressure in the central retinal vein is abnormally high in relation to that of the central retinal artery, papilledema develops and then slight pressure fails to elicit the normally induced venous pulsation on the optic disc. The papilledema associated with orbital tumor gives further support to the view that stoppage of venous drainage is an important factor in its development. With brain tumor, venous obstruction ensues from the increased pressure transmitted by the cerebrospinal fluid to the central retinal vein where it traverses the perineural space about the optic nerves. As marked retinal edema is infrequent, obstruction to venous outflow is apparently not the sole cause. Van Heuven showed that the brain and optic nerves have an extraordinary water-binding capacity and suggested that papilledema is part of a generalized cerebral edema. The swelling of the disc which may reach 7.00 D. is due to accumulation of fluid between the nerve fibers and to swelling of the nerve fibers. The spread of edema into the retina accounts for the frequently seen fan-shaped figure at the macula.

Reference

Walsh, F. B.: *Clinical Neuro-Ophthalmology,* chap. VI. The Williams & Wilkins Company, Baltimore, 1947.

Biographical Note

John Hughlings Jackson (1835–1911) was the son of a farmer and was born in a village near York, England. Jackson, who had only a grammar school education, began his medical studies at York Medical School and completed them at St. Bartholomew's Hospital where he qualified in 1856.

Jackson was largely self-educated and believed that the meagerness of his formal education had stimulated his progress, but much of his writing betrays this deficiency by being oppressively meticulous, overly qualified and overburdened with footnotes. At age 24 Jackson had served three years as house surgeon at the York Dispensary and decided to practice in London. Sir Jonathan Hutchinson, also from Yorkshire, was most helpful and secured his appointment as assistant as Moorfield's Eye Hospital, where Jackson speedily became expert in the use of the ophthalmoscope, which Hemholtz had invented just eight years before. From the start his primary interest was neuro-ophthalmology and one of his earliest publications dealt with the ocular and visual conditions observed in the course of intracranial tumors. Jackson observed that in diseases of the nervous system defects of sight exceeded in frequency those of all the other special senses put together. He invariably made an ophthalmoscopic examination of every patient under his observation. Jackson joined also the staffs of the National Hospital for the Paralysed and Epileptic at Queen's Square, the Metropolitan Free Hospital and the London Hospital in Whitechapel. In 1860 he was elected to the Royal College of Physicians and in 1878 to the Royal Society. He and Hutchinson regularly contributed a clinical column to the *Medical Times and Gazette.* Jackson illuminated the subject of epilepsy with 32 articles, spurred on by his wife's affliction with this hitherto mysterious disease. He was especially interested in that type of epilepsy, now named after him, in which the convulsive movements begin always in the same group of muscles and spread in a definite march to other groups. From a meticulous examination of his patients, supplemented by post mortem when available, Jackson advanced far-reaching conclusions regarding neurophysiology. His evolutionary view implied that the most lately developed level controls and inhibits the lower levels, and hence a loss of inhibition from the highest level results in discharge from lower centers.

Jackson wrote more than 300 articles, of which 90 were on some phase of neuro-ophthalmology. His frequent contributions to ophthalmology appeared in the *Transactions of the Ophthalmological Society of the United Kingdom, Royal London Ophthalmic Hospital Reports, Ophthalmic Review, British Medical Journal, Lancet* and other journals. Jackson delivered the Croonian Lecture, the Hunterian Oration, and the Harveyan Society Lecture. He was invited to give the Bowman Lecture in 1885 and was elected president of the Ophthalmological Society of the United Kingdom in 1889. He was awarded an honorary M.D. from the University of Bologna. His portrait, commissioned by his colleagues, now decorates the Royal College of Physicians in London; and his marble bust stands in the entrance hall of the National Hospital. Hutchinson, his lifelong friend, spoke of Jackson as his greatest discovery, the nearest to a genius that it was his privilege to know.

Reference

Chance, B.: *Hughlings Jackson, the neurologic ophthalmologist.* Arch. opht. *17:* 241–289, 1937.

The State of the Arteries in Bright's Disease

W. R. GOWERS, M.D.

BRIT. M. J., 2: 743–745, 1876

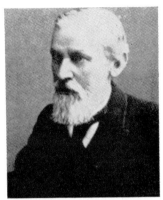

The object of the following paper is to bring forward certain facts concerning the retinal vessels in Bright's disease, and the facts warrant this conclusion; that, in chronic Bright's disease, the arteries of the retina are sometimes of normal size and sometimes very distinctly lessened in size; that this diminution in size depends upon contraction; and that this visible contraction stands, as a rule, in direct proportion to the tension of the arterial blood, as measured by the incompressibility of the radial pulse.

A few words are necessary as to the manner in which the size of the arteries is estimated. Their condition can only be seen under considerable magnifying power. Now and then, if the eye be hypermetropic and the vessels very distinct, the indirect examination with a lens of three-or-four-inch focus will suffice; but as a rule, it is necessary to employ the direct method of examination. If the pupil be small, it must be dilated with atropine, since it is often necessary to trace the vessels for some distance from the disc.

There is unfortunately no method of applying any gauge to the vessels; their size must be estimated by the eye. The change in size may be judged absolutely or by comparison with the veins. For an absolute estimate of their size, familiarity with their normal appearance under direct examination is, of course, necessary. Further, as the degree of magnification varies with the refractive power of the eyeball, this must be allowed for. It may generally be estimated by noticing the apparent size of the disc.

The change in the size of the arteries is frequently such as to be recognized at once; there is no need for comparison with the veins. The reduction in size may be so considerable, that even the primary branches of the central artery are so small that their double contour is recognized with difficulty, and it may be unrecognizable even by direct examination, the arteries being as in one example visible only as lines.

In other cases where the diminution in size is slighter, it can be most conveniently estimated by comparing the arteries with the veins. The distribution of the arteries and veins corresponds approximately, not exactly. Sometimes two arteries accompany one vein, sometimes one vein corresponds with two arteries. But in each eye there are usually some single branches of arteries and veins which have an identical course and distribution, run side by side, and are available for comparison. When this is the case, it will be found that, as a rule, the width of the artery is about two-thirds or three-quarters that of the vein. When the artery bears less proportion to the vein than this, it is usually due to one of three causes: 1. General venous distension, as in cyanosis; 2. Impediment at the sclerotic ring, by which the entrance of blood into the arteries is impeded, and its exit from the veins is also hindered, in which case the arteries are narrow and the veins distended as in certain stages of optic neuritis; 3. Contraction of the arteries. In the two former cases, the veins are, of course, abnormally large, and their abnormal size is generally easy of recognition. In the latter case, the veins may be normal in size or may be smaller than natural. If they be smaller, the diminished proportionate size of the arteries is of still greater significance. It is necessary, therefore, to be familiar with the normal size of the veins, in order to estimate the size of the arteries by comparison. From their darker colour, their size is easily noted, and the size of the arteries is readily estimated by comparison.

The arteries may be of normal size upon the optic disc, and yet present very marked reduction in size on the retina, a little distance from the disc. An artery may leave the disc beside a vein to which it bears its normal proportion, and, after a little course, without giving off any visible branch, may diminish to one-half or one-third of the size of its accompanying vein.

From what has been said, it will be obvious that these changes in the relative size of the vessels possess most significance when the retina has not undergone the special changes to which it is liable in chronic Bright's disease. Exudation within the sclerotic ring, compressing the vessels, alters their relative and absolute dimension, as I have stated. This is well seen in ordinary optic neuritis. I believe that it is rare in Bright's disease for the neuritic change to be sufficient to produce this effect. Certainly, in cases of albuminuric retinitis, the actual contraction may often be recognized as something quite out of proportion to the retinal change.

As I have said, the rule that, when the arterial tension is increased, the retinal arteries may be seen to be contracted, is general, but not universal. This is in accordance with what might be expected from the various conditions which are known to influence, on the one hand, blood-tension, and, on the other, arterial contraction. Moreover, local influences may cause local modifications. The most notable exceptions to the rule, which I have met with, have been in cases of local retinal disease. The incompressibility of the radial pulse was employed as the estimate of arterial tension. When practicable, my estimate has been corroborated by a sphygmographic tracing.

On the opposite sides of a ward in University College Hospital, there recently lay two patients whose cases illustrated the relation of blood-tension and the state of the retinal arteries. The one case was that of a man, fifty-eight years of age, whose illness had commenced gradually, with shortness of breath and weakness, two years before. Slight edema of the legs had existed for only one month before his admission. His urine contained one-third of albumen; had a specific gravity of from 1.005 to 1.008, and contained numerous casts, granular and hyaline, with some degenerated epithelium, both free and within the casts. His retinae were normal in appearance; the arteries of full size, presenting not the slightest evidence of contraction. His pulse was full, but very soft and compressible. There was no evidence of cardiac change. The other case was that of a man, aged forty-six whose symptoms resembled those of the first. They began with shortness of breath and swelling of the legs nine months before. His urine had a specific gravity of 1.007 to 1.010, and contained from one-third to one-half albumen; its quantity was from two to four pints, and it contained many casts, granular, hyaline, and epithelial. His retinae presented evidence of slight disease. The optic discs had softened outlines, and their surface was reddish-grey, paler in the vicinity of the vessels. There was little, if any swelling. The veins were smaller than normal; in the left eye, one only approached the average size. The arteries presented a greater reduction in size than in any case I have seen. Even on direct examination, they were visible only as lines, no double contour being recognizable, although they were quite distinct. A few minute white dots existed in each eye near the macula lutea, and in each there were a few small extravasations. The vessels were similar in the two eyes. The disc in the right was a little less grey than in the left. Vision: R. 1/6; L. 1/20. There was no peripheral limitation of the fields of vision. The pulse was extremely hard; the artery felt like a whipcord under the finger, and was almost absolutely incompressible.

I shall now describe the sepia drawing of the fundus oculi in a case of chronic Bright's disease, the sequel of an acute attack twelve years previously, the patient having in the meantime had at least two other acute attacks. The urine was loaded with albumen and contained granular and fatty casts. The retina presents abundant soft-edged white areas and also many striated extravasations; most of these had appeared during the preceding ten days. The disc is concealed by edema. The veins are of normal size; the artery at the papilla is rather smaller than natural, its branches being not more than half the size of the veins; but, a little distance beyond the limits of the papilla, they disappear. The veins can be followed distinctly on the retina, but the arteries can only be seen as dim lines here and there. The fact that they can be dimly seen here and there as lines suggests that their indistinctness is due in part only to the opacity of the retina, in part also to their reduction in size. The greater extent of this reduction on the retina than on the disc suggests that it is not due to their obstruction at the lamina cribrosa, but to their active contraction. The facts of other cases give support, I think, to this view. This patient's pulse was also very hard and incompressible. He died comatose a few days afterwards. A post mortem examination was obtained. The kidneys were found lessened in bulk, increased in consistence, and moderately granular on the surface. The heart was hypertrophied.

The next two sketches represent the optic disc of a patient suffering from acute Bright's disease passing into a chronic state. The first was made six weeks after the onset. The retina presented a few small haemorrhages, white dots around the macula lutea, with a few larger white areas. The arteries and veins were normal in size, the former being just two-thirds the diameter of the latter. The pulse was soft and compressible, giving no evidence of increased blood-tension. When the second sketch was made, six weeks later, the patient's general condition had improved, the albumen in the urine was less, but the casts had become fatty; the retinal changes had become considerably less; the white areas had lessened. The retinal arteries, however, presented distinct diminution in size compared with their previous condition. The veins were apparently of the same size as when the former sketch was made, while the arteries had diminished to one-half the size of the veins. The pulse also presented a marked alteration. It had become distinctly harder and less compressible.

I have repeatedly formed, from an inspection of the retinal vessels, an opinion as to the arterial tension, which, I afterwards found, on examining the pulse, was correct. In order, however, to obtain some evidence which might be without even unconscious bias, I asked my friend Dr. Coupland to be good enough to examine the pulse in a series of cases of Bright's disease whilst I examined the retinal vessels. Each wrote down independently the result of the examination. Five cases were examined, and the results agreed in four. In one case, they differed; but in this the fact that there were many retinal haemorrhages may, as I have already said, explain the absence of arterial contraction, although the pulse was hard.

In the case in which the retinal arteries were smallest, the arterial tension was greatest; that in which the arteries and the retina were normal presented no excess of arterial tension; the two others, in which there was a moderate contraction of the arteries, presented a moderate increase in the arterial tension.

There is nothing new in the fact that the retinal arteries are small in Bright's disease; it has long been remarked as a common feature in albuminuric retinitis, and is shown plainly in the best illustrations of this change (as in those of Liebreich). But it is usually regarded as a consequence of the retinal change, and the points on which I would insist are that it occurs also quite independently of the retinal change, and stands commonly in direct relation to another condition—the blood-tension.

It is hardly necessary for me to point out the bearing of this conclusion on the theory which ascribes the increased tension of the blood in Bright's disease, in part at least, to contraction of minute arteries. It constitutes a direct proof of the correctness of the theory, which has hitherto derived its chief support from indirect inference from pathological facts. If the tension of the arterial blood and the arterial contraction occur in common proportion, they must stand in a causal relation to one another. But the blood-tension cannot be the cause of the arterial contraction, because it is well known from physiological experiments that the tendency of increased blood-tension is, through the depressor nerve, to cause relaxation of the arterioles. But, on the other hand, as the immediate effect of contraction of the arterioles must be an increase in the arterial blood-pressure, it is reasonable to conclude that the contraction of the arteries, seen in those of the retina and inferred to exist elsewhere, is the cause of the increased blood-tension.

The practical use of inspection of the retinal vessels is considerable. It is true we can generally ascertain the amount of arterial tension more rapidly and more surely by feeling the pulse than by looking at the retinal vessels. As affording definite information regarding the pathological processes in different cases of Bright's disease, retinal inspection will have considerable value; and some facts which have come under my observation, at present too few and isolated for more than mention, make me hope that ultimately it may help us better to distinguish between morbid states included under the term and at present imperfectly distinguished.

Comment: Renal retinopathy is an almost inevitable accompaniment of chronic diffuse glomerulo-nephritis with high blood pressure, while the gravity of nephrosclerosis with hypertension is revealed in the ominous picture of malignant hypertensive retinopathy. Richard Bright was the first to comment on visual failure in renal disease (1836), and 20 years later the retinal changes were first observed in the living eye ophthalmoscopically by Heyman. The label "albuminuric retinitis" originated from the view held by von Graefe (1860) that the retinal lesions were related to retention of nitrogenous waste products, and was discarded after Gowers (1876), Gunn (1892) and Volhard (1921) established that the retinal changes in renal disease depended primarily on hypertension and arteriolar constriction. In nephritis without elevation of blood pressure (acute glomerulo-nephritis) normal fundi are the rule. Goldblatt (1934) discovered that experimental interference with the renal circulation, induced by clips on one or both renal arteries, resulted in a steady rise in blood pressure, producing a benign or malignant type according to the severity of the ischemia. The humoral agent released is renin, a proteolytic enzyme extractable from the cortex of the kidney, discovered by Tigerstedt and Gergman in 1898. The actual pressor substance, however, is hypertensin, a polypeptide produced by the action of renin on hypertensinogen, an α_2-globulin of the plasma. Since hypertension follows the removal of both kidneys, other mechanisms are probably involved in the production of primary hypertension. Hence Grollman would explain the dominating influence of the kidney in hypertension by the assumption that the kidneys normally destroy a pressor substance elaborated elsewhere in the body.

The differential diagnosis must be made between chronic glomerulo-nephritis with hypertension and primary hypertension. If the hypertensive patient shows the kidney function greatly reduced and little arteriolar sclerosis is seen in the retina, the diagnosis is chronic glomerulonephritis; but if the eye ground shows severe arteriolar sclerosis and the kidney function is good, the diagnosis is primary hypertension. Wendland found that in primary hypertension the degree of arteriolar sclerosis seen in the retinal vessels equals or exceeds that in the kidney in 85 per cent of cases. The malignant phase of hypertension may supervene, regardless of cause, provided the blood pressure rises high enough in the diastolic phase. If, by drugs or other measures, the diastolic pressure can be kept below the critical level of about 130 mm. Hg, the malignant phase with its attendant retinopathy can be prevented or reversed.

References

Wendland, J. P.: The relationship of retinal and renal arteriolosclerosis in living patients with essential hypertension. Am. J. Ophth., *35:* 1748–52, 1952.
Scheie, H. G.: Evaluation of ophthalmoscopic changes of hypertension and arteriolar sclerosis. A. M. A. Arch. Ophth., *49:* 117–138, 1953.

Biographical Note

Sir William Richard Gowers (1845–1915) was born in London, received his preliminary education at Christ Church School, Oxford, and studied medicine at University College Hospital in London. He graduated M.B. in 1869, with gold medals in botany, physiology, anatomy and materia medica. Gowers was adept at shorthand, and later, in his inaugural address as first president of an organization devoted to writing skills, he urged students to learn shorthand before beginning a medical career. His own writings were notable for perfect observation, precise description and easy prose. He was also an able artist and illustrated his numerous books himself, including his detailed *Manual and Atlas of Medical Ophthalmoscopy*. He also painted pictures that were invariably accepted by the Royal Academy of Arts. While a medical student, Gowers became private secretary to Sir William Jenner, who assisted his brilliant progress. Although Gowers was expert in general medicine, his special interest centered on the diseases of the nervous system and the diagnostic value of ophthalmoscopy. After he was awarded his M.D. in 1870, also with a gold medal, Gowers was appointed medical registrar at the outstanding center for neurology, the National Hospital for the Paralysed and Epileptic, Queen Square, London, later receiving a staff appointment there as a junior colleague of J. Hughlings Jackson. At the same time he taught at the University College Hospital. By his early forties he had already become famed for his neurologic accomplishments and was advanced to Professor of Clinical Medicine. In 1879 he discovered "Gowers' tract" of the spinal cord by following the ascending degeneration in a case of crushed cord in which sensation was greatly impaired.

Gowers devoted detailed study to every case and in time accumulated more than 20,000 full records, all written by himself in shorthand, on the basis of which he wrote his two-volume *Manual of Diseases of the Nervous System* (1886–1888). Gowers was the first to indicate the clinical difference between supranuclear and infranuclear ocular palsies, pointing out that conjugate movements were affected in the former situation, while individual muscles were involved in the latter. He also observed that, before the total loss of the light reflex in tabes dorsalis, some cases showed, with the light test, an intermittent and abrupt oscillation of the iris, since called "Gowers' pupillary sign." His other notable publications included *The Diagnosis of Diseases of the Spinal Cord, Diagnosis of Diseases of the Brain, Syphilis of the Nervous System,* and two books on epilepsy (1881, 1907). In his philosophic *Dynamics of Life* are many quotable sentences, such as "Words have a strong tendency to cause opacity if they be numerous."

Gowers was recognized in his day as one of the great clinical neurologists of all time. He was a fellow of the Royal Society, and an honorary member of many societies, including the American Neurological Society and the Russian Medical Society. On the occasion of Queen Victoria's Diamond Jubilee in 1897, he was knighted.

Reference

Critchley, M.: *Sir William Gowers. A Biographical Appreciation.* London: William Heinemann, 1949.

Remarks on Lipemia Retinalis Occurring in a Case of Diabetes Mellitus

ALBERT GALLATIN HEYL, M.D.

Philadelphia, Pennsylvania

PHILADELPHIA MEDICAL TIMES, 1880, *10:* 318–319

It is well known that diabetes mellitus is frequently accompanied by abnormal conditions of the eye: this fact was noticed far back in pre-ophthalmoscopic times. Rollo, in his monograph on Diabetes, London, 1798, refers to two cases of the kind, probably the first mentioned in literature in which there is reason to infer that the diabetes was the cause of the eye affection. It is true that Blankaart, of Amsterdam, in 1688, mentions the occurrence of blindness in a case of diabetes; whether the case were one of diabetes mellitus or insipidus does not appear. Possibly Blankaart was unaware of the distinction, as it was only fourteen years previously that Thomas Willis called attention to the sweet taste of the urine of certain cases of diabetes. However, as Blankaart ascribes the blindness of his case to a tumor found after death pressing upon the optic nerves, we must look upon the blindness rather as a coincidence than a sequel of the diabetes. Since Rollo's time numerous instances of eye affection in diabetes mellitus have been observed, and in later years the ophthalmoscope has enabled us to study them more closely. These eye affections are disturbances of refraction and accommodation, lens opacities, vitreous clouds and hemorrhages, certain affections of the optic nerve, and certain affections of sight apparently depending on central lesions. It is, however, to none of these that I invite attention tonight. The appearance I bring before you has, I believe, never been described or copied.

The patient from whom this picture was copied was an inmate of the male medical ward of the Episcopal Hospital, under the care of Dr. Louis Starr. Owing to his complaining of defective vision, I was asked to examine his eyes. I saw him for the first time November 11, 1879. Examination, under atropia, revealed a nuclear cataract, with partial involvement of the cortical, on each side. The appearance of the fundus of each eye was quite peculiar; that of the left was more visible than that of the right, owing to the left lens being less involved than the right;

still the right fundus was clearly enough visible. The peculiar appearance which attracted my attention was the color of the bloodvessels. Those of you who are familiar with the normal fundus know that one of the most striking objects seen in ophthalmoscopic examination is the retinal vessels,—that the retinal veins are characterized by their larger size and the dark color of their blood, the arteries being smaller and lighter in color. In the picture of the fundus which I present to you, you will notice at once a great difference from the normal appearance. The vessels are very light in color, both veins and arteries, and the color very closely approximates that of the fundus; the veins are very large in size, and at the same time not tortuous; the artery is seen branching off from the trunk and running downward and inward for a short distance, and is then lost, by reason partly of similarity of color, in the fundus. Whether a branch also ran upward could not be told. A vessel in the upper half of the fundus is seen stopping, apparently, at the edge of the excavation; it could not be traced farther: very possibly it was a branch of the artery.

The color of the vessels is represented as they appeared when the light was thrown on them directly; when the mirror was shifted by a slight rotary motion the veins could be distinguished by their slightly darker color. There was no retinitis in either eye, nor were any hemorrhages seen.

I will now pass around this accurate painting of the fundus of the right eye; it was very skilfully copied for me by my friend Dr. Nancrede, and recalls the case very vividly to my mind. While the picture is being examined we may briefly discuss its nature.

1. Was it due to any structual change in the vessel-coats, by reason of which the contained blood was partially obscured from sight? There are morbid processes which attack the tunica adventitia of the vessels, which may almost render the blood invisible to the eye. The appearance of this condition is totally different from that under consideration. Those acquainted with the two could not mistake the one for the other.

2. We may, then, turn to the character of the blood itself. To be as brief as possible,—for I am only presenting this picture, not attempting to do more,—the blood was examined: the finger was pricked, and a small quantity of blood obtained. The character of the blood was very peculiar: it had a milky-red hue, approximating that of a piece of pink coral. Examination with the microscope revealed the presence of fat globules. The number of red globules was carefully counted by Dr. F. P. Henry, and it was found that the blood was not leucocythemic. This was, therefore, one of those cases of diabetes mellitus accompanied by lipemia, or a condition of blood characterized by a milky hue, arising

276

from the presence of an abnormal quantity of fat. Cases of the kind have been described by Virchow, Griesinger, Kussmaul, Sanders, and others.

This peculiar appearance of the retinal vessels was then, doubtless, due to abnormal presence of fat in the blood, and I may properly apply to it the name of retinal lipemia.

I have thus presented to your notice this picture of the fundus oculi of this case, without going into the details. The condition is interesting from its novelty, but it may also have some practical bearings. Without, however, alluding, at this time, to points which might be of interest to the specialist, I have presented this picture as showing one feature of an obscure complication of an obscure disease. I though also it would be of some interest to the Society, as the attention of the profession has recently been called to this condition of lipemia in diabetes mellitus: I refer to the able and interesting paper on Lipemia in Diabetes Mellitus and Fat Embolism, written by Professor Sanders and Mr. Hamilton, published in the Edinburg Medical Journal for last July.

Comment: Since Heyl first described lipemia retinalis some 80 cases have been reported, including 14 in nondiabetics. Lipemia retinalis comes from a very excessive concentration of neutral fats in the blood, the other lipids being of no significance in this connection. In normal serum the neutral fat content ranges from zero to 150 mg. per 100 cc. according to the stage of digestion. The serum assumes a milky appearance when the concentration of neutral fat reaches 0.5 per cent, but lipema retinalis is only seen with a neutral fat content of over 2.5 per cent and disappears when the level falls below 2 per cent. In lipemia retinalis the milky appearance of the arteries and veins is first seen in the far periphery and gradually extends centrally to the disk. The arteries and veins then become difficult to differentiate and the vessels appear larger and ribbon-shaped. As less sugar is utilized in diabetes more fat is mobilized from the storage depots for migration to the liver. Insulin reverses the process by making sugar available for combustion; fat then disappears from the blood and liver and returns to the storage depots. In a diabetic, lipemia retinalis indicates poor control of the disease, but the condition in itself causes no organic damage to the retina nor any disturbance of retinal function. This transportation hyperlipemia may occur also in chronic alcoholism, severe anemias and leukemia, lipid nephrosis, and poisoning by phosphorus, chloroform and carbon tetrachloride. Lipemia retinalis may also occur in retention hyperlipemia where the mechanism by which the blood fat is removed to the storage depots is disturbed. In these cases the lipemia retinalis disappears by drastically reducing the fat in the diet; insulin, in this situation, does not affect the level of blood fat.

Reference

Davies, W. S.: Idiopathic lipemia retinalis. Arch. Ophth., 1955, *53:* 105.

Biographical Note

Albert Gallatin Heyl (1847–1895) was born in Philadelphia and attended the University of Pennsylvania, from which he received his medical degree in

1870. After a year of internship he devoted the next three years to the post-graduate study of ophthalmology in London, Heidelberg, and Vienna. On his return to Philadelphia he was appointed to the eye staff of the Episcopal Hospital, becoming in time Senior Ophthalmic Surgeon. In 1886 he also joined the Pennsylvania Eye and Ear Infirmary, a private, free dispensary supported by Dr. George Strawbridge. He was regarded as a brilliant eye surgeon. A profound student, he contributed numerous papers to the Transactions of the American Ophthalmological Society and other publications, the most important being on uremic amblyopia, hyphema, coloboma lentis, metastatic tenonitis, intraocular lipemia, acute glaucoma induced by duboisin, operative treatment of glaucoma, diffusion circles of ametropia, and spontaneous rupture of the choroid. According to S. D. Risley, who was his colleague for 10 years, he was very much of a recluse.

Reference

Risley, S. D.: Tr. Am. Ophth. Soc., *32:* 471, 1896.

Cases of Retinal Hemorrhage, Associated with Epistaxis and Constipation

H. EALES, M.D.

Birmingham, England

BIRMINGHAM MED. REV., *9:* 262–273, 1880

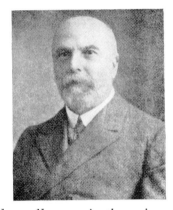

The following facts have characterised the first four cases. All are lads; all have been troubled more or less with sluggish and even constipated bowels; none having daily movements of the bowels without the aid of medicine. While under treatment, all have had symptoms of high arterial tension, such as slow pulse, accentuation of the sounds of the heart. None has been subject to polyuria. Two have had very slight traces of albumen in the urine, while two have had no albumen in the urine. In the two cases in which albumen was found casts were looked for but not discovered. All have been subject, more or less, to epistaxis. In all there has been profuse hemorrhage from the left retina, while, in one case only, a few small hemorrhages were found in the right eye also. In all the cases the hemorrhages have been roundish and diffused, as though situated in the granular layer of the retina, while, in one case only, a few of the hemorrhages were striated, i.e., in the nerve fibre layer of the retina. In all the cases the retinal vessels have been full, tortuous, and distended, especially the veins, in both eyes. In none has there been any other evidence of structural disease in the retina besides the hemorrhage and distended state of the vessels. In one case only the whole retina was visible, namely, the one that had a few hemorrhages in the right eye; and in this eye I would especially point out that not only were the hemorrhages in the granular layer, but they were found only at the periphery; that is, at the most distal end of the branches of the retinal artery and veins. In two cases complete recovery occurred, no trace of retinal disease being left; though in one a recurrence of the hemorrhages took place, which is not uncommon in my experience of these cases. The same thing occurred in the case which terminated in glaucoma.

In no case was there any evidence of primary retinitis, or any constitutional disease, such as syphilis, leucocythemia, anemia, etc., to account for the hemorrhage. I think, therefore, that we are compelled to look on high arterial tension, with dilated arterioles, and capillaries, and consequent distended venous system (all increasing the tension in the capillaries) as the cause of the hemorrhages, both in the eyes and from the nose, in both of which places the hemorrhage probably occurred from the capillaries. The seat of retinal hemorrhages in the granular layer, and at the periphery, are in accordance with this view.

I consider the constipation, however, produced, as the starting point of all the other phenomena in these cases. It surely may be said that local hemorrhages demand a local cause. We are not certain the hemorrhages do not occur elsewhere, though probably not; for in the mucous membrane of the air passages and meninges of the brain, and in the secreting membranes generally, the capillaries probably relieve themselves, either by serous transudation, or are saved from rupture by some counter-posing force, such as is found in the contraction of the intestine on its contents, and similar state of tension in most gland ducts; but in the nose there is no counter-posing force; hence epistaxis seems to be the commonest form of hemorrhage.

In the retina there is a great want of supporting connective tissue, and the retinal arteries and veins cannot relieve themselves through any other channels, having no collateral anastomoses, as most vessels do, hence the wonder at first is that rupture does not occur here more often; the explanation is to be found in the tension of the ocular contents, vitreous, etc., supporting the vessels, and so in spite of their unfavorable conditions, we find hemorrhage from the retinal vessels comparatively rare, while epistaxis is very common: however, the retina is undoubtedly one of the commonest seats of hemorrhage in high arterial tension from all causes. The occurrence of the hemorrhage in three of these cases on the left side, and in the fourth worst on the left side, is I think, more than mere accident, and I cannot help thinking that the left carotid artery coming off direct from the aortic arch, and the greater length and more indirect course of the left innominate vein, which joins the others almost at right angles, may cause a slightly higher tension in the capillaries on this side, and so account for the greater frequency of hemorrhage on this side. Possibly too, the fact of the right arm being supplied by the innominate artery, through the subclavian, and being in constant use, tends to lessen the tension in the carotid: because when muscles are used their capillaries are dilated, and there is local diminution of tension.

I do not propose to discuss here the occurrence of glaucoma in case I, though it is very interesting, and I believe unique in so young a lad; but the fact that this case is the worst, and the patient is suffering from mitral regurgitation, is strongly in favor of the overloaded state of the venous system being a factor in these cases telling back on the already over distended capillaries.

Case V is introduced as a contrast. Here the patient is older, the bowels are habitually loose, there is polyuria, and all the history and evidence of chronic alcoholism, with probably light increase of arterial tension (shown by accentuation of the aortic second sound) and gastro-intestinal catarrh. Here I imagine, in spite of a general vasomotor dilation in the alimentary and all other areas, the tension is raised by the stimulant to the heart, and possibly by the blood being altered in some way, that makes its passage through the capillaries more difficult—as would appear to be likely in these cases. Of course it is possible that some blood changes may be a factor in the other cases also. It is curious too that in this case the hemorrhage was limited to the right eye and not the left. Possibly some unknown local peculiarity in the arrangements of the vessels might explain it; possibly a transposition of the innominate artery to the left side. I would particularly draw attention to the fact that the epistaxis in this case, and in case I, was usually from the same side as that on which the retinal hemorrhage occurred, as this appears to me to be strong presumptive evidence of both being due to the same cause, and would point to this cause being the general state of the vessels on one side, and not to a local retinal disease, or to accident.

Comment: A tuberculous retinal periphlebitis is the most common cause of recurrent intraocular hemorrhages in young adults, though a similar picture is occasionally produced by other disease processes such as septic foci and anemia. Henry and Chapman recently reported nine cases of sickle-cell disease with retinal involvement in which four showed localized areas of chorioretinal atrophy and five had retinal hemorrhages. Eales' disease affects predominantly young males of an average age of 27 years. The tuberculin skin test is nearly always positive. The hemorrhages are originally confined to the retina and occur usually in the periphery—nearby veins showing perivascular exudation. Eventually a hemorrhage bursts through the internal limiting membrane into the vitreous obscuring all fundus details. In favorable cases the vitreous cloud may clear between attacks but in the less fortunate the sequence may be permanent vitreous opacities, retinitis proliferans, chronic uveitis or secondary glaucoma. In most cases the period of recurrent hemorrhages averages about three years after which the disease becomes inactive. The left eye is usually the first affected but the other eye becomes involved in about half the cases, generally within 18 months. The visual prognosis for the first eye with hemorrhages is rather poor while that for the second eye is almost invariably good. Bed rest for one to two weeks is indicated at the onset of a retinal hemorrhage. Elliot believes that the exudate and hemorrhages are the reaction of a hypersensitive vessel wall and found that in three patients given prolonged cortisone or ACTH no further hemorrhages occurred. Combined anti-tuberculous chemotherapy, including isoniazid, streptomycin and p-aminosalicylic acid, may be of value.

Henry, M. D. and Chapman, A. Z.: Vitreous hemorrhage and retinopathy associated with sickle-cell disease. Am. J. Ophth., *38:* 204–209, 1954.
Elliot, A. J.: Recurrent intraocular hemorrhage in young adults (Eales's disease). Trans. Am. Ophth. Soc., *52:* 811–875, 1954.

Henry Eales (1852–1913) was born in Devonshire, the son of a vicar. During his medical course at the University College of London he was awarded silver medals in anatomy and materia medica. He settled in Birmingham and for a time was Demonstrator in Anatomy at Queen's College. He started in ophthalmology as house-surgeon to the Birmingham Eye Hospital in 1873, and in 1878 became a staff member. He served as chairman of the section of ophthalmology, British Medical Association and as president of the Midland Medical Society. Being particularly adept in ophthalmoscopy, his principle writings were based on fundus observations. Besides giving the first adequate description of the entity now known as Eales disease, he contributed an important account of "The state of the retina in 100 cases of glomerular kidney." He was noted for his amiable, loyal and kindly character. He was so engrossed in his large consulting practice that he never indulged in a vacation.

Obituary. Brit. M. J. 1913, *1:* 368.

Amaurotic Family Idiocy

BERNARD SACHS, M.D.

New York, New York

The Eye and Nervous System Edited by W. C. Posey, M.D. and W. G. Spiller, M.D., pp. 532–537, Lippincott Co., Philadelphia, 1906

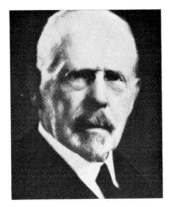

The above title was given by me to a rare disease affecting several members of the same family, and characterized by a distinct lack of mental development, by a progressive weakness of all the muscles of the body, and by a defect in vision (associated with changes in the macula lutea and optic nerve atrophy) terminating in complete blindness. The disease is generally fatal, the children dying as a rule in a condition of complete marasmus before the end of the second year of life.

History.—In 1881 Waren Tay described a case presenting "symmetrical changes in the region of the yellow spot in each eye of an infant. The child was twelve months old. It was deficient in holding up its head or moving its limbs. There was weakness but no absolute paralysis of any part. Its cerebral development was slow and poor. At the first examination, March 7, 1881, the optic disks were apparently healthy, but in the region of the yellow spot of each eye there was a conspicuous, tolerably diffuse, large white spot more or less circular in outline, and showing at its centre a brownish-red, fairly circular spot contrasting strongly with the white patch surrounding it. This central spot did not look at all like a hemorrhage, nor as if due to a pigment, but seemed a gap in the white patch, through which one saw healthy structures." The author likened these appearances to those one is familiar with in cases of embolism of the central artery of the retina. He believed the changes in the retina to be "possibly congenital." Five months later another examination was made, showing that the disks had become atrophied, but that the changes in the macula lutea were the same as before. In the same family, according to Waren Tay's later reports, three similar cases had occurred, each one of the children presenting ocular symptoms and exhibiting physical conditions that were similar in all respects, and all three dying before the age of two years. This peculiar ophthalmoscopic finding was noted by Magnus, Goldzieher, Wadsworth of Boston, Hirschberg of Berlin, and H. Knapp.

In 1887, without any knowledge of the cases described by the oculists, I published the history and the postmortem record of a patient suffering from what appeared to be a peculiar form of idiocy associated with blindness. The family character of the affection was not evident until a sister of my first patient became similarly affected. In still another family I saw another instance of this affection, and received the history of three other children who had been afflicted with and had died of this disease.

Kingdon, of Nottingham, called attention to the fact that the rare condition reported by the oculists was part of the disease which I had described. In 1894 Carter collected all cases of this disease known up to that time, and in 1896 I was able to give a list of nineteen cases of which eight had come to my own notice. Since the publication of this last paper other cases of this sort have been described and published by American and some European writers. In Europe cases have been published by Kingdon and Russell, Higier, Falkenheim, Shaffer, Frey, and others. In 1901 Falkenheim analyzed a series of sixty-four cases and since that time others have been reported both here and abroad.

Symptomatology.—As a rule, the children affected with this disease are born at full term and apparently in perfect health. They do well until the first three to six months of life, when they become listless and apathetic, move their limbs very little, and show the first signs of visual disturbance which ultimately leads to blindness. The child is not able, as the months go on, to hold up its head or to sit up. Its muscles are either flaccid or spastic; the reflexes are normal, a trifle subnormal, or exaggerated. In some cases there is an unusual sensitiveness to touch and to sound (hyperacusis), the child being startled by the slightest noise occurring in the room. Convulsions are present in some cases but are not an integral symptom of the disease. All the functions of the body are in a low state of activity. The children are subject to frequent bronchial attacks and soon show gastro-intestinal disturbances. An examination of the fundus reveals the peculiar condition so well described by Tay. There is a gradual increase of all the symptoms, the mental defect becomes more and more noticeable, the palsy more extreme, complete blindness is established and the child gradually lapses into a condition of marasmus in which it dies as a rule before the end of the second year. The chief symptoms may be summed up as follows: (1) Mental impairment observed during the first months of life and leading to absolute idiocy; (2) paresis or paralysis of the greater part of the body, and this paralysis may be either flaccid or spastic; (3) the reflexes may be normal, deficient or increased; (4) a diminution of vision terminating in absolute blindness (the cherry-red spot in the region of the macula lutea and later optic nerve atrophy); (5) marasmus and a fatal termination, as a rule, before the age of two years; (6) the occurrence of the affection in several members of the same family.

The changes in the macula lutea are so striking that they constitute a very important symptom of the disease. But it is to be noted that the disease can be diagnosticated even in the absence of this one symptom, and that in some of the cases the general cerebral symptoms are developed some months prior to the retinal changes. Koller has reported a case in which at the first examination the changes in the macula lutea were not in evidence although they appeared later on, and in Higier's case the optic nerve atrophy was much more pronounced than the changes in the macula lutea.

Etiology.—The causes underlying this disease are still obscure. In some of the families there has been blood relationship between the parents, in many others no such relationship existed. Injury to the mother during pregnancy has been noted in several of the cases and the tendency to mental derangement in the families of one or both parents is also suggestive of another possible factor. The family predisposition is evident from the fact that twenty-eight cases have occurred to my knowledge in fifteen families. Carter was the first to call attention to the fact that all of the cases reported have occurred among Hebrews, and even at this day I can say that I know of no indubitable case occurring in others. The racial feature of the disease is all the more astounding, because other diseases to which it must necessarily be more or less closely allied have been observed and recorded among all races and all nationalities.

The disease runs its course, as was intimated above, in a little less than two years. I have encountered but a single prominent exception to this rule, and in this instance the child had attained the age of five and a half years when I examined it, and it is, so far as I know, still living. The characteristic symptoms of the malady were present, and the same symptoms had been presented by two or three other members of this family. Spiller threw out the hint that the symptoms and the anatomical changes may vary somewhat if some of these children should live beyond the usual term of years. Many of these children are extremely well nourished at birth and for the first few months of life. By degrees they lapse into a state of marasmus to which they slowly succumb. I wish to insist on marasmus as a very important symptom of the condition, and the emaciation observed in such cases is so extreme that it unfortunately makes of the child a most disagreeable object. One writer has referred to sudden death as characteristic of the disease, but the very opposite of this has been observed in my experience.

Pathological Anatomy.—In my first case of palsy, in 1887, the outer surface of the brain exhibited abnormalities which we were accustomed to associate with brains of inferior development. There was a confluence of the central and Sylvian fissures and a complete exposure of the island of Reil. There was unusual hardening, the knife grating on removing a small section of the cortex. On microscopical examination the most important changes were found in the cortex, and sections were taken from the frontal lobes, motor areas, from the base of the 3d convolution, from the first temporal, and from a part of the apex. The same changes were found practically throughout the cortex. It was possible to make out the various layers of cells, but examination and a most careful search on removal of the sections showed that there were scarcely half a dozen pyramidal cells which presented anything like their normal appearance. The contour of the cells was either rounded or elongated, and the cell protoplasm exhibited every possible change such as we note in degenerated cells. In some cells the nucleus and nucleolus were entirely wanting or were relegated to the margin of the cell. In later examinations further changes had been noted. Hirsch was the first to point out that these same cellular changes occurred not only in the gray matter of the cortex, but in the gray matter of the entire central nervous system, in the cortex of the brain, in the basal ganglia, in the gray matter of the spinal cord, and even in the spinal ganglion. I was able to corroborate this finding by a later examination in another case of my own, and in 1903 I felt warranted in declaring amaurotic family idiocy to be a disease chiefly of the cortex and of the gray matter of the entire central nervous system. These findings have received further and most satisfactory corroboration in careful studies recently published by Spiller. Kingdon, Schaffer, and others, including Hirsch and myself, who found degeneration in the pyramidal tracts, yet this degeneration does not seem to be as marked as we would expect it to be from the very considerable involvement of the gray matter.

There is no doubt in my own mind that the disease is developed as the result of a congenital defect. The nervous system of such a child is able to perform tolerably normal functions until the age of four or six months, then it is no longer able to meet the strain put upon it, and an active process of degeneration sets in. This degeneration is, to my thinking, a natural result of an arrest of development. Gowers has claimed very much the same for some of the scleroses that have developed very much later in life, and the fact that the first symptoms of amaurotic family idiocy become evident about six months after birth, does not militate against the theory of a congenital defective development.

Amaurotic family idiocy should not be regarded as an isolated though interesting disease, but all the symptoms and anatomical findings suggest a relationship to other hereditary family affections.

Treatment.—Unfortunately, little can be said in favor of any therapeutic measures. It would be natural to infer that the wisest thing to do would be to avoid bringing such children into the world; but, as several healthy children have been born to parents who have had one or two children afflicted with amaurotic family idiocy, advice bearing upon this point cannot readily be given. In conclusion I consider it necessary to remind the oculist that these patients can no longer be regarded as afflicted with a rare ocular condition, but that the ocular condition, interesting as it is, is merely one symptom of an easily recognizable family affection.

Comment: The London ophthalmologist, Waren Tay, was the first to describe the fundi in infantile amaurotic family idiocy, but Sachs investigated thoroughly also the associated lesions of the central nervous system. The fundus in a recent occlusion of the central retinal artery shows also a milky opacity of the retina with a cherry-red spot at the macula, attributable here to edema and subsequent necrosis of the ganglion cell layer; but in infantile amaurotic family idiocy the similar ophthalmoscopic picture reflects a lipoid degeneration of the ganglion cells with sequential atrophy of the nerve fibers. In both instances the red spot at the macula is due to the choriocapillaris shining through the thin tissue of this area. In contrast to Tay-Sachs disease, late infantile and juvenile amaurotic family idiocy show no racial predilection. These conditions are characterized likewise by widespread lipoid degeneration but the retinal picture combines features of primary pigmentary degeneration with those of Tay-Sachs disease. Instead of a cherry-red spot the macula presents a finely mottled pigmentation. In all types of amaurotic family idiocy the lipoid disturbance is limited to the ganglion cells of the nervous system, but in Niemann-Pick's disease the lipoidosis involves also the reticuloendothelial system, including the liver, spleen, lymph nodes and skin and the fundus may show the typical picture seen in Tay-Sachs cases. Klenk identified the prelipoid substance that accumulates in the ganglion cells in the amaurotic family idiocies as a phosphorus-free lipid containing carbohydrate to which he gave the name, ganglioside. The ganglioside content of the total solids of the normal brain is 0.3 per cent, while in Tay-Sachs disease the concentration reaches 4 to 8 per cent, and in juvenile amaurotic family idiocy, 1.5 per cent. In Niemann-Pick's disease the prelipoid that accumulates is sphingomyelin.

Reference

Elwyn, H.: Heredodegenerations and heredoconstitutional defects of retina. A.M.A. Arch. phth., *53:* 619–33, 1955.

Biographical Note

Bernard Sachs (1858–1944) was born in Baltimore and educated at Harvard. Inspired by William James, he made psychopathology his major interest. His postgraduate work in Europe included study under Waldeyer, Goltz, Kussmaul, von Recklinghausen, Meynert, Hughlings Jackson, Charcot and Westphal. Shortly after entering private practice he identified and investigated infantile amaurotic family idiocy. Another milestone in his career was his *Treatise on the Nervous Disease of Children* (1895). He was at times president of the following societies: American Neurological Association, New York Neurological Society, New York Academy of Medicine, and the 1931 First International Neurological Congress at Berne. At the age of 84 he was honored by his confreres for the half-century he had served as chief and consulting neurologist of Mount Sinai Hospital of New York City.

Reference

Kennedy, F.: Obituary. Am. J. Psychiat., *100:* 853–54, 1944.

Part Ten

Ocular Motor Disorders

A New Test for Heterophoria

ERNEST E. MADDOX, M.D.
Edinburgh, Scotland

OPHTHALMIC REVIEW, *9:* 129–133, 1890

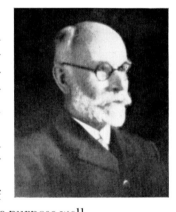

There is a simple test for latent deviations of the eyes which is within the easy reach of all who are interested in their study, since the only apparatus absolutely requisite is a glass rod, such as most will have already in their possession.

Any glass stirring rod will do, provided it does not taper. The rod supplied by Messrs. Burroughs, Wellcome & Co. in their hypodermic case, for the purpose of crushing their small tabloids, often serves the purpose well.

The principle of the test depends on the property of transparent cylinders to cause apparent elongation of any object viewed through them, so that in looking at a distant flame, with a glass rod before one eye, it appears converted into a long thin line of light, so dissimilar from the flame itself, as seen at the same time by the other naked eye, that there remains practically no desire to unite the two images, whose relative position indicates the conditions of equilibrium in the two eyes. The length of the rod is immaterial if not less than a third of an inch: the best thickness is a quarter of an inch.

The importance of avoiding a rod that tapers at any part likely to be used is, that it would have a conical effect, and thus a prismatic action in addition to its cylindrical one. Freedom from this defect may be ensured by testing the rod itself, as follows: Hold it a little to one side, so that it only covers part of the pupil; the flame is then seen partly through the rod as a line of light, and partly past it, as a flame; or, in other words, the flame and line are both seen by the same eye. If the rod is free from tapering at the part tested, the line passes exactly through the flame; if otherwise, the rod tapers towards the direction in which the line appears displaced, in accordance with fact that prisms cause apparent displacement of objects towards their edge. Though not essential, it is better to choose a rod with a smooth and regular surface, free from longitudinal grooves, which cause the line of light to appear broken and interrupted by unsightly notches. Transverse grooves are of course inadmissible in the portion of the rod used, as they come under the head of local taperings. The line of light is always exactly at right angles to the axis of the rod; so that to produce a vertical line with which to test horizontal deviations, the rod is held horizontally, and to produce a horizontal line with which to test vertical deviations, it is held vertically.

Care must be taken that the rod covers the entire pupil, so that the flame is not seen by the same eye as that which sees the line of light. The difficulty of always ensuring this in practice makes a little accessory to the rod almost indispensable. It consists of a disc of thin metal or cardboard, which is most conveniently made of a size to fit into any ordinary trial-frame, and punched out with a rectangular slit in the centre about half an inch long, and slightly narrower than the rod, which is fixed close to the slit, or in it. To permit of free rotation in a trial-frame, the rod should be so short as not to reach quite to the edges of the disc. The test is made prettier, and any desire for single vision still further reduced by holding the rod before one eye and a piece of coloured glass before the other.

To test for heterophoria, stand the patient at six metres from a small flame, such as a gas jet turned down till it is only a quarter of an inch high (or a more distant street-lamp will do as well), and place the rod horizontally before one eye, a coloured glass before the other. If the line passes through the flame, there is orthophoria as far as the horizontal movements of the eyes are concerned. Should the line lie to either side of the flame, as in most people it will, there is either latent convergence or latent divergence manifested; the former, if the line is the same side as the rod (homonymous diplopia); the latter, if to the other side (crossed diplopia).

If relative convergence should be demonstrated, the patient may be made to advance towards the light till the line passes through the flame: the flame then lines at his "point of coincidence" if he has one, and its

290

distance can be measured. On advancing still further, the line will probably cross to the other side, showing relative divergence, until the near point of accommodation is reached, when it may again given way to convergence, though this is less easily demonstrated by this test than by the scale test described elsewhere. There may, of course, be no point of coincidence, but convergence throughout, for all distances, as in some hypermetropes, and some few myopes, though rarely in emmetropes. It is very rare to find any point of coincidence (except that at the near point) in cases where there is ever so little divergence for distance; indeed, I have not met with a case. The significance and frequency of these differences may be left for another paper.

So much for horizontal deviations, now for vertical ones. Hold the rod vertically, so as to produce a horizontal line of light. If the line pass through the flame there is no tendency to vertical deviation, but if it appear above or below it there is "hyperphoria" of that eye which sees the lowest image; that is, if the flame is lowest there is a tendency to upward deviation of the naked eye; if the line is lowest, of the eye before which the rod is.

These deviations, whether vertical or horizontal, may be measured in two or three ways. Prisms of increasing strength may be placed in succession before the naked eye, till that prism is found which brings the line and the flame together. In testing for hyperphoria the edges of the prisms should be up or down: up if the flame appear lower than the line; down if the flame appear higher than the line. In testing for horizontal deviations, their edges should be in or out: in if the diplopia is homonymous; out if it is crossed. The deviation is half the refracting angle of the prism.

Another way is, in testing for hyperphoria, to place a prism before the naked eye in a trial frame with its edge in or out, and slowly rotate it till the flame and the line meet. This method is a very good one, but has the disadvantage of needing a calculation, from a table of sines. The sine of the deviating angle of the prism, multiplied by the sine of the angle of its rotation, gives the sine of the deviation of the eye. A trial frame, however, could easily be marked with degrees of deviation for different rotations of a known prism, and thus calculation be saved.

Another method still, the principle of which is, I think, a new one, is to use two flames instead of one, such as two candles, or two movable gas jets; on looking at these with a rod before one eye two lines and two flames are seen. If both flames have a line passing through them there is no deviation, but if otherwise, the flames are made to mutually ap-proach or recede from each other till the central flame and line meet, when their distance apart measures the heterophoria. The efficiency of the rod test is least manifest in uncorrected myopia, since the line of light becomes a diffusion band, in the centre of which the flame lies, if there is no deviation. The test is of course still available, but its delicacy is impaired. It is for vertical deviations especially that the tests already in use are most unsatisfactory, since greater accuracy is needed, and yet stronger prisms (with proportionate risk of accidental errors) must be used than in testing for horizontal deviations. The rod test is as good for one as the other, and possesses the great advantage over prism tests, except with the obtuse prism, that the result is not appreciably affected by slight rotations of the rod, or small inclinations of the head. The time spent in securing exact rectitude of position is thus saved.

The obtuse prism to which I have just referred has been described elsewhere, but, since its use led to the rod tests, may be briefly mentioned again. It may be regarded either as a single obtuse prism with an angle of about 174° or as two weak prisms of 3$^\Delta$ united by their bases. On looking through the line thus formed, at a distant flame, two false images of it are seen, one higher and the other lower than the real image seen by the other eye, the position of which to the right or left of the line between the two false images indicates the equilibrium of the eyes. A faint band of light, of the same breadth as the two false images, is seen extended between them, the explanation of which was shown by Dr. George Berry to be that the edge of the obtuse prism is not a mathematical line, but, from imperfect manufacture, a rounded ridge. He noticed that the band was transversely striated with exceedingly fine dark stripes, evidently due to "interference" similar to that which Fresnel obtained with mirrors, but which is in this way obtained by refraction. The rod test was an easy deduction for me from the effect of the rounded ridge. It is, I believe, the only existing test for latent deviations dependent on alteration in the shape of the images.

Comment: To detect and measure heterophoria demands the prevention of fusion of the uniocular impressions. Von Graefe (1867) depended on prisms to create a vertical or horizontal diplopia. The same result is better achieved by rendering the retinal images so dissimilar that fusion will not be attempted. With either method, the eyes tend to oscillate about the passive position. With the Maddox rod, greater accuracy is obtained when the test is performed in a dark room to remove the influence of the surroundings and if the eye having the Maddox rod is covered for a few seconds and the result noted immediately on uncovering. The Maddox rod is the simplest and most precise means of measuring small deviations. In the measurement of lateral phoria, the dissociation test of von Graefe gives a lesser measurement than the Maddox rod or the cover test. In both tests, the primary stimulation in heterophoria is macular in one eye and eccentric in the other. The Maddox rod originally consisted of a glass rod, 3 mm. in diameter. A brighter and better defined streak is obtained by the multiple Maddox rod, introduced by Aikin in 1894, which consists of a parallel series of grooves. In that same year, Norton effected a design with grooves at right angles, through which a cross of light was seen, so that both lateral and vertical deviation could be measured simultaneously. This useful device is now marketed as "the heterodisk" by Uhlemann Optical Co. An occasional defect in the Maddox rod is the unintentional incorporation of a prism. This can be readily detected by noting whether any change occurs when the previous top and bottom of the Maddox rod are reversed. Measurements with Maddox rod that are ordinarily within the physiologic range are: for distance, 2^Δ esophoria, 5^Δ exophoria, $\frac{1}{2}^\Delta$ hyperphoria; and for near exophoria, up to 8^Δ. If the streak is not horizontal when the Maddox rod is in the exact vertical position, cyclophoria is evident. With the Maddox rod before the right eye, if the temporal end is tilted up, incyclophoria is present; if it is tilted down, excyclophoria is present. By rotation of the rod in the trial frame, the streak can be rendered horizontal and the degree of cyclophoria measured.

Why does a Maddox rod give an image at right angles to its axis? Linksz demonstrated the mechanism of this apparent paradox on the optical bench. A collimating lens is placed in front of the light source, to produce parallel rays. At some further distance is set $+4.00$ C $\times$ 90. A screen of 25 cm. from the cylinder shows a sharp vertical line of light, as a result of the convergence of the horizontal rays. At the screen, the curvature of the wave front of the horizontal rays is reduced to a point with the power of infinity. If the screen is replaced by $+5.00$ S, the surface of the lens shows the same sharp focal line of light, because nothing can alter the power of infinity, which the horizontal wave front then possesses. But the vertical rays are still parallel with a wave front of zero power, and only these can be influenced by the lens. This is demonstrable by the horizontal line of light focused on a screen set at 20 cm. from the $+5.00$ S. The $+5.00$ S with a screen 20 cm. behind is practically an optical replica of the eye on a 10:1 scale. Similarly, the strong cylinder of the Maddox rod placed at Ax. 90 produces a real vertical line in front of the cornea. The refracting power of the eye acts on the parallel rays of light to produce a horizontal focal line on the retina, the length of which is determined by the width of the pupil. It is psychologically projected to the same distant plane in which the other eye views the muscle light and hence appears several feet long.

No form of optical compensation for anisometropia should be prescribed without first considering the influence of any intrinsic hyperphoria that may be present for distance or for near. Hyperphoria is usually incomitant, that is, greater in the primary position than at the reading level, or *vice versa*. Friedenwald called this condition anisophoria and found that even 0.5^Δ of verticle anisophoria may be clinically significant. The induced anisophoria created by the anisometropic correction may correct the intrinsic anisophoria of the eyes. On the other hand, when hyperphoria is present in the primary position but not at the reading level, the prism that corrects the distant hyperphoria frequently neutralizes or mitigates the prismatic differential of the lenses. After the refraction is completed, the dominant eye is determined while the patient wears the correction. The hyperphoria tests are then made with the corrective lenses removed, as hyperphoria is not affected by accommodation and errors in its determination are avoided if the anisometropic correction is omitted. In even the lesser degrees of hyperphoria, the involved muscle shows a paretic attribute: hence, it is essential that the red glass be placed over the dominant eye and the white-ribbed Maddox rod and measuring prisms over the other eye, so as not to shift fixation from the dominant eye. A change in fixation will give unequal measurements in more than half the cases. The eye that elicits the greater vertical imbalance when fixing has the involved muscle, and this may be either the dominant or nondominant eye. Hyperphoria for distance is determined in the primary position and for near with the patient holding a small fixation light in the habitual reading position with the eyes turned down about 20°. The data obtained with the dominant eye maintaining fixation are, of course, of primary importance.

References

Linksz, A.: *Physiology of the Eye*, Vol. 1. pp. 206–209. Grune & Stratton, New York, 1950.
Lebensohn, J. E.: The management of anisometropia. Am. Orthopt. J., 121–128, 1957.

Biographical Note

Ernest Edmund Maddox (1860–1933) was born in Shipton, England, and was educated at the University of Edinburgh, where he received his M.B. in 1882 and his M.D. in 1889. In 1884, his contribution on accommodation and convergence secured the award of the Syme Surgical Fellowship at the Royal Infirmary, and for 10 years he was assistant surgeon in the department of ophthalmology, where he was associated with Argyll Robertson and Berry. His career was interrupted by a long period of poor health after which he settled at Bournemouth, where he received appointments as ophthalmic surgeon to three local hospitals, including the Royal Victoria Hospital, and built a large and successful ophthalmic practice. Throughout his professional life, he was preoccupied with the elucidation of the problems of ocular motility. His books included *Tests and Studies of the Ocular Muscles* (1895), *Clinical Use of Prisms and the Decentering of Lenses* and *Golden Rules of Refraction*—all of which went through several editions. His ingenuity in devising new instruments led to numerous inventions: the double prism, Maddox rod (1890), Maddox tangent scale (1898), Maddox prism verger (1907), Maddox wing test (1912), duochrome test for near (1928), the V-test for astigmatism and the cheiroscope for orthoptic training. Toward the end of his career, he became interested in orthoptics. The clinics now established for this work in the major centers of England owe their origin primarily to him. The subject of his Doyne lecture before the Oxford Ophthalmologic Congress in 1921 was another masterpiece, on "Heterophoria." He was a corresponding member of the French Ophthalmologic Society and, in 1931, was elected president of the Ophthalmic Section of the British Medical Association.

Reference

Burdon-Cooper, J.: Obituary. Brit. J. Ophth., *18:* 55–58, 1934.

Congenital Deficiency of Abduction, Associated with Impairment of Adduction, Retraction Movements, Contraction of the Palpebral Fissure and Oblique Movements of the Eye

ARCH. OPHTH., *34:* 133–159, 1905

Attention has been repeatedly called to a special class of congenital deficiency of movement of the eye characterized by all or some of the following peculiarities:

1. Complete, or less often partial, absence of outward movement in the affected eye.

2. Partial, or rarely complete, deficiency of movement inward of the affected eye.

3. Retraction of the affected eye into the orbit when it is adducted.

4. A sharply oblique movement of the affected eye either up and in or down and in when it is adducted.

5. Partial closure of the eyelids (pseudoptosis) of the affected eye when it is adducted.

6. Paresis, or marked deficiency of convergence, the affected eye remaining fixed in the primary position while the sound eye is converging.

The findings in these cases may be summarized as follows:

Objective Symptoms

(a) *Restriction of Abduction.* In 41 of the cases abduction was altogether absent while in 12 it was deficient. It is further to be noted that in spite of the completeness of paralysis of abduction that obtains in most cases, there is rarely any contracture of the internus.

(b) *Restriction of Adduction.* Out of 49 cases, adduction was normal in only 2, diminished slightly in 2, diminished considerably in 37, and practically absent in 8.

(c) *Oblique Movements Upward or Downward.* In 31 cases, oblique movements were noted in the affected eye. In 24 the eye when it was adducted moved up and in, in 3 it moved down and in, and in 4 it moved up and in when the eyes were directed up, and down and in when the eyes were directed downward.

(d) *Torsion Movements.* In 5 cases, when the affected eye was carried in, or up and in, its vertical meridian rotated strongly outward (spasmodic action of inferior oblique). In one case at adduction the eye went up and rotated inward (spasmodic action of the superior rectus). In 3 cases torsion movements, indicating spasmodic action of the obliques, took place when attempts were made to abduct the eye.

(e) *Retraction Movements.* Retraction movements were very slight in 3, slight in 6, and well-marked in 32. It may be present, as in 2 cases, when there is no adduction, but the patient simply makes an effort to adduct. The retraction varied from 1 to 10 mm. To determine the amount, it is a good plan, as Weeks suggests, to put a spectacle frame containing a diaphragm on the patient and measure the distance between the diaphragm and the eyeball when the eye is turned in various positions.

In at least 2 cases in which retraction was produced by voluntary adduction of the eye, it could not be produced when the eye was drawn inward with forceps. Not only is there recession of the affected eye when adducted, but it may be sunken when the eyes are looking straight ahead. This was noted in 14 cases.

(f) *Protraction in Abduction.* In 9 cases it was noted that the affected eye protruded somewhat when abducted.

(g) *Narrowing of the Palpebral Fissure.* Closure of the palpebral fissure when the affected eye was adducted was present in 40 cases and absent in 2. It was present in one case when, although adduction was impossible, yet contraction of the lids occurred whenever the attempt at adduction was made.

When the eye is abducted the palpebral fissure often dilates somewhat. This was noted in 14 cases.

The narrowing of the palpebral fissure is evidently not a ptosis but due to contraction of the orbicularis, the closure being effected as much by an ascent of the lower lid as by a descent of the upper.

(h) *Insufficiency of Convergence.* In 20 cases in which the power of convergence was examined, it was normal in 4, subnormal in 7, and absent in 4.

The objective symptoms just described constitute the characteristic features of the syndrome. Other features of less significance are the following:

(i) *Restriction of Passive Movement.* In most of the cases in which traction with forceps has been tried, there is more or less restriction of passive movement, either outward or inward. Such restriction indicates the existence of an obstacle, probably an inelastic band, preventing the movement in a given direction.

(j) *Deviation in the Primary Position.* In the primary position there may be orthophoria, divergence or convergence. If there is convergent squint in the primary position, there will be orthophoria when the gaze is directed toward the side of the unaffected eye. In any event, the range through which equilibrium is maintained is usually narrow, the condition changing quickly into convergent squint when the eyes are turned in one direction and into divergent squint when the eyes are in the opposite direction.

(k) *Secondary Deviation of the Sound Eye.* When the affected eye is made to fix, and the sound eye is covered, the latter usually shows a pronounced secondary deviation.

(l) *Position of the Head.* In many cases the patient carries the head to one side either to avoid diplopia or to avoid the tension when not in the position of equilibrium.

(m) *False Projection.* False projection appears to be infrequent.

(n) *Nystagmus and Pseudonystagmus.* Slow nystagmoid twitchings may occur when the eyes are carried towards the limits of their movement.

(o) *Relation to Ametropia.* Most cases are hypermetropic, but few extremely so. Nor does there seem to be any undue number of high astigmatism or marked anisometropia.

(p) *Frequency in Women.* Out of 51 cases, 31 were women. This preponderance is the more striking since the other congenital motor anomalies are more frequent in males.

(q) *Frequency in the Left Eye.* Out of 54 cases, the left eye was affected in 38, the right in 11, while 5 were bilateral. The comparative infrequency of bilateral cases is surprising, since other congenital motor anomalies are as a rule bilateral. That the left eye is more prone to be affected than the right agrees with what we find in congenital anomalies in general.

(r) *Absence of Involvement of Pupil or Ciliary Muscle.* In none of these cases is there noted any impairment of accommodation or any derangement of the pupil. In those cases in which the convergence is weak the convergence reaction of the pupil will be absent, just as it is in any convergence insufficiency.

Subjective Symptoms

The subjective symptoms are not very marked. They are:

(a) *Imperfect Vision.* In some cases the affected eye was more or less amblyopic. In 16 the affected eye had normal vision, in 7 the vision was 20/40 or better, and in 11 less than 20/40.

(b) *Asthenopia, Headache, and a Sense of Strain* when the eyes are used are sometimes complained of, and in some cases are due to the abnormal condition of the eye muscles.

(c) *Diplopia.* Sometimes the patient observes that diplopia occurs when he turns his head in a certain direction. If diplopia is not present it can almost always be elicited by tests. In cases like these, when the abducens is completely powerless we find an homonymous diplopia occupying almost the entire half of the field of vision; but it is not so obvious why we should have almost all the rest of the field occupied by a crossed diplopia and but a narrow strip in which true single vision obtains. This fact and the occurrence of an excessive secondary deviation of the other eye when the affected eye fixed an object toward its inner side indicated that the internus, however effective apparently, was relatively weak. In the area within which the patient sees single, he has true stereoscopic vision.

Explanations Offered to Account for the Phenomena

Theories advanced to account for this singular combination of symptoms must explain why we have (a) the absence of abduction, (b) the restriction of adduction, (c) the retraction movements of the eye, (d) the oblique movements observed in adduction, (e) the peculiar lid movement observed in adduction, and (f) the deficiency of convergence.

(a) *The Absence of Abduction* is most probably accounted for by the fact that the external rectus is replaced by an elastic or inelastic connective-tissue cord. In spite of this complete absence of abduction, there is no contracture of the internus, since secondary contracture is usually absent in congenital paralyses.

(b) *Restriction of Adduction* may be ascribed to two causes: First, the internus may be normal, but its contraction may be opposed by an extensible cord replacing the externus. Second, the internus may be inserted too far back. This condition may be inferred to exist if on traction with forceps the eye can be adducted fully and fails to retract.

(c) *To Explain the Retraction Movements* of the eye five theories have been advanced. Indeed when the retraction is very marked it is probable that it may be due to several causes combined.

(d) That *the Oblique Movements* are due to spasmodic action of the inferior or superior oblique has been confirmed in my mind by the observation of a number of cases.

(e) The peculiar *Closure of the Palpebral Fissure* when the affected eye is directed inward cannot be due to the enophthalmos since it occurs in cases in which retraction is absent and on the other hand may be absent when the enophthalmos is extreme.

(f) The *Insufficiency of Convergence* seems to be due to the mechanical hampering of the action of the affected internus. The patient, finding it difficult to make the affected eye move inward as fast as its fellow, gives up the attempt at converging and lets the faulty eye diverge.

Treatment

In view of the pathological condition which underlies most of these cases, advancement by increasing the tension, and hence the retraction, would do more harm than good.

In cases where there is inward squint, tenotomy of the internus may help. In the opposite sort of case, where the eye tends rather to diverge by an inextensible band replacing the externus, an operation for lengthening this band might be serviceable. In one case, however, it did no good; nor did tenotomy of the externus in another case. The proper operation would be tenotomy of the externus of the other eye.

In general an operation is not required, and is to be avoided when possible.

Comment: Although the retraction syndrome had been previously described by Stilling in 1887 and by Türk in 1896, Duane's paper was the most definitive. Its opening paragraph emphasizes the six cardinal features of the condition. The syndrome has been classified as a congenital mechanical squint and grouped with strabismus fixus, fibrotic muscles and abnormalities of fascial attachment. Recent electromyographic studies, however, have revealed in Duane's syndrome a paradoxical synergistic innervation between the medial and lateral recti muscles that accounts for the perverted ocular movements. The electric potential of the lateral rectus increases when the eye turns in and decreases when thet eye turns out. The co-contraction of the horizontal muscles explains the retraction of the globe in adduction and the consequent enophthalmos and pseudoptosis. Hence advancement of the apparently paretic lateral rectus would aggravate the retraction. Simultaneous innervation to one of the obliques accounts for the intorsion or extorsion with upward or downward movement of the globe, respectively, that frequently accompanies adduction. In a unilateral case, when the gaze is in the primary position, the innervation of the horizontal muscles is practically equal and binocular single vision is then usually present; but adduction results in simultaneous increased innervation to both muscles while in the attempt to move the globe laterally the simultaneous relaxation of the medial and lateral recti prevents abduction. As in the Marcus Gunn phenomenon the motility disturbance is caused by an abnormal supranuclear innervation. The not infrequent association of the Duane syndrome with the Klippel-Feil deformity (congenital brevicollis) and other posterior fossa disorders or with the Möbius syndrome (congenital paralysis of sixth and seventh nerves) likewise supports the idea of a central mechanism.

In true abducens paralysis, the domination of the internal rectus results in a convergent strabismus in the primary position of gaze, but neither retraction of the globe nor pseudoptosis is elicited. The rare case of bilateral Duane's syndrome shows convergent strabismus in the primary position with amblyopia and abnormal retinal correspondence. The logical operation for Duane's syndrome when an improved appearance is desired is tenotomy of the lateral rectus of the affected eye, combined with the Hummelsheim procedure. A subsequent operation may be necessary if oblique muscle overaction in adduction was present.

Females are more affected with Duane syndrome than males (3:2) and the left eye is affected more than the right. Birth injury is not a factor, as Gifford noted the syndrome in a baby born by uncomplicated Cesarean section.

References

Papst, W., and Esslen, E.: Symptomatology and therapy in ocular motility disturbances. Am. J. Ophth., *58:* 275–291, 1964.

Blodi, F. C., Van Allen, M. W., and Yarbrough, J. C.: Duane's syndrome: a brain stem lesion. Arch. Ophth., *72:* 171–177, 1964.

Biographical Note

Alexander Duane (1858–1926) was born in Molone, New York, of an illustrious ancestry. His great-great-grandfather, Judge James C. Duane, the first mayor of New York City, was a veteran of the American Revolution and helped to found Union College in Schenectady, N. Y. His father, General J. C. Duane, served in the Civil War and his mother was the daughter of General Brewerton, superintendent of West Point at the time of their marriage. Duane graduated from Union College, where he made both the baseball team and Phi Beta Kappa, and then studied at the College of Physicians and Surgeons, now the University of Columbia Medical School. While an intern at the New York Hospital, he began an avocation as medical lexicographer, supplying the medical terms for *Webster's Dictionary*. After performing the same function subsequently for the *Oxford Dictionary, Murray's New Dictionary of the English Language and Foster's Encyclopedic Dictionary of Medicine,* he published his own *Student's Dictionary of Medical Terms.* Duane began ophthalmology as an assistant to Dr. G. T. Stevens, a renowned contributor to the surgery of strabismus, and then worked with Dr. Hermann Knapp for more than 2 years. His impressive ophthalmic contributions started in 1889 with new tests for insufficiencies of the ocular muscles. In 1896 he submitted a new classification of motor anomalies, which is still accepted. During the Spanish-American War, Duane served in the U. S. Navy as signal officer and from his experience published a text on rules for signalling on land and sea. In 1901 his initial monograph on accommodation appeared, a subject that continually occupied his attention after that time. In 1903 Duane launched the first American edition of *Fuchs' Textbook of Ophthalmology,* and his masterly translations continued through eight editions—the last made in 1924, 2 years before his death. As a recognized authority he was invited to contribute on ocular muscles in the textbooks of Weeks, of de Schweinitz and Randall, and of Posey and Spiller. His eldest son, Alexander Galt Duane,

300

was killed in service in France during World War I. Duane was awarded the honorary degree of Doctor of Science and made alumni trustee by Union College in recognition of his devotion to his alma mater, and his professional eminence. In 1917, he was Chairman of the Ophthalmic Section of the A.M.A. and in 1924 he was President of the American Ophthalmological Society.

Reference

White, J. W.: Obituary. Arch. Ophth., *56:* 66–73, 1927.

Hyperphoria, Diagnosis and Treatment

JAMES WATSON WHITE, M.D.

New York

ARCH. OPHTH., MAY, 1932, 7: 739–747

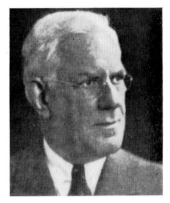

In no branch of muscle work is there as much uncertainty and confusion, both as to diagnosis and as to treatment, as in the subject of hyperphoria. Diagnoses vary as widely as the test by which the diagnoses are made, and the treatment varies still more widely. These tests and treatments have all been successful part of the time; else they would not be persisted in, but the chief difficulty seems to be in the proper use of the tests, the correct interpretation of the findings, the correct diagnosis and the best choice of treatment for the particular case at hand. The common mistake is to have a more or less pet plan of procedure and to make each case conform to this plan.

When speaking of hyperphoria as opposed to hypophoria, one is saying that the hyperphoric eye is higher than it should be and that the hypophoric eye is lower than it should be. But these terms are being used before it has been proved which is correct. In my experience, at least 98 per cent of cases showing a difference in level of the eyes are due to a weakness of one or more of the elevators or depressors, with usually some secondary contraction of the direct antagonist and secondary deviation of the associate antagonist. Nothing can be intelligently done in the diagnosis and treatment in such a case until the offending muscles are determined. Then, instead of a diagnosis of right hypophoria, one has a diagnosis, for example, of paresis of the right superior rectus. This tells at once that the right eye is lower than it should be. But the cause of this is not known until the paretic muscle is determined. When this fact is learned, neither the term hyperphoria nor hypophoria is wanted, but the diagnosis is given by naming the affected muscle.

For simplicity in working and teaching, I do not use the terms hypophoria or hypotropia but right and left hyperphoria or hypertropia.

This does not commit me to an opinion until I have made the diagnosis; then the affected muscle is stated in the diagnosis as paresis of the right superior rectus, right superior oblique, etc. After using this simplification for some years in teaching at the New York Post-Graduate Medical School and Hospital and elsewhere, the results with untrained men have been very satisfactory. More mistakes are made by the experienced men, who continue to use these terms as opposed to each other.

The amount of the hyperphoria is no indication of the amount of trouble it can give. Slight amounts may be the source of marked symptoms, while decidedly larger amounts may be entirely without symptoms. The amount, too, has but little bearing on whether the deviation is a hyperphoria or a hypertropia, as slight amounts are often the latter, while larger amounts are overcome in one way or another. The normal function of sursumvergence no doubt helps overcome small amounts of hyperphoria, while a head tilt will correct marked differences in level.

The difference between hyperphoria for distance and near has often been noted. The explanation of this, I believe, is as follows: The majority of cases of hyperphoria are due to a paresis of a superior or an inferior rectus muscle, the superior oblique and inferior oblique muscles being much less frequently affected and in the order mentioned. When measured at 20 feet, the eyes are in the eyes front position, in which position the vertical recti are the main elevators or depressors. At the distance of from 25 to 35 cm. the oblique muscles are the main elevators and depressors, and hence, when the superior or inferior rectus is paretic, hyperphoria is greater for distance and less for near. However, in paralysis of a superior oblique or an inferior oblique muscle, hyperphoria is found to be more for near than for distance. This may not be so, however, if a marked secondary deviation is present. These points must be considered when prescribing prisms for relief of hyperphoria, as will be spoken of later.

The relation of hyperphoria to exophoria and esophoria has been variously stated. The two conditions may be brought about independently, but more often the esophoria or exophoria are a result of hyperphoria. One evident proof of this is seen in the reduction of an esophoria or exophoria when the hyperphoria is corrected by prism or operation.

When operation is indicated, if this difference is found in testing either a hyperphoria or a hypertropia, it is better to correct the difference in level before attacking the lateral muscles. There are exceptions to this rule, but with the findings given this is the better procedure. In hypertropia, when correction of the vertical deviation by prism influences but little the lateral, then the lateral deviation may safely be corrected first.

Tests

The tests used first are the screen and parallax. A deviation of less than 0.5 Δ may be observed by the former, while an observing patient will note an amount as low as this in the parallax test. These tests are made for distance and near in the eyes front position.

Next the deviation is measured in the six cardinal directions.

In most instances this will determine definitely the paretic muscle or muscles.

Primary overacting muscles are rarely seen, but they frequently over-act due to a secondary deviation or a secondary contraction.

As a further check, I use the screen-Maddox rod test as described by Maddox and later by Dolman. Place the Maddox rod before one eye and find the amount of deviation at 20 feet. Then cover and uncover the eye slowly, placing prisms before the eye until the line of the rod crosses the spot light when the eye is first uncovered. It is usually found that the hyperphoria increases as the test is continued, and when the screen is left off, that the deviation becomes less and less. This is not always so, but is a very frequent observation and gives an idea of the patient's ability to overcome his hyperphoria.

The tangent curtain is used to map out the field of diplopia, after the foregoing tests are made; this is rarely necessary for a diagnosis. It is, however, further confirmation and is an important record to compare with later tests made to show the effect of treatment, whether it is operative or otherwise.

The common directions for use of the Maddox rod is to use it as a routine measure before the same eye, but much is lost if this is adhered to. It is often possible to demonstrate only double hyperphoria in the primary position by placing the Maddox rod before first one eye and then the other. Primary and secondary deviations are also usually brought out best by this method, primary deviation being shown when the prism is before the paretic eye, and secondary deviation when placed before the sound eye. The primary and secondary deviations may also be brought out on the tangent curtain by placing the red glass first before the paretic eye, then before the sound eye.

When the tests are made in the primary position only, as is so commonly done, it is often overlooked that a hyperphoria in this posi-tion may be a hypertropia in one field and not even a hyperphoria in some other field, and other cases showing so little hyperphoria in the eyes front position that they are considered normal may, by increasing in a certain field, be the whole cause of the patient's symptoms.

When examining in the primary position for distance or at the near point with either screen and parallax or Maddox rod, the tests should be made both with and without glasses if the vision will permit, as a poorly centered glass may produce a false hyperphoria.

A head tilt is a common finding in hyperphoria and affords some interesting study. A hypertropia with the held straight is often only a hyperphoria with the head tilted. It is evident that in many cases this is the reason for the tilting of the head. On the other hand, the head may be tilted in exactly the same way when it is definitely proved that fusion is not present and when suppression is complete. One case was seen in which, due to injury, the right eye had a complete optic atrophy. The vision in the left eye was normal, but there was complete paralysis of the external rectus muscle. The head was turned well to the left, and the secondary deviation of the blind eye was so marked that the eye was constantly at the inner canthus. In this case and in total suppression, a sense of muscle imbalance must be the explanation of the marked secondary deviation and head tilt.

As a general rule, when an elevator is paretic, the head is tilted back, and, when a depressor is involved, the tilt is forward. In this the general rule is followed, *i.e.,* to tilt the head toward the paretic muscle. Not infrequently the head is tilted so as to increase the separation of the images and so make suppression easier. This was observed in a juggler who had paresis of the superior oblique muscle. He could continue his work when the separation of the images was wide enough to make the false image so faint there was no chance of mistaking it for the true image.

When examining a case of hyperphoria, the head must be held straight for the first tests both for distance and near and in the upper and lower corners. However, an interesting and often helpful finding is next to measure the deviation with the head tilted in its usual position and then exaggerated by tilting the head to the opposite field. In mapping diplopia on the tangent curtain, the head should likewise be held straight for the first test, but at times additional information is to be had by allowing the head to be tilted into the chosen position and then exaggerated by tilting to the other side.

The treatment of hyperphoria varies as the ophthalmologist's experience increases. Often the symptoms are due to ametropia, which, when properly corrected, relieves the symptoms, hyperphoria being overcome by the power of sursumvergence, by head tilt or otherwise.

The rule to correct two-thirds of the hyperphoria by prism has so many exceptions that it is unsafe to follow. A great percentage of ordinary vision is in eyes moderately down; for this reason, if the hyperphoria is due to a paresis of an elevator, the correction by prism may be two-thirds or even less; however, if the hyperphoria is due to a paretic depressor, a full correction is often required, and, at times, even more to correct the increasing hyperphoria in looking down. In low amounts the prism is usually added equally to each lens; in the higher amounts, however, a better correction is often made by putting more prism on the sound eye to correct better the secondary deviation. This applies also to lateral correction by prism when due to a paretic externus or internus.

In correcting a simple hypophoria or a double hyperphoria in which one predominates over the other, the test is usually made in the position of eyes moderately down. The light is placed from 30 to 45° down to about 3 feet distance. The distance below the eyes front position varies as that particular person's use of his eyes. For a person who uses his eyes more in the upper field, the test is made with eyes moderately up.

On the results of these tests, I prescribe the prism I think to be best for the case in hand. The more noncomitant hyperphorias, either single or double, usually require special consideration. Here a portion of one or both lenses may be frosted. Prism pasters are sometimes used with good results. In those patients who cannot be made comfortable in any other way, the whole lens may be frosted or the association of the eyes otherwise discouraged.

Operative Procedures in Phorias

Operative procedure should not be resorted to until other means of relief have been thoroughly tried, such as treatment of constitutional causes, prism for wear or for exercises and the various other methods of relief. No operation should be undertaken unless there is a reasonable chance for improvement of symptoms.

Many operative cases are not relieved, not because an operation was contraindicated or was improperly performed, but because the wrong muscle or muscles were chosen on which to operate.

As a general rule, in hyperphoria a resection or tucking of the paretic muscle is preferred over an advancement, first, because of the relatively small amount of correction desired and secondly, because the old insertion is used and a torsion is less liable to result. In some cases tenotomy of the associate antagonist is a better procedure. An example of this is tenotomy of an inferior oblique muscle for paresis of the superior rectus of the opposite eye. The lowest amount of hyperphoria corrected by me in this way was 5^Δ in the primary position, which increased rapidly in looking up into the field of the paretic muscle. In some of these cases, however, a resection of the superior rectus is preferable; for example, when the paresis is not marked and the secondary deviation is slight.

In paralysis of a superior oblique muscle, the operation of choice is

306

tenotomy or recession of the inferior rectus of the other eye. I have done this and have advised it in several cases with uniformly good results. Here again operation was done on the associate antagonist.

Cases in which the wrong muscle is chosen for operation are commonly seen. Given a case, for example, of right hyperphoria. As the right eye is the higher, tenotomy of the right superior rectus is done. But the right hyperphoria is due to a paretic right inferior rectus, and following the operation there is a paretic superior rectus of the same eye added to the previous condition.

Cases have been observed in which the left superior rectus was advanced to bring the left eye up to the right, where the original trouble was a paretic right inferior rectus. The way to ward against this is by the careful measurement in the upper and lower corners, the only way to be sure of the correct diagnosis.

Conclusion

In conclusion, may I emphasize the following:

1. Most cases of hyperphoria are due to a paretic elevator or depressor.

2. In examining every case of hyperphoria the amount should be measured for distance and near, but more important than this, it should be measured in the six cardinal fields, especially the upper and lower corners.

3. The screen and parallax test with the amount of deviation measured by prism is the test best adapted for the corner.

4. The deviation for distance and near may be made by any of the multitude of tests, but, since the screen must be used in every case, it is more convenient to use this method for the primary position also. In this position the screen-Maddox rod, Maddox rod alone, phorometer or any favorite test may be used when desired.

5. When the diagnosis has been made, determine the etiology and institute treatment, systemic or otherwise, as indicated.

(a) In prescribing prisms for wear, each case must be considered as to amount of hyperphoria, the field in which the hyperphoria increases and whether prism can be used for the correction of this or not. These tests should be made with prisms in the trial frame, and the usual habits simulated as closely as possible.

(b) Always keep in mind that some patients with hyperphoria have learned so well how to overcome it, that it may not be the cause of symptoms and should be disregarded. Often the only way to decide this is to prescribe prisms with the proviso that they are to be taken off if not well borne.

(c) Frosting some portion of one or both lenses often gives marked relief. To experiment with this, in the office, cover the desired area with adhesive. This often gives a very definite idea as to the wisdom of frosting, and if frosted, how much.

In those cases in which relief is not to be had in any other way, it may be best to frost the whole lens or in some other way dissociate the eyes.

6. Contraindications for operation are:

(a) When there is still a possibility of a change in the amount or character of the hyperphoria. This may be due to a change in the course of the disease or as a result of treatment, systemic or otherwise.

(b) When the patient has not suppression of the false image, but because it is so far from the true image, it does not annoy. When an operation is performed in this case, the false image may approximate the true image so closely that it would be very troublesome, if for any reason the patient was unable to fuse the images.

7. When operation is decided on, determine whether to (a) resect the paretic muscle, (b) tenotomize the associate antagonist or (c) tenotomize the direct antagonist. The choice will depend on the amount of paralysis and also on the amount of the secondary deviation and the secondary contracture. Not infrequently, the operator may have to resort to any two or all of these procedures.

Most important of all is to study well the corners in all cases of hyperphoria.

Comment: White demonstrated that the predominant cause of hyperphoria was a weakness of one or more of the elevators or depressors. In the measurement of hyerphoria a shift of the Maddox rod from one eye to the other produces a shift in fixation and unequal findings in a manner comparable to the primary and secondary deviations characteristic of paresis. The paretic attributes manifested in hyperphoria frequently result from an induced motor inhibition due to a functional response to some coexisting aberration such as anisometropia or aniseikonia. In contrast to true paretic hyperphoria, such innervational hyperphorias have these characteristics: elevation or depression is not excessive; the disparity between primary and secondary deviation is moderate; the variation with conjugate movement of the eyes in the different directions is small; and effective control can be achieved with a properly selected prism. Hyperphoria, though rare in isometropia, is prevalent in anisometropia. In adults anisometropia is linked with intrinsic hyperphoria with even more frequency than hyperopia is associated with esophoria or myopia with exophoria. Optical compensation for anisometropia should not be prescribed before considering the influence of any intrinsic hyperphoria that may be present for distance or near. As little as 0.5^Δ of vertical anisophoria may be significant in this respect. Hyperphoria is anisophoric, that is, greater in the primary position of the eyes than at the reading level or *vice versa*. Extensive studies have demonstrated that in 2 of 3 patients with anisometropia the determination of the intrinsic anisophoria simplified the handling of the case by rendering optical compensation unnecessary. As hyperphoria is not affected by accommoda-

308

tion, errors are avoided if the measurements are made without corrective lenses. Both the Maddox rod and measuring prisms must be placed on the nondominant eye to assure continued fixation by the dominant eye.

In the following hypothetical case, R.E. −4.00 S., L.E. −1.00 S. Add +2.00 D., the following situations may occur:

1. Tested without lenses, no hyperphoria for distance, $2\frac{1}{2}^\Delta$ R. hyperphoria at the reading level. As the prismatic disparity of the lenses at the reading level is 2.4 Δ base down R.E., no optical compensation is needed here; and such compensation would not be tolerated.

2. Or, this patient may have $2\frac{1}{2}^\Delta$ R. hypophoria for distance and no hyperphoria at the reading level. Incorporating $2\frac{1}{2}$ Δ base up in the right eye-lens would then correct the vertical muscle imbalance for distance and neutralize the prismatic disparity of the lenses at the reading level.

3. Or, the patient may have no hyperphoria for either distance or near. This situation demands optical compensation. Flat-top bifocals should be prescribed with a slab-off of 2.4 Δ in the right lens.

4. Or, the patient may be using the less myopic eye for distance, and the more myopic eye for near vision. With this habituation the patient is happiest with lenses that are fitted to this alternating vision: R.E. −1.75 S., L.E. −1.00 S.

In cases of anisometropia, the tests for hyperphoria are most reliable if done in the following manner:

1. The dominant eye is determined while the patient is wearing the indicated correction for distance, after which the lenses are removed.

2. A red glass is placed over the dominant eye, and a white-ribbed Maddox rod over the other. The measuring lenses must be placed over the Maddox rod.

3. Hyperphoria for distance is determined with the eye in the primary position and for near with the patient holding a fixation light in the habitual reading position with the eyes turned down about 20°.

References

Lebensohn, J. E.: Anisophoria, anisometropia and the final prescription. Am. J. Ophth., *36:* 643–649, May 1953.
Lebensohn, J. E.: Nature of innervational hyperphoria. Am. J. Ophth., *39:* 854–858, June 1955.
Lebensohn, J. E.: The management of anisometropia. Am. Orthoptic J., *7:* 121–128, 1957.

Biographical Note

James Watson White (1877–1946) was a native of Dutchess County, New York and taught school there for 5 years before attending Albany Medical College from which he graduated in 1905. He spent 8 years in general practice before he embarked on the specialty of ophthalmology. White worked with Duane from 1914 till Duane's demise in 1926, and from this association he developed an abiding interest in the anomalies of the extraocular muscles. Eventually his practice became limited to this field, and he became recognized as an international authority on the subject. White was attached to the staff of the department of ophthalmology of Columbia University since 1919 and was appointed professor and executive officer of the department in 1939. He was also associated with the New York Eye and Ear Infirmary and the Herman Knapp Memorial Hospital and served as con-

sultant to several hospitals in New York and New Jersey. In 1938 he was
elected chairman of the Section of Ophthalmology of the New York Academy
of Medicine. White was a brilliant teacher and for 25 years devoted much
time to teaching both elementary and advanced courses in the ocular-muscle
anomalies at his office and hospitals and before various groups around the
country. He popularized the teachings of Duane and stimulated widespread
interest in all phases of his subspecialty. His most significant surgical innovation was the recession of the insertion of the inferior oblique muscle,
which initiated further developments in the surgery of the oblique
muscles by his many disciples.

References

Dunnington, J. H.: Obituary. Arch. Ophth., *36:* 231–233, 1946.
Brown, H. W.: Obituary. Am. J. Ophth., *29:* 1039–1041, 1946.

Paralysis of the Trochlear Nerve

ALFRED BIELSCHOWSKY, M.D.

Excerpts from Chapter 8 of *Lectures on Motor Anomalies,*
Dartmouth College Publications, 1940

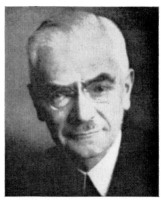

By far the most frequent and important type of paralysis of a single vertical muscle is trochlear-nerve palsy—most important because not infrequently there are variations which lead to a wrong diagnosis. From my material comprising several thousand cases of ocular paralyses, I can state that isolated trochlear palsies occur at least half as often as abducens palsies. Most statistics give too small a number of trochlear palsies, obviously because frequently these palsies are not recognized or are misconstrued. The most striking sign in many cases is habitual torticollis; that is, a tilting of the head toward one shoulder. The ocular origin of torticollis is often not recognized, especially in cases of congenital trochlear-nerve palsy or those acquired in early childhood. The general practitioner or the surgeon who is first consulted about torticollis frequently takes it for a contracture of the sternocleidomastoid muscle, although there is neither a contracture which can be felt nor a resistance to the passive straightening of the head or to its being tilted toward the opposite side.

I have observed many such cases in children who had to endure various kinds of orthopedic treatment for several years, naturally without the least effect. As soon as the physicians or the parents discontinued the forced straightening of the child's head, it was tilted toward the same side as before the treatment. At last the physician advised the parents either to punish the child because of the "bad habit" or to divide the sternocleidomastoid muscle. But when the operation was done, the child did not cease to tilt the head. In several cases the child's mother was the first to discover the ocular origin of the position of the head by observing that the child closed one eye during the forced upright posture of the head, whereas both eyes were opened as soon as the child was allowed to keep the head tilted in the habitual way. This observation was correct; the habitual position of the head helped the child to secure binocular single vision, whereas to avoid a disturbing diplopia arising from straightening the head the child closed one eye. These children discard the anomalous position of the head spontaneously as soon as the balance of the vertical motors of the eyes is restored by the required operation.

The ocular origin of this kind of torticollis was first recognized by Cuignet in 1873; he could not, however, explain the connection between the ocular disorder and torticollis. A. Nagel in 1871 supposed that in cases of slight paresis of an elevator or depressor muscle a vertical and rotary deviation would be caused by tilting the patient's head toward one side, a supposition based on the discovery that a parallel rotation of the eyes around the visual axis is produced by tilting the head towards the opposite side. As we now know, parallel rotation of the eyes is due to a reflex innervation of vestibular origin. The parallel rotary movement could only be performed, as Nagel presumed, by both the inferior muscles of one eye (inferior rectus and inferior oblique) and at the same time by both superior muscles of the other eye (superior rectus and superior oblique). The combined action of the two superior muscles as well as that of the two inferior muscles cannot cause a deviation of one of the visual lines provided the two muscles of each pair are equally strong, for in that case the antagonistic components of those muscles will compensate each other and there can result neither a vertical nor a lateral deviation of the visual axis. The only effect of the combined action of these two muscles is the rotary movement which they produce in the same direction.

Let it be supposed that in a case of right trochlear-nerve palsy the head is tilted toward the right shoulder. From this will arise a vestibular excitation of those muscles that are able to produce a parallel rotary movement of the eyes to the left. This movement is produced in the left eye by the two inferior muscles, and in the right eye by the two superior muscles. The paralyzed right superior oblique muscle can no longer compensate the elevating and adducting component of the right superior rectus, from which a vertical and lateral deviation of the right visual line must result, whereas in a normal person both the visual axes would be stationary. And what will happen if the head of the patient with the paretic right superior oblique muscle is tilted toward the left side? Both inferior muscles of the right eye and the superior muscles of the left eye receive the vestibular innervation to rotate the eyes around the visual axis to the right. This movement can be performed without the cooperation of the paretic muscle; hence no deviation of the visual axis will result. As mentioned before, the more the sound muscles are burdened the more favored will be the paretic muscle. Now one can understand the reason for the habitual tilting of the head that is observed in so many cases of trochlear-nerve palsy. If the head is tilted toward the shoulder of the sound side, a cooperation of the superior oblique muscle is not called for, so that binocular single vision is obtained.

Nagel's supposition has been proved correct by the investigations made by Hofmann and me in 1900. In that publication the explanation given by other authors concerning the tilting of the head in cases of trochlear-nerve palsy was discussed and proved wrong. But, strange to say, that wrong explanation has found currency to this day in many later articles on the subject. It is said that the paretic eye, deviated upward, by tilting the head is depressed as far as necessary to bring both visual axes to the same level, so that the vertical distance between the double images is removed and only a small lateral distance remains, which can be easily corrected by a convergence or divergence innervation. The error of this explanation can be recognized at once. In cases of paresis of the superior or inferior rectus muscle the tilting of the head does not influence this distance between the two images. This peculiar posture of the head will be found only if the balance of the oblique muscles is disturbed, provided that the patient can get binocular single vision at all. According to my experience, paresis of the superior or inferior oblique is in all cases at the bottom of ocular torticollis, since only by this posture can binocular single vision be obtained.

For an exact investigation of the influence that the position of the head just discussed exerts, one may use a simple apparatus. While the patient's head is fixed by his taking between his teeth a little plate at one end of a rod, he looks at a horizontal black stripe on a piece of white cardboard fixed to the other end of the rod 30 inches away. When the patient tilts his head it rotates around the same axis and through the same angle as the head. In this way it is insured that the visual line keeps its direction during the tilting of the head, since the cardboard with the fixed stripe keeps pace with the movement of the head in respect to both the amount and the direction. A patient with a left trochlear-nerve palsy using this apparatus will see, while the head is erect, two images of the black stripe, the image belonging to the left eye being below the other image and both converging to the left side. When the head is tilted toward the left shoulder, the vertical distance and the obliquity will increase considerably, whereas tilting of the head toward the right shoulder makes the two images come to fusion.

The deviation caused by a trochlear palsy is made up of several components, the vertical one being the most important in point of diagnostic value. In typical cases the vertical deviation increases in look-ing down as well as in looking to the sound side, according to the physiologic function of the superior oblique, which has the main in-fluence on the depression of the eye while the visual line is turned in; whereas, if the latter is turned out, the only effect the superior oblique has on the eye will be an inward rotation of the vertical meridian. Bearing this in mind one has to expect that the vertical distance of the double images will increase in looking down because the paretic eye will lag behind, while in looking up there will be the minimum, if any, vertical diplopia. In looking to the sound side, the disturbance of balance between the oblique muscles will become more and more noticeable. The paretic eye will deviate upward under the influence of the inferior oblique which is not, or insufficiently, counterbalanced by its antagonist. In looking to the paretic side, the vertical position of the paretic eye depends less and less on the oblique muscles. There-fore, the vertical deviation will decrease more the more the paretic eye is turned out. But in that position the loss of the rotary component of the superior oblique will bring about the maximum of obliquity of the double images; whereas, the latter will appear parallel in the opposite part of the field of fixation where the function of the oblique muscles is confined to the vertical component.

From what was said about the behavior of the paretic deviation in the various parts of the field of fixation, it is easily understood that a patient with trochlear-nerve palsy will instinctively try to bring the objects that attract his attention into that part of the field of fixation where he will see them singly. He can achieve this either by rotating his head around the frontal axis so that the chin is pressed against the chest, or by turn-ing the head around the vertical axis toward the sound side. In either case, the object looked at may be seen single since the eyes are brought into a position where the paretic muscle is considerably unburdened. A habitually depressed position of the head in cases of trochlear-nerve palsy is very seldom met with because it is rather inconvenient. More frequently, the head is turned habitually toward the sound side so that the patient looks at an object straight in front with the visual line of the paretic eye abverted. But this position of the head will be satisfactory only in cases with very slight trochlear-nerve palsy because it does indeed do away with the vertical deviation, but not with the meridianal disclination due to which disturbing diplopia, particularly in reading, may remain, double images of the vertical lines crossing each other at acute angles. Hence, the majority of patients with trochlear-nerve pareses will show a habitual tilting of the head toward the shoulder of the sound side, sometimes combined with a rotation of the head around the vertical axis toward the same side. By that position of the head, the paretic superior oblique is unburdened completely and the patients do not feel any discomfort. Patients with ocular paralysis will demonstrate an anomalous position of the head only if it relieves them of diplopia. If binocular single vision cannot be obtained by any vicarious position of the head or if unilateral amblyopia prevents a disturbing double vision, the head is held in its ordinary position. Sometimes anomalous positions of the head are given up if the paretic deviation increases to an insuperable degree.

Not infrequently trochlear-nerve palsy gradually loses its typical features by the development of a secondary contraction of the inferior oblique muscle, the antagonist of the paretic muscle, while the latter is recovering. In such a case the vertical distance of the two images no longer increases on looking down or decreases on looking up. Changes in the amount of vertical divergence take place only when the patient is looking from left to right; the vertical divergence increases in the direction of the sound side and decreases in the opposite direction, whereas the contrary is found with respect to the rotary deviation. Why does the change in the type of the paresis not extend to the influence of the lateral movements on the vertical divergence, so that the deviation becomes concomitant in the whole field of fixation as in abducens-nerve palsy? The influence of the vertical motor muscles on the position of the eye depends on the angle between the visual line and the muscle planes of those muscles. If the visual line is abducted, the oblique muscles have no influence on the vertical position of the eye, whereas their influence increases the more the visual line is adducted. These conditions are not altered when an originally paretic vertical deviation is maintained later by a contracture of the antagonist of the paretic muscle. If such a case is encountered and the first stage of the paresis is not known, it is difficult to decide whether the deviation is to be connected with a palsy of the left trochlear nerve or with a paresis of the right superior rectus muscle. In either case the behavior of the vertical deviation is the same, increasing if the patient looks to the right and decreasing if he looks to the left.

In such cases the head-tilting test will help to find the origin of a paresis. The patient observes the two images of the black stripe on the cardboard screen. If, for instance, the vertical distance between the two images increases when he tilts his head toward the left shoulder and decreases or disappears when he tilts it the other way, one may conclude that the change in the vertical distance is caused by a disturbed balance of the left oblique muscles, the superior oblique being too weak in relation to its antagonist. If in the head tilting test vertical distance does not show the aforementioned difference, one may take it for granted that the muscles of the left eye are intact, but the right superior rectus muscle is too weak in relation to its antagonist. Since this test has proved true in several hundred cases of the palsy under discussion which I saw before the atypical stage developed, I know that it is absolutely reliable, positive results always indicating that the change in the vertical distance between the images is caused by the oblique muscles.

Comment: In the primary position the efficiency of intorsion of the normal superior oblique is about twice that of the superior rectus (56 per cent *vs.* 25 per cent), but the reverse holds in vertical movement, the effectivity of the superior oblique as a depressor being 43 per cent, while that of the superior rectus as an elevator is 75 per cent. Since both muscles are intorters, paralysis of either is followed by a head tilt to the opposite shoulder by which means the vertical meridian is kept upright and the diplopia minimized. The head tilt is large in paralysis of a superior oblique but only slight in paralysis of a superior rectus. If the examiner tilts the head to the shoulder on the side of the affected eye, the result in paralysis of a superior oblique is an increase in vertical diplopia and an upward movement of the eye is observable due to the unopposed action of its superior rectus. In paralysis of a superior rectus, the movement, if any, will be slightly downward, due to the unopposed action of the superior oblique.

In paralysis of the left superior oblique, if the sound eye fixates, an increasing separation of the diplopia images down and in can be seen. When the affected eye is used for fixation, the separation down and in is even greater, and in looking up and to the right, the right eye lags. The left inferior oblique, the direct antagonist of the paralyzed muscle, then requires less than the normal innervation, and consequently its yoke muscle, the right superior rectus, also receives less innervation, according to Hering's law, and so underacts. However, if the left eye is covered, the right eye moves up fully, demonstrating that the muscle was not actually paretic. Similarly, if the right superior rectus is paralyzed and that eye is used for fixation, the opposite superior oblique appears to underact. Chavasse labeled this phenomenon inhibitional palsy of the yoke muscle to the antagonist of the paralyzed muscle. In this situation the differential diagnosis between paralysis of a superior oblique and paralysis of a superior rectus can be determined by the following observations:

1. In the primary position the affected eye is the higher in paralysis of the superior oblique and the lower in paralysis of the superior rectus.

2. If the patient tilts his head slightly toward the shoulder of the higher eye, the superior rectus of the opposite eye is paralyzed; if the head is greatly tilted on the shoulder of the lower eye, the paralyzed muscle is the superior oblique of the other eye.

3. If the patient's head is tilted to the shoulder on the same side as the paralyzed eye, the eye will make an upward movement if the superior oblique is paralyzed; if the superior rectus is paralyzed, the movement if any will be slightly downward.

References

Adler, F. H.: *Physiology of the Eye. Clinical Application.* 2nd Edition, Chap. X. C. V. Mosby, St. Louis, 1953.
Hardesty, H. H.: Diagnosis of paretic vertical rotators. Am. J. Ophth., *56:* 811–816, 1963.

Biographical Note

Alfred Bielschowsky (1871–1940) was born near Breslau and educated in Germany. He was one of the five famous assistants to Sattler, head of ophthalmology in Leipzig; the other assistants were Carl von Hess, Kruckman, Birch-Hirschfeld and Seefelder. While in Leipzig, Bielschowsky worked also with Ewald Hering, the great investigator of visual physiology, and this association inspired his scientific approach to the study of the anomalies of ocular movements to which he devoted his professional life. In 1900 Bielschowsky employed Hering's mirror haploscope to measure fusion movements, a principle now embodied in the major amblyoscope. In 1907 he contributed a major monograph on disturbances of ocular motility to the Graefe-Saemisch *Handbuch der gesamten Augenheilkunde*. He filled with distinction the chair of ophthalmology at Marburg and later at Breslau. He soon became one of the great figures of ophthalmology and was made an honorary member of the Hungarian Ophthalmological Society and of the Swedish Medical Society. He was coeditor of both Archiv für Ophthalmologie and Zentralblatt für Ophthalmologie till his name was stricken from the list by the Nazi government because of his Jewish origin. In 1934, at the invitation of Arnold Knapp, Bielschowsky visited the United States and gave a series of lectures in New York, Chicago and other cities. Lancaster introduced him to Ames, who invited him to the Dartmouth Eye Institute of which he became the director in 1937. His zeal as a teacher was remarkable; during his stay in this country he delivered 123 lectures besides the papers read at various medical meetings.

Reference

Lancaster, W. B.: Obituary. Arch. Ophth., *23:* 1354–1358, 1940.

Part Eleven

Diverse Surgical Innovations

Operation for Making an Artificial Pupil

WILLIAM CHESELDEN, F.R.S.

PHILOSOPHICAL TRANSACTIONS, *35:* 452, 1729

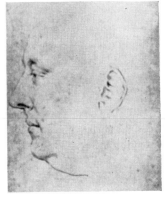

A new Operation was performed, by making an Incision through the Iris, which had contracted itself in both cases so close, as to leave no Pupil open for the admission of light.

The Perforation in the Eye *A* was made a little above the Pupil, the closing of which ensued upon the putting down a Cataract, which, not knowing how it might be lodged, I made the Incision a little higher than the Middle, lest any part of it should be in the Way.

The Eye *B* was one I couched not long before, where the patient had been blind but a few Years. At first he thought every Object further from him than it was; but he soon learned to judge the true Distances.

C is a sort of Needle with an Edge on one Side, which being passed through the Tunica Sclerotis, is then brought forward through the Iris. This done, I turn the Edge of the Needle, and cut through the Iris as I draw it out.

F is an instrument to keep open the Eyelids.

Addenda

The Anatomy of the Human Body. Appendix, Ed. 4, 1730

The Distemper for which the Operation is performed is either a total closure of the Pupil which is sometimes natural and sometimes happens from Inflammation; or else when the Pupil is extremely contracted, and the inner Edges of the Iris growing to a Cataract, or part of a Cataract after couching.

When this Distemper is without a Cataract it is best to make the Operation in the Middle; but if there is a Cataract or part of a Cataract, then to make it higher that the Cataract may not obstruct the Light. These Cataracts are generally very small, and sometimes by reason of their adhesion not to be removed.

In the operation great care must be taken to hold open the lids without pressing upon the eye; for if the aqueous humour is squeezed out before the incision is made in the iris, the eye grows flaccid and renders the operation difficult.

Comment: Peter Kennedy in his Ophthalmographia (1739) discusses an interview with a woman on whom Cheselden had made an artificial pupil. She said that she had been blind and was given sight, and that otherwise her husband would not have married her. Cheselden's original procedure soon fell into disuse because of ignorance as to its limitations and contra-indications, but this pioneer effort in iris surgery was not without ultimate results. In 1798 Joseph Beer introduced iridectomy as a better method of forming an artificial pupil and this led eventually to the glaucoma iridectomy of von Graefe. The reintroduction of iridotomy by Demours in 1801 revived interest in the surgical production of an artificial pupil and a wide variety of techniques have been developed since. The principal indication is the drawn up or occluded pupil after extraction of cataract. Contra-indications to such intervention are active iridocyclitis and pathological hypotension.

Reference

Sorsby, A.: *A Short History of Ophthalmology.* Dale Sons and Danielson, London, 1933.

Biographical Note

William Cheselden (1688–1752) was born in the village of Burrough, England. At age 15 he went to London to become a barber-surgeon. An intense interest in anatomy was inspired by the instruction of William Cooper and on the completion of his apprenticeship he himself embarked on the systematic teaching of anatomy. In 1712 he was elected to the Royal Society and in 1713 published a handbook on anatomy that was a standard student's manual for more than a century. A German edition was published in 1790, an American edition in 1795. After Cheselden joined the surgical staffs of St. Thomas's Hospital and the Westminster Infirmary, he soon became the most eminent general surgeon of his time. He was noted likewise for his skill in ophthalmic surgery. On one occasion his friend, Alexander Pope wrote from Bath that three cataracts were awaiting his arrival. He was the first to actually make an artificial pupil. He trained many pupils including several from the American colonies. His most distinguished disciples were John Hunter and Samuel Sharp. The clever quack, Chevalier Taylor boasted of his study under Cheselden. Cheselden was a leading figure in obtaining the legal separation of surgeons from barbers by Parliament in 1745.

Reference

Cope, Z.: *William Cheselden*. E. & S. Livingstone, London, 1953.

A New Method of Performing Plastic Operations

J. R. WOLFE, M.D.

Glasgow

BRIT. M. J., 2: 360–361, 1875.

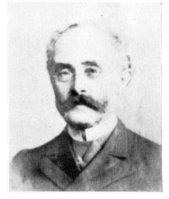

It is now nearly three hundred years since Tagliacozzi published his great work on Plastic Operations; and, notwithstanding the admiration which the work of the Bologna professor had elicited, it is remarkable how comparatively little has since been done for the cultivation of plastic surgery. The reasons are obvious. The fact is that, in operations on the nose, eyelids, and face —the most interesting regions for improving deformities—Tagliacozzi's method of taking flaps from the arm has been generally abandoned, on account of the extreme discomfort which it involves; and the practice of taking flaps from the forehead or face having been the only one in vogue, the procedure came to be considered more serious. In addition, when we take into account the elements of failure, from shrinking of the flap, from erysipelas or gangrene, it is not to be wondered at that surgeons are generally chary of resorting to the expedient, except in great emergencies. It amounts to this: we are to cut skin off the face to repair the face; and, in doing so, we run great risk of failure. To render plastic operations on the face more acceptable, and to bring them within a wider scope of utility, the following conditions must be fulfilled. 1. We must take a flap from the arm, or from any other part but the face. 2. We must seek to eliminate the elements of failure. I propose, in this short communication, to indicate the means of fulfilling both these conditions.

First, Tagliacozzi laid down the rule, which has ever since been considered as the primary law, and *sine qua non* to the success of the operation, that the flap must retain its connection to the adjacent living structure by a pedicle which is to be severed only after complete union and cicatrisation of the raw surfaces. This pedicle has, in my opinion, been a source of great embarrassment to surgeons, and tended rather to retard the progress of plastic surgery. From my observations on transplantation of structures from the lower animals and on skin grafting, as well as on plastic operations, I have long held it demonstrated, that in most cases the pedicle is not essential, if indeed it does contribute anything, to the vitality of flap. This being once established, we are henceforward free to choose our bit of skin from any part of the body we may find suitable.

My next endeavour has been to eliminate the elements of failure. The principal cause of failure I find to be in the subcutaneous structures. If we wish a skin-flap to adhere to a new surface by first intention or agglutination, we must be sure that it is cleared of all areolar tissue, and properly fixed in its new place. The following case will illustrate the points referred to.

Formation of the Lower Eyelid with Skin from the Forearm

P. C., aged 25, a quarrier, was admitted into the Glasgow Ophthalmic Institution, with his face, eyes, and eyelids injured by an explosion of powder. I showed the man recently to the Edinburgh meeting of the Association, as an instance of conjunctival transplantation from the rabbit. The right upper eyelid, which was strongly everted, I partially succeeded in correcting by skin-grafting. The lower right eyelid being completely everted, its integument totally destroyed, and the skin of the face consisting of discoloured cicatrices not by any means suitable for plastic operations, I formed a new lower eyelid in the following manner. The edges of the upper and lower eyelids having been vivified, I introduced three ligatures into the border of the lower eyelid, which I entrusted to my assistant. By means of these ligatures, he used traction, whilst I dissected the whole of the cicatricial tissue, and thus liberated the subjacent structure. The ligatures were then introduced into the upper eyelid, and the edges of the upper and lower eyelids were thus united. I then elevated the edges of the wound, preparing them to receive the new flap like a watch-glass. The skin required for the formation of this eyelid was two inches in length and one inch in breadth, which I took from the forearm. To test the principles above indicated, I divided my flap into three portions. The first I removed, along with the cellular tissue, as close to the dermis as compatible with the integrity of the flap. The other two portions, after removing them from the forearm, I turned up; and with a cataract-knife I sliced off the areolar tissue, leaving a white surface, which I applied to the eyelid. The difference between these flaps was very remarkable. The two flaps, which were previously prepared, healed by agglutination, without exhibiting even the slightest tendency to desquamation of the cuticle. Twenty-four hours after the operation, the surfaces looked pale; but the next day the temperature was normal, and appearance healthy; whilst that part which was applied without previous preparation looked rather livid the first day, improved the next two days; the fourth day, it began slightly to suppurate; and, after a hard struggle for life, a portion of it only remained, while the rest shrank. This, however, will not compromise the result of the operation, which may be considered satisfactory.

The dressing consisted of gutta-percha tissue applied next to the skin, a graduated lint-compress, and a bandage to maintain immobility of both eyes. The union was so rapid and so perfect, that I separated the upper from the lower eyelid on the fourth day.

In conclusion, I would recommend this method to the profession, from its simplicity and safety, for trial, not only in similar cases, but also for the cure of congenital blotches on the skin of the face, which are not amenable to any other treatment.

Comment: Reverdin, in 1869, demonstrated the possibility of successfully transplanting living pieces of epidermis to a granulating area, but healing was slow and the results were unsightly. To overcome these disadvantages Thiersch in 1886 used large strips of epidermis after the granulations had been removed. Even this improvement was not wholly satisfactory—the epithelial cover did not prevent contraction, slight pressure caused ulceration, and the color was poor. These drawbacks led to the revival of the full thickness free skin graft introduced by Wolfe in 1875. The Wolfe graft more nearly matched the surrounding skin in color, texture and pliability and provided a freely movable cover resistant to pressure. The Wolfe graft survives at first only through the absorption of plasm. Intimate contact between the graft and its host is essential; otherwise the graft succumbs before its circulation is re-established. A mucous membrane graft applied on a stent mold according to the method developed by J. F. Esser in 1917 is particularly valuable in reconstruction of the socket. The use of grafts of the Wolfe type is limited to sterile operative wounds in areas capable of complete immobilization.

Reference

Foman: S.: *Surgery of Injury and Plastic Repair.* Williams & Wilkins Co., Baltimore, 1939.

Biographical Note

John Reissberg Wolfe (1823–1904) had an unusually adventurous career. He was botn in Breslau of Hungarian-Jewish ancestry, but he himself was a fervid Protestant and originally intended to enter the Church. Sometime after 1848 he came to Glasgow, possibly as a refugee, and became a Hebrew Tutor of the Free Church of Scotland. In 1853, he published a *Practical Hebrew Grammar.* He studied medicine at Glasgow University, and after graduation in 1856 practiced in Salonica for 2½ years, probably as a medical missionary. He then studied ophthalmology in Paris under Desmarres, but before embarking on this specialty spent an interlude with Garibaldi's army as a volunteer medical officer. In 1863 he was appointed Ophthalmic Surgeon to the Aberdeen Royal Infirmary, and in 1868 established, as a private venture, the Glasgow Ophthalmic Institution, which in 1892 was amalgamated with the Glasgow Royal Eye Infirmary. In 1875 he reported the successful repair of a lower lid by a free skin graft taken from the forearm and freed from areolar tissue. The idea met with a favorable reception only after Dr. Wadsworth of Boston took it up in the following year. In 1882, Wolfe published a 450-page illustrated handbook on *Diseases and Injuries of the Eye* which gave a good summary of contemporary clinical ophthalmology. In 1889 Wolfe left Anderson College, where he had been teaching ophthalmology for 20 years, to become Professor of Ophthalmology at the new St. Mungo's College. Both schools were amalgamated with the University of Glasgow recently (1947). In 1893 Wolfe visited Melbourne, Australia and practiced there until his return to Scotland in 1901, where he passed away 3 years later.

Reference

Riddell, W. J. B.: John Reissberg Wolfe. Brit. J. Plast. Surg., *3:* 153–164, 1950.

The Application of Cocaine to the Eye as an Anesthetic

KARL KOLLER, M.D.

Vienna, Austria

Wien. med. Bl., October 23, 1884, 7: 1352–1355*

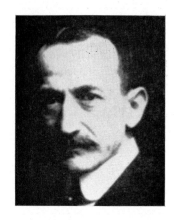

This paper will report the results of some experiments relating to the anesthesia of the eye. A preliminary communication was sent to the Convention of German Oculists which met in Heidelberg, September 15–16, 1884, in order to claim priority. Dr. Brettauer of Trieste had the kindness to forward my paper and demonstrated my experiments, which since have been repeated and verified quite often in different places in Germany.

That cocaine, the alkaloid contained in the leaves of the Erythroxylon coca, possesses the characteristics of anesthetizing the mucous membrane of the tongue upon local application was discovered in 1859 by Nieman, a student of Whöler. This property was mentioned by Prof. Schroff in a paper read before this very society in 1862. It is furthermore known that cocaine when injected diminishes the caliber of the peripheral blood vessels and produces dilatation of the pupil and this also occurs after local application. The instillation of cocaine in the eye has therefore been studied before but the observations which form the object of to-day's paper have thus far escaped attention.

The experiments made with the internal administration of cocaine have been disappointing so that the remedy fell into discredit and was eventually forgotten. In 1880 von Anrep published an extensive work on experiments with cocaine at the end of which he hinted at the possibility of cocaine becoming a useful local anesthetic (Pflüger's Arch. ges. Physiol., Vol. 21). My colleague, Sigmund Freud of the Allgemeines Krankenhaus, brought cocaine into prominence by his thorough

* Based on the translation of Boerne Bettman, M.D., Chicago. Chicago M. J. & Examiner, February, 1885, 50: 91–100.

compilation and interesting therapeutic work (Centralbl. Therapie, August, 1884).

I started out with the supposition that a substance which paralyzes the terminations of the sensitive nerves of the mucous membrane of the tongue would produce the same effect upon those of the cornea and conjunctiva and made a series of experiments in Prof. Stricker's laboratory based on these conjectures. My results were in short as follows:

If a few drops of a 2 per cent aqueous solution of cocainum muriaticum be applied to the cornea of a guinea pig, squirrel or dog or instilled in the cul-de-sac of the conjunctiva, the animal will wink a short time, presumably in consequence of a slight irritation, but within one-half to one minute will again open its eye, which has gradually assumed a strange staring appearance. If the cornea be now touched with the head of a pin, taking care not to come in contact with the lashes, no reflex closure of the lid ensues, the eyeball remains immobile, the head is not drawn backwards as would have otherwise followed, the animal remains perfectly quite, and the application of stronger irritants proves conclusively that both cornea and conjunctiva are entirely anesthetized. Thus I scratched and punctured the cornea with my needle and then irritated it by an induced current which was so strong that it pained my fingers and was unbearable to my tongue. I also cauterized the corneae with lunar caustic until they became milky white but all this did not elicit the slightest movement from the animal.

The experiments convinced me that the anesthesia affected not only the surface of the cornea but the entire structure. But if after the cornea was cut the aqueous escaped and the iris prolapsed, the animal gave vent to lively manifestations of pain. I was unable to determine in these animal experiments whether the iris could be anesthetized by instilling some of the solution into the corneal wound or by continued application into the conjunctival sac for experiments relating to tests of sensibility, if only comparatively complicated, are very unsatisfactory on animals.

I tried to ascertain whether cocaine could induce anesthesia of an inflamed cornea. This was decided affirmatively through experiments made on animals on whom I had previously produced a traumatic keratitis. Their corneae were as thoroughly anesthetized as healthy ones. The complete anesthesia effected by a 2 per cent solution lasts on an average ten minutes.

After these successful experiments upon animals I no longer hesitated to test its action on the eyes of human beings, and applied it to my own eyes, to that of my colleagues, and later on used it on numerous other individuals. All, without exception, testified to the complete anesthesia of their corneae and conjunctivae. The following manifestations occur: if a few drops of a 2 per cent solution be instilled into the conjunctiva or allowed to flow over the cornea a slight burning sensation and quite a copious flow of tears ensues, which ceases in one-half to one minute, to be succeeded by a dull sensation of dryness. To an observer the eye appears dull and staring as noted in the experimental animals. This expression is due to a decided expansion of the lid fissure. If, now, the cornea be touched with a needle, no sensation either of pain or touch is experienced, and even the reflex action fails to appear. The same applies to the conjunctiva, where also the sensation due to change of temperature is affected. The conjunctiva bulbi can be grasped with a mouse-toothed forceps without causing the patient the slightest discomfort, or the cornea may be indented with a probe without cognizance of this manipulation. The complete anesthesia last from seven to ten minutes, and gradually passes into the normal state through a long transition stage of diminished sensibility. The pupil begins to dilate about fifteen to twenty minutes after the instillation. The dilatation reaches its maximum during the first hour, diminishes visibly in the second, and a few hours later all traces of mydriasis have disappeared. The dilatation is never maximal, and the pupil reacts promptly to light and to convergence during the entire time, in consequence of which the dazzling sensation which accompanies atropine mydriasis is either not experienced or only in very moderate degree. The mydriasis is accompanied by a transitory and slight paralysis of accommodation; in my case and in another individual the near point receded one-half inch.

I have noticed furthermore a decided ischemia of the normal conjunctiva, especially of the conjunctiva palpebrarum, but am unable to state anything definite regarding its duration. The application of cocaine during my entire observations has never been followed by symptoms of irritation. I regard the dilatation of the lid fissure as due to the loss of sensibility of the cornea and conjunctiva, rendering them insensitive to the irritation which in the normal state affects them, and which thus regulates the width of the lid fissure.

There are a few practical points relating to the anesthesia which I wish to emphasize:

1. If, on the abatement of the anesthesia, cocaine be newly instilled a second anesthesia in induced which lasts longer than the first. I have obtained complete anesthesia lasting from 15 to 20 minutes by repeating the instillation every five minutes.

2. The anesthetic action is purely local.

3. Since it is known that cocaine is absorbed and on every instillation a minute amount enters the anterior chamber, one might surmise that the more remote parts of the eye would be anesthetized if it were

possible to introduce a large enough quantity of the remedy. I produced a decided diminution of the sensibility of the eye, against strong pressure, after having instilled a five per cent solution of cocaine, repeated every five minutes for a half-hour period.

Through the liberality of Prof. von Reuss, director of the clinic, and his assistants, Drs. Dimmer and Bochner, I have been enabled to test the action of the remedy on inflamed eyes. Cocaine might be put to two therapeutic uses: first, as a local narcotic in painful diseases of the eye, and secondly, as an anesthetic in operations on that organ.

With reference to the first mentioned usage I have employed cocaine, in 2 per cent solution, on a number of patients afflicted with eczematous conjunctivitis, ulcers of the cornea and fascicular keratitis. All patients treated expressed a few moments after instillation an amelioration subjectively with diminution of pain and photophobia. But they unanimously complained of the return of symptoms two to three hours later. The pain consequent to the cauterization of the lids with nitrate of silver may be controlled or diminished by previous instillation of cocaine.

I will now consider the second applicability of cocaine, as an anesthetic in operations on the eye. In the removal of foreign bodies from the cornea I induced anesthesia as follows: I dropped on the cornea of the patient two drops of a 2 per cent solution, which was repeated 3–5 minutes later. All kept their eyes perfectly quiet during the digging out of the foreign body, and when questioned as to their sensations, replied that they had felt absolutely nothing. Cocaine was applied with the same good results in a case of tattooing of corneal scars and in a pterygium operation. Prof. von Reuss did staphyloma operations upon a boy and girl, aged 7 and 8 years respectively, not narcotized, but anesthetized with cocaine. Both kept quiet and experienced no discomfort.

Prof. von Reuss kindly permitted me to apply cocaine in several cases for iridectomy and cataract operations. Almost perfect results were obtained with the following method of application: for a half-hour prior to the operation two drops of a 5 per cent solution were instilled in the eye at intervals of 5 minutes. The upper lid was raised, and while the patient was looking down, the solution was dropped on the sclerotica above the cornea. One of the numerous cases thus treated, a woman, upon whom the extraction of a cataract was undertaken, when asked at each step of the operation as to her sensations, asserted that she was not cognizant of the corneo-scleral section; the grasping and excision of the iris was felt, but produced only slight pain. A man with seclusio pupillae of both eyes was iridectomized on the left eye after cocaine instillation. The man was perfectly quiet during the operation and stated that he had felt nothing of the corneo-scleral section made with a keratome. He experienced tactile sensation when the iris was grasped and excised but no pain. A week later the patient underwent a similar operation on the other eye without local anesthesia. This time he wriggled and squeezed the eyelids so violently as to render the operation very difficult.

Comment: Possibilities of cocaine were first explored in ophthalmology. Though Moréno in 1868 and von Anrep in 1879 had suggested that cocaine might be of value in surgery, it remained for Kóller, then but two years out of medical school, to furnish tangible proof. In less than three months after his demonstration almost every conceivable eye operation had been attempted under local anesthesia by distinguished ophthalmologists the world over, including von Reuss, Becker, Hirschberg and Horner of Germany, Panas, Vulpian and Abadie of France, Gunn and Nettleship of England, and Noyes, Agnew and Knapp of America. In 1885, Halstead initiated conduction anesthesia by performing a mandibular block for the extraction of a tooth; and in 1899 Bier showed the feasibility of spinal anesthesia on man in an operation for the removal of hemorrhoids. Adrenalin, isolated by Takamine in 1901, furnished an ideal adjuvant for the local anesthetic —a chemical tourniquet—which increased the duration of its action and minimized toxic reactions. Elucidation of the chemical constitution of cocaine by Willstätter in 1898 inspired attempts to synthesize less toxic substitutes. The first such products were insoluble (benzocaine, orthoform), but in 1905 Novocaine was developed by Alfred Einhorn and though the first of its type it remains the most popular local anesthetic for injection. And tetracaine, available since 1931, has in turn almost displaced cocaine as a surface anesthetic. Cocaine, however, is still the only drug for instillation in the eye that combines anesthetic, mydriatic and astringent actions.

Reference

Lebensohn, J. E.: 1934—The semicentenary of local anesthesia. Am. J. Ophth., *17:* 949–952, 1934.

Biographical Note

Carl Koller (1857–1944) was born at Schuettenhofen, Bohemia, studied in Vienna, graduated in medicine in 1882 and then entered the Allgemeines Krankenhaus as a resident in ophthalmology under Arlt. While a medical student, he became interested in embryology and in Stricker's laboratory contributed a new conception of the origin of the mesoderm. During his residency he still continued his laboratory work vainly trying now to find a local anesthetic, adequate for ophthalmic surgery. At this juncture Sigmund Freud wanted to test a recent reported treatment of morphine addiction by the substitution of cocaine, and knowing of Koller's laboratory connections, asked him to cooperate in experiments with the new drug. The numbness of the tongue that followed a taste of a cocaine solution suggested to Koller that he had chanced at last upon a true local anesthetic agent.

Koller's further training under Snellen and Donders instilled an interest in optics. Besides contributions on astigmatism and telescopic lenses he designed the lighting system now used in most electric ophthalmoscopes. He arrived in New York City in 1888, became a member of the American Ophthalmological Society in 1889, and since 1901 was connected with the Mount

Sinai Hospital. For his discovery of local anesthesia he was elected to honorary membership in a number of societies in America and Europe and received also a scroll of recognition from the International Anesthesia Research Society and medals of honor from the University of Heidelberg (1920), American Ophthalmological Society (1922), New York Academy of Medicine (1930) and American Academy of Ophthalmology and Otolaryngology (1934).

Reference

Bloom, S.: Obituary: Carl Koller. Arch. Ophth., *31:* 344–345, 1944.

The Nature and Treatment of Pterygia

JOHN O. MCREYNOLDS, M.D.

Dallas, Texas

J.A.M.A., *39:* 296–299, Aug. 9, 1902

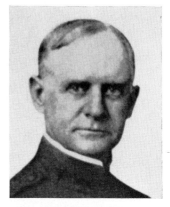

Before proceeding to a discussion of the treatment of pterygium it would be well to consider the nature of the growth and the circumstances under which it develops. So eminent an authority as Prof. Fuchs speaks of pterygium as a growth peculiar to those past middle life, and while this may be true of Vienna and the country surrounding that city, it certainly is not true of the southwestern part of the United States, where I have been practicing ophthalmology for a number of years.

In this region, where we have the combination of summer heat from April to November, with a dry atmosphere agitated by high winds and impregnated with alkaline dust, we will find the ideal conditions for the development of pterygia. Consequently, it is not at all infrequent to see boys in that country afflicted with pterygia of small size, while among those who are older we see pterygia growing from both the inner and the outer canthus until they practically cover the entire cornea, reducing the vision to the dim perception of large objects. This tendency to pterygium is by no means the same throughout the region of the southwest, but is found especially in those districts where the conditions mentioned above are so abundantly supplied. In the southwest, embracing that territory lying between the Mississippi river and the Pacific ocean and between the Gulf of Mexico and the Mexican Republic on the south and the continuation of Mason and Dixon's line on the north, we have a vast variety of climates and of soils. And it has been my observation that patients coming from the still, warm, humid regions of the south are not so frequently nor so seriously affected with pterygium as are those coming from the warm, dry, windy and dusty regions of the same latitude. Heat, a dry atmosphere and high winds will cause the maximum degree of evaporation of moisture from any surface, and the combined influence will be felt upon any exposed

mucous membrane. And when these factors are exerted almost continuously on the structures in the palpebral opening for many years and are
reinforced by enormous quantities of alkaline dust, which clings to the
eyeball about the sclero-corneal junction and the inner canthus and the
outer canthus, and is not wiped away by the motion of the lids, but
rather heaped up in the axis of the palpebral fissure, and when the
evaporation of the tears is so rapid that they do not accumulate in sufficient quantity to wash away the foreign particles accumulating on the
globe, then we have conditions most favorable for the development of
pterygia, as experience has shown. And not only do we observe the
difference in liability to pterygia among the inhabitants of different
localities, but in any given locality pterygia will be far more frequent
or much more severe among those who are exposed to the irritating effects of direct sunlight and wind and dust. And thus I find that I have
many more cases of pterygia among ranchmen and farmers than I do
among women and men of sedentary occupations, although the later
class will apply much earlier for relief on cosmetic grounds.

I would conclude, then, from my experience, that pterygia are produced by the prolonged irritating action of several factors, chief among
which are heat, a dry atmosphere, high winds, exposure to sunlight and
an abundance of dust, especially if alkaline in character. Then, with
these facts of causation before us, we must recognize that an important
part of the postoperative treatment will consist in the removal, as far
as possible, of those conditions which favor the development of the
growth in the beginning. And we must recognize that a pterygium that
would prove harmless in New York or Vienna, might prove distinctly
injurious on the plains of western Texas or New Mexico. We must also
recognize that a method of operation which would give satisfactory results in New York or Vienna might not succeed to the same degree on
the plains of the far southwest.

All forms of simple abscission requiring a break in the conjunctiva
along the axis of the palpebral fissure must be more or less unsatisfactory, because this will demand one or more sutures, bringing the
divided parts in apposition, and the line of union is apt to be associated
with some thickening of the tissues and seldom is altogether as smooth
as the normal conjunctiva, and the irritation consequent upon these
conditions will serve to invite the neighboring subconjunctival vessels
and thus cause a return of the growth in some cases. In my own experience, among a people who are afflicted with pterygium as frequently
as the inhabitants of any part of the world, I must say that my results
have been far more satisfactory with the method of transplantation
than with any method of simple abscission. But the exact way in which

this transplantation is accomplished has much to do with the success of the operation, and after a very thorough trial of the various procedures along this line I have finally adopted a plan which has never disappointed me a solitary time within the last few years. It is a modification of the old operation originally devised by Desmarre, but it differs in some very important features from Desmarre's operation, and these differences constitute the most important elements of its value.

The details of the operation are the following: 1. Grasp completely the neck of the pterygium with strong but narrow fixation forceps. 2. Pass a Graefe knife through the constriction and as close to the globe as possible, and then with the cutting edge turned toward the cornea shave off every particle of the growth smoothly from the cornea. 3. With the fixation forceps still hold the pterygium, and with slender, straight scissors divide the conjunctiva and subconjunctival tissue along the lower margin of the pterygium, commencing at its neck and extending toward the canthus, a distance of one-fourth to one-half of an inch. 4. Still hold the pterygium with the forceps and separate the body of the growth from the sclera with any small non-cutting instrument. 5. Now separate well from the sclera the conjunctiva lying below the oblique incision made with the scissors. 6. Take black silk thread armed at each end with small curved needles and carry both of these needles through the apex of the pterygium from without inwards and separated from each other by a sufficient amount of the growth to secure a firm hold. 7. Then carry these needles downward beneath the loosened conjunctiva lying below the oblique incision made by the scissors. The needles, after passing in parallel directions beneath the loosened lower segment of the conjunctiva until they reach the region of the lower fornix, should then emerge from beneath the conjunctiva at a distance of about one-eight to one-fourth of an inch from each other. 8. Now, with the forceps, lift up the loosened lower segment of conjunctiva and gently exert traction upon the free ends of the threads, which have emerged from below, and the pterygium will glide beneath the loosened lower segment of the conjunctiva, and the threads may then be tightened and tied and the surplus portions of thread cut off, leaving enough to facilitate the removal of the threads after proper union has occurred.

It is very important that no incision should be made along the upper border of the pterygium, because it would gap and leave a denuded space when downward traction is made upon the pterygium. On the contrary, the elasticity of the conjunctiva is such that when this downward traction is exerted upon the head of the pterygium the conjuctiva becomes thinned out and smoothly applied to the sclera corresponding to the former site of the body of the growth and the margin of the conjunctiva coincides accurately with the sclero-corneal junction. Thus, when the operation is completed and the speculum removed, no stitch is seen, because it is hidden by the lower lid; the only denuded area is on the cornea. The former site of the body of the pterygium is covered by a thin and comparatively non-vascular conjunctiva, and what blood vessels remain are directed downward and not horizontally, and hence do not tend to encroach again upon the cornea. In fact, the whole vascular activity is concentrated beneath the lower lid, where it is not only removed from view, but protected from the irritating influences of dust and exposure, and the process of atrophy naturally and surely follows. In the meantime, the corneal wound heals quickly and the thin conjunctival tissue becomes closely adherent to the sclera in the palpebral opening. After a few days the single stitch can be removed and the old pterygium will be found firmly adherent to the sclera and hidden beneath the loosened lower segment of conjunctiva. If the head of the pterygium is very large it may be cut off before the growth is drawn down beneath the loosened lower segment of the conjunctiva.

The general direction of the traction threads is vertical, but generally it is best to incline them in such a way that they will emerge from that part of the conjunctiva which lies below the cornea. This may be necessary many times in order that all of the denuded sclera may be completely covered by smooth conjunctiva, and if the conjunctiva should slightly overlap the cornea at any point it can easily be trimmed smoothly away without interfering with the desired result. If the head of the growth is very large so that it covers something like a third of the cornea, and if the body is also very thick and fleshy, it may be best to dissect away the head from the cornea with a sharp knife and then remove with scissors the head and a part of the subconjunctival portion of the body of the growth and then proceed with the rest of the pterygium according to the method already described.

Comment: The McReynolds operation was immediately accepted with enthusiasm and until recently received unchallenged endorsement. The recurrence rate prompted further investigations which demonstrated that the active disease was in the underlying tissue. On this basis D'Ombain of Australia proposed a more effective procedure (1948). He dissected off the subconjunctival tissue from the head of the pterygium to the caruncle and left a perilimbal strip of bare sclera, 4 mm. wide, so that the denuded cornea would epithelialize before the conjunctiva reached the limbus. Sugar modified the operation by removing instead the underlying Tenon's capsule which he maintained was the source of the disease. Later, Walter combined this technic with the McReynold's procedure. The average rate of recurrence after McReynold's original operation is 16 per cent and after the bare sclera technique 9 per cent. β-Radiation effectively prevents recurrences but, because of its narrow margin of safety, must be used with

334

caution. Immediate reaction is usually of short duration and self-limited. Delayed complications are telangiectasia of the conjunctiva and cataracts. The smallest dose which produced equatorial vacuoles in the lens was 4 gm.-sec. with radon and 5000 rep with the Sr-90 applicator. With this dosage, telangiectasia of the conjunctiva occurred in 50 per cent after 1 year, and the earliest cataracts were seen 2.5 years after treatment. The advisability of applying β-radiation after the first operation for pterygium depends on its type; but following a recurrence β-radiation is definitely indicated. In the prevalent method the Sr-90 applicator is placed directly on the limbus with its center in contact with the area where the head of the pterygium was removed. Depending on the vascularity 1000–2000 rep are applied a week after surgery; and repeated 2 weeks later. An alternative schedule is three applications of 1000 rep at weekly intervals.

References

Sugar, H. S.: A surgical treatment for pterygium based on new concepts as to its nature. Am. J. Ophth., *32:* 912–916, 1949.
Walter, W. L.: Pterygium surgery. Am. J. Ophth., *51:* 441–450, 1961.
Hughes, W. F.: Beta radiation, uses and dangers in treatment of eye. J.A.M.A., *170:* 2096–2101, 1959.

Biographical Note

John Oliver McReynolds (1865–1942) was born in Elkton, Kentucky, and attended Transylvania University from which he later received the honorary degrees of LL.D. and Sc.D. After completing his medical education in Baltimore, McReynolds located in Dallas, Texas, in 1892. He became widely known for his skill in ophthalmic surgery and frequently visited the ophthalmic centers in London, Paris, Berlin and Vienna to learn first-hand newly developed techniques. His personal contributions were concerned chiefly with surgical problems. During World War I, he served as director of aviation research and retired with the rank of Colonel. In 1922 McReynolds was elected chairman of the Section of Ophthalmology of the American Medical Association. His activity in civic affairs was appropriately recognized by the Dallas Chamber of Commerce in 1930. As a reward for his interest in Latin American ophthalmology, he was decorated in 1934 with the order of Carlos Finlay by Cuba and received the Venezuela Medal of Honor. Always influential in the promotion of hemispheric solidarity, he became the first president of the Pan-American Medical Association.

Reference

Gifford, S. R.: Obituary. Arch Ophth., *28:* 762–764, 1942.

The Treatment of Detached Retina by Searing the Retinal Tears

JULES GONIN, M.D.

Lausanne, Switzerland

Arch. Ophth., 1930, *4:* 621–625

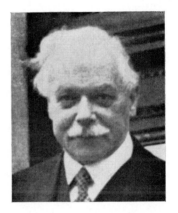

As I was entrusted by my teacher, Prof. Marc Dufour, with the preparation of the chapter on the diseases of the retina for the French *Encyclopedia of Ophthalmology*, I felt obliged to recognize the truth of the explanation given by Leber of Heidelberg for the sudden forms of retinal detachment. Leber emphasizing the fact that an exudation from the choroid should necessarily increase the intra-ocular tension (while it is known that hypotomy is rather more frequent in eyes with detachment), admitted that the source of the subretinal fluid was the liquid part of the vitreous which passed into the subretinal space. This explanation was based on the frequent presence of a crescentric or horseshoe-shaped tear in the retinal tissue, the flap always projecting into the vitreous body with its apex toward the papilla and its base to the periphery, these peculiarities showing that the tear was due to traction on the retinal tissue from behind, forward and inward.

The anatomic examination of some relatively recent cases of detachment enabled me in 1904 to complete with greater precision Leber's theory, and in a report for a symposium which the French Ophthalmological Society asked me to write in 1920, I gave the following conclusions on the basis of a greater anatomic and clinical material:

(a) In most, if not in all cases of so-called "spontaneous" or "idiopathic" detachment, one or several tears may be seen in the retina.

(b) The production of the tears is due to the vitreous humor dragging on the retina at the site of previous adhesions between both tissues, those adhesions having been formed near disseminated foci of chorio-retinitis, which are frequent in myopic and senile eyes.

(c) The presence of a hole, allowing the fluid of the vitreous to pass

335

behind the retina and maintaining thus the subretinal collection of liquid, explains the ophthalmoscopic appearance of the "spontaneous" detachment much better than the hypothesis of an exudation from the choroid. In the forms caused by such an exudation (detachment of pregnancy, in Coat's disease or associated with tumors or acute inflammations, etc.), the clinical course is also different.

As the retinal tear was the determining cause of the "spontaneous" detachment and prevented it from healing, it was obvious that it was impossible to secure permanent cure by any of the therapeutic methods hitherto in use, the danger of a recurrence lasting as long as the hole in the retina remains open. Particularly the many treatments the purpose of which is to give exit to the subretinal fluid or to promote its resorption, such as scleral punctures or draining, diaphoresis, subconjunctival injections, etc., were condemned as useless, as they did not hinder the continual passing of liquid through the rent in the retina. This explains the habitual failures of those treatments and the general skepticism that is met with among most ophthalmologists, many of whom think that it is not even worthwhile to make an attempt at cure. Professor Haab of Zurich, has lately written me that when he was in America he asked one of the most prominent oculists what treatment he generally used for patients with retinal detachment. "I send them to the most disagreeable of my colleagues," was the answer. That this special method did not prove to be sufficient as a rule is shown by the well known statistics of Dr. Vail, of Cincinnati, who in 281 replies from oculists in the United States whom he asked for information found that 250 of them never cured a single patient; of the 31 who obtained cures, 25 obtained a single cure each, so that permanent success occurred in hardly 1 in every 1,000 cases. Dr. Vail's conclusion, therefore, was that any vigorous treatment was to be refrained from until a "cure" should be found that really cures.

The British ophthalmologist who, I think, is at present the best informed on retinal detachment, Sir William Lister, has come to the same pessimistic conclusion as our American colleague, judging from the address he gave in 1927 before the British Medical Association (Brit. M. J. 2: 1127, 1927). Holes in the retina, he said, are often seen, and they probably occur more often than they are found even by those who look for them, but it would seem that in such cases treatment is practically valueless, and "should not be urged except as a last clutch at a straw of hope."

I was of the same opinion as Sir William Lister, until I thought of the possibility of closing up the tear and checking at the same time the dragging force of the vitreous on the retinal flap. I then succeeded in doing so by means of a thermopuncture through the sclera, first in some cases of rather old detachment, and obtained a complete reposition of the retina, although, of course, its visual function was not restored. With greater courage, I then tried the same operation in more recent cases and even in cases in which the patient had vision in one eye, and obtained the astonishing result that not only the progress of the detachment was stopped and the retina reapplied near the cauterization, but that even in widely spread detachments, the whole fundus of the eye had recovered a normal appearance with no further trace of folds or of grayish discoloration. In a certain number of cases, central vision and peripheral field were restored to normal so that the formerly detached eye remained the better one, being used even for watchmaker's work.

These unexpected successes were first referred to before the Swiss oculists at Bâle in 1919, with, of course, great reserve, then in some Swiss or French reviews, such as Annales d'oculistique, 1921, and Revue générale d'ophtalmologie, 1923, later, with a short description of some typical cases presented before the French, Swiss and German Societies in Brussels, Zurich and Heidelberg in 1925 and 1926. In 1927, there was shown at Bern several patients, the complete disappearance of whose detachments lasted for several months, and in the following year, at Lucerne, my colleagues, Siegrist of Bern and Vogt of Zurich, referred to their own confirmatory experiences; this was the first occasion on which credit was given to me by ophthalmologists other than my own fellow-workers and assistants. Later descriptions of cases or of the method were published in Italian, French or German in the reports of the ophthalmologic meetings held at Palermo, Paris and Heidelberg in 1928, and a more detailed account was published in the Annales d'oculistique (May, 1930).

My actual experience on about 250 patients and in more than 300 operations can be summed up as follows:

1. In more than 95 per cent of the cases, whenever ophthalmoscopic examination is possible, one or several holes may be detected in the retina if looked for with sufficient care.

2. In about 10 per cent of these cases, the hole is not in the retinal tissue, but consists of a rupture or tearing away from its insertion at the ora serrata ("disinsertion of the retina").

3. In all recent cases, when the hole or tear has been closed, cure is immediate, complete and permanent.

4. In older cases (several weeks or months), closing the tear stops the detachment and may produce a more or less complete reposition of the retina, but restoration of the vision generally remains incomplete.

5. If the detachment relapses, it is found that the tear has not been completely closed or that there was another tear which had not been previously seen.

6. A recurrence of detachment in a different region of the eye is due to formation of a new hole in the retina.

It may appear curious that all my communications on that matter, numbering more than twenty, remained unknown to the English-speaking ophthalmologic world until the International Congress in Holland, no mention of them even being made either in an article in the Lancet (Operation for detachment of the retina, 2: 1202, 1929), or in an article by Stallard (Brit. J. Ophth., 14: 1, 1930) in the British Journal of Ophthalmology. Only following a recent visit to me at Lausanne by five members of the staff of the great eye hospitals in London were my ideas set forth in two papers published by Juler (Brit. J. Ophth., 14: 73, 1930) and by Ormond (Brit. M. J., 1: 940, 1930). The observers described accurately the preliminary procedures (J. B. Lawford in the British Journal of Ophthalmology, 14: 359, 1930), and the operation of the thermopuncture; the latter dealt adequately with the anatomic side of the question.

As both of these papers gave a sufficient account of my ideas, I will not repeat the particulars but I wish to emphasize the great importance of being acquainted with the conditions causing a detachment rather than with the routine procedure of the operation itself. I fancy the latter could be done in a different manner than mine, but the pathogenesis of the detachment is not a matter of personal preference, for truth must be accepted such as it is. Some of the visitors seemed to have an insufficient knowledge of the facts underlying the method, so that I could not imagine what benefit they might derive from their visit. It is surely of little value to witness an operation if one is unable to understand not only the how but also the why of the procedure. Before inquiring about the technic of, and performing the thermopuncture, it is necessary to be well aware of anatomic and clinical reasons (Gonin, J.: Ann. ocul., 132: 30, 1904; Encyclopedie francaise d'ophtalmologie, Paris, O. Doin, 1906, vol. 6; Ann. ocul., 156: 281, 1919; Bull. et mém. Soc. franç. opht., 23: 1, 1920; Ber. deutsch. ophth. Gesellsch., 45: 114, 1921).

Summary

In summarizing my experiences to date, I should say that definite cure may be obtained in about 60 per cent of recent cases, this percentage diminishing with the age of the detachment. Not only is this proportion of cures an improvement in comparison with the former rarity, but the length of the treatment is far shorter than the many weeks or months of absolute rest in bed with both eyes bandaged, which was up to this time the most usual torment for the patient.

In the Lancet of December, 1929, it was said that: "There are few ophthalmic surgeons who cannot count on the fingers of one hand the cases of cure of detached retina within their own personal experience."

I should be very unhappy and quite unable to operate if I had on my two hands as many fingers as I can count patients who for the last three years have been completely and lastingly cured as rapidly as if they had simply been operated on for cataract. I trust these facts will offer my honored colleagues, Vail and Lister, more than "a straw of hope" for the benefit of their patients, and that even "away from the magnetic personality" of the writer, all oculists will find a new courage for the treatment of detached retinas, so that they may soon acquire with their own experience many successful cures.

Comment: The first ophthalmoscopic observation of retinal detachment was reported by Coccius in 1853. Leber in 1887 noted a rent or rents in the separated membrane. Nordenson suggested that vitreous traction produced the rent through which a posthyaloid effusion entered. Gonin clinched the significance of retinal tears by accomplishing cures with their closure. Until then the diagnosis of retinal detachment was practically a condemnation to blindness. The standard diathermy procedure (a modification of Gonin's technique) proved successful in 75 per cent of uncomplicated cases. To help the complex cases, Linder revived in 1946 the operation of scleral shortening proposed by Müller in 1903, in order to nullify the traction effects of vitreo-retinal adhesions by bringing the diathermied choroid to the detached retina. Vitreous traction is diagnosed by fixed folds, frequently star-shaped, which do not undulate with ocular motion or flatten after bed rest and binocular occlusion or by the observation of tears with rolled up, convex edges. Experience has shown that scleral shortening is indicated also for retinal detachments associated with large or multiple breaks, or with high myopia or aphakia, and for detachments sequential to penetrating wounds, intraocular foreign bodies or vitreous hemorrhage. To enhance the effect of lamellar resection, Schepens in 1955 advocated the incorporation of a scleral buckle. He now makes a segmental scleral groove just posterior to each retinal tear, around which light diathermy is applied, and folds a grooved silicone implant into the groove. To make the buckle permanent, he adds an encircling silicone band, 2 mm. wide, which is tightened after the release of subretinal fluid to create an ocular pressure of 20 mm. Hg.

Simple diathermy is still indicated for retinal tears with less than a quadrant of detachment and without signs of vitreous traction. In a a total detachment with small tears and some evidence of vitreous traction, Schafer prefers a vitreous implant, following drainage, to provide support for the diathermied choroid. Fluid silicone in a viscosity of 500 to 1000 centistokes may serve as a substitute for vitreous. Armaly demonstrated complete tolerance in animals to intraocularly injected silicone fluid. In 5 patients with detachments refractory to previous surgery, the subretinal fluid was drained and silicone fluid was injected. The retina reattached, and the retinal folds disappeared. The silicone fluid pressed against but did not flow through the retinal tears.

Meyer-Schwickerath's apparatus for photocoagulation has made the prophylaxis of retinal detachments possible. Even in the absence of symptoms, all superior holes and all inferior holes displaying traction should be photocoagulated. If a detachment has occurred in one eye, potentially dangerous areas of lattice degeneration are similarly treated. Peripheral flat holes should also be treated with photocoagulation if there is a family history of retinal detachment.

The past 15 years has witnessed a variety of improvements in the management of retinal detachment, but regardless of the procedure used, Gonin's principles must be fulfilled to attain success. In summary: (1) An exudative choroiditis must be produced in the proper place; (2) the retina must be brought in contact with the induced choroiditis so that the edges of the tear or hole touch the exudate; (3) the retina must be allowed to remain in contact until firm adhesions form.

References

Regan, C., Schepens, C., Okumura, I., Brockhurst, R., and McMeel, J.: The scleral buckling procedures. Arch. Ophth., *68:* 313, 1962.
Armaly, M. F.: Ocular tolerance to silicones. Arch. Ophth., *68:* 390, 1962.

Biographical Note

Jules Gonin (1870–1935) was born, educated and achieved fame in Lausanne, Switzerland. He graduated from the medical school of the University of Lausanne and trained at the ophthalmic hospital directed by Professor Marc Dufour, a former assistant of von Graefe. In 1900 Dufour and Gonin collaborated in preparing the chapter on diseases of the retina and optic nerve for the French Encyclopedia of Ophthalmology. This task initiated Gonin into the challenging problem of retinal detachment. Leber's writings convinced him of the causal relationship between tears in the retina and retinal detachment. In 1908 Gonin helped in establishing the Swiss Ophthalmological Society, and in 1918 he succeeded Eperon in the Chair of Ophthalmology at the University of Lausanne and became chief surgeon of the eye hospital. In 1923 Gonin published the first of his papers on the cure of retinal detachment by the thermocautery method. His ideas failed to attract attention until 1929, when he reviewed his results before the International Congress of Ophthalmology at Amsterdam. His cures of retinal detachment were astounding—22 of 30 cases of less than 3 weeks' duration, and 15 of 35 cases of longer than 3 months' duration, a success rate of 57 per cent. Gonin, a proficient linguist, spread his gospel in 34 papers published in Swiss, French, Belgian, English, American and German journals. His operating room became the mecca for ophthalmologists from every country. Schoenberg, who visited the vivacious Gonin in 1926 and 1928, performed the first Gonin operation in the United States on January 10, 1929. Gonin was honored in Switzerland with the Marcel Benoist prize in 1929 and gave the William Mackenzie Memorial Lecture in Glasgow in 1934. In that same year, a few months before his death from cerebral hemorrhage at the age of 65, he published his final work, a large monograph recording in detail his work on retinal detachment. Certainly the most significant surgical contributions to the preservation of vision are the operations of cataract extraction by Daviel, iridectomy for acute glaucoma by von Graefe and the cure of retinal detachment by Gonin.

References

Schoenberg, M. J. Obituary. Arch. Ophth., *14:* 643, 1935.
Lewis P. Obituary. Am. J. Ophth., *18:* 769, 1935.

Orbital Tumors

WALTER E. DANDY, M.D.

Baltimore, Maryland

EXCERPTS FROM *Orbital Tumors,* OSKAR PIEST, NEW YORK, 1941

Introduction

In 1921 the writer encountered, by the cranial route, an intracranial tumor that had extended through the optic foramen into the orbital cavity. The orbital roof was removed in order to follow and extirpate this portion of the tumor. So simple was the operative attack, and so perfectly could the intraorbital contents be exposed, that this method suggested a very marked improvement in operative attack upon the great 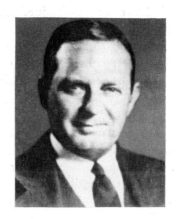 group of intraorbital tumors. No matter in which direction the intracranial portion of the tumor extended, or in which part of the orbit the tumor was situated, this approach appeared to be far superior to the usual frontal or lateral (Krönlein) routes by which these tumors had heretofore been attacked.

Even for tumors confined to the orbit alone, this approach has been found far superior to those hitherto used by ophthalmologists. The great advantage of this approach lies in the much fuller and safer exposure of the intraorbital contents. The optic nerve, the eyeball, three of the extraocular muscles, the ophthalmic veins and arteries can be well exposed and avoided during the dissection of the orbital tumor.

From the clinical findings on patients with exophthalmos it is not usually possible to tell whether or not there is an intracranial extension of the orbital tumor. And too often the orbital tumor is but a small fraction of the large but silent intracranial tumor which is usually the primary growth. Since intracranial tumors are present in approximately three-fourths of the orbital tumors in this series, it should be assumed on the law of probabilities that the tumor extends into the cranial chamber. And anything less than the combined intracranial and intraorbital approach will offer no surgical solution of the problem. All too frequently the orbital contents have been exenterated in a radical attempt to remove the tumor from the front of the orbit, with an infected granulating wound resulting. Such a result forever precludes the intracranial approach because of the certainty that infection will follow. In safe hands the intracranial approach involves very little risk, offers the maximum hope of cure, and is without cosmetic defects. Even when the character of the tumor prevents a permanent cure, the maximum period of relief and extension of life is afforded by subtotal removal of the extensive tumor.

Although the best available evidence of an intracranial component of the tumor is obtained from the roentgenograms, this proof is often lacking. The optic foramen is occasionally enlarged or reduced in size, but the vast majority of tumors are not continous through this opening. The dural tumors (meningiomas), which comprise almost one-half of the series, usually but not always show a diffuse hyperostosis of the walls of the skull and orbit. In these cases there is usually no gross defect in the orbital roof, but the extension of the tumor is due to diffuse invasion of the bone. At times calcification may be detected in the intracranial part of the tumor, entirely unsuspected from the clinical data; or a bony prominence may indicate an underlying growth. In none of the tumors has enlargement of the sphenoidal fissure indicated intracranial participation in the tumor.

From symptoms alone, intracranial extension of the tumor would have been suspected in perhaps two cases. In case 12 there was headache but no papilledema, and in case 14 there were uncinate attacks.

The Operative Procedure

For exposure of the orbital roof, the regular hypophyseal approach is made. The concealed incision has for many years been employed in all operations upon the brain, with no loss of room or increased difficulty of approach. The cutaneous incision begins about 2 cm. anterior to the ear passes straight toward the midline and, when about 3 cm. from it, makes a sharp curve forward and ends anteriorly at, or slightly in front of, the hairline. The galea and skin are then stripped from the bone and temporal muscle and retracted anteriorly.

The bone flap is made so that the anterior border misses the frontal sinus and skirts the supraorbital ridge as far laterally as possible. When turned back and broken under the temporal muscle it is retracted laterally and is well out of the way. The dura is opened just within the bony margin and the roughly circular incision is so complete that it becomes practically an autotransplant, thus being a factor in preventing postoperative extradural bleeding. The frontal lobe is elevated and the cisterna chiasmatis evacuated, thus reducing the volume of the intracranial contents and providing room for attack upon the roof of the orbit. The head is then lowered to permit the frontal lobe to fall away without the need of traction.

If the cisterna chiasmatis is not opened, the brain so completely fills the operative field that undue pressure would usually be necessary to retract the frontal lobe to a degree sufficient to permit the attack upon the orbit and its contents.

From the optic foramen the dural covering of the orbital roof is incised in a curve sweeping laterally around the outer margin of the orbit, then curving anteriorly almost to the cribriform plate. The dural flap is stripped toward the midline with a periosteal elevator.

The initial opening in the orbital roof can frequently be made by applying slight force with the periosteal elevator at the thinnest point of the bone. The remainder of the roof is removed with rongeurs, care being taken not to extend the defect into the ethmoidal cells. At times the bone is so thickened (by an osteoma) that the chisel is required to make the primary defect, and it may then be necessary to complete the removal of the roof with numerous applications of this instrument.

The capsule of the orbit then presents and is incised longitudinally and the edges retracted. Either the tumor or orbital fat presents, depending upon the position of the growth. If fat presents, it is under pressure and extrudes and must be excised. Identification of the superior rectus muscle is usually immediate, unless the tumor is superimposed. This muscle is surrounded by a silk suture and retracted to one side, thus providing inspection of the entire superior half of the orbit. From this view tumors in any part of the orbit would be found and their extirpation can be carried out deliberately. The optic nerve, the posterior part of the eyeball, and the ophthalmic artery and vein are readily identified. In closing, the dura is snugly resutured, the bone flap replaced and wired, the galea and skin closed without drainage.

The thought doubtless occurs whether a pulsating exophthalmos does not follow removal of the orbital roof. I have looked carefully for such a sequela but have never found it, despite the fact that pulsating exophthalmos is known to occur when the orbital roof is congenitally absent.

Although I have never done a lateral Krönlein operation for an orbital tumor, it does not seem possible that it can provide the exposure for the deliberate painstaking dissection of a tumor needed in order to avoid injury to important structures within the orbit. And for tumors that extend beyond the orbital cavity, the Krönlein operation would, of course, be perfectly futile. When an orbital tumor is small and protrudes anteriorly beyond the orbital ridge, the attack upon the tumor by an incision under the supraorbital ridge is doubtless adequate; but when the tumor extends back of the eyeball, the intracranial approach is advisable.

Before the operation is begun, the size and position of the frontal sinuses should be known. In making the anterior bony incision, it is important that the frontal sinus be avoided. Entry into a frontal sinus is a potential source of infection and of subsequent rhinorrhea. If a frontal sinus is opened, a flap of dura should be tightly sutured over the opening. If an ethmoidal cell is opened, it can be covered with wax and the dural flap replaced over it. A small opening in the frontal sinus may also be covered with wax, but the larger openings would require a dural flap. In none of the cases in this series has the frontal sinus been opened.

The method of attack upon the intracranial part of the tumor is dependent upon the nature and position of the growth. Usually the hypophyseal approach affords ample room. If the middle fossa or temporal lobe contains a large dural growth, it may be necessary to rongeur away an additional area of bone beneath the temporal muscle. This was done in two of our cases. It has not been necessary to enlarge the cutaneous incision or to turn down an additional bone flap, either of which, however, is easily possible if the situation should demand. Retraction of the temporal muscle with or without transverse division of its fibers will, after the underlying bone has been removed, expose most of the temporal lobe and even permit its resection in large part if necessary. The removal of a large dural endothelioma is always a difficult feat and requires ample room. Since the arterial bleeding is from the middle meningeal artery, the tributaries of which cover the middle fossa to the foramen spinosum, it is essential that access to this area be unimpeded by inadequate exposure. The dural attachments should, when possible, be totally excised. As long as the dura along the floor of the middle fossa is the site of origin, this is not difficult; in fact, the removal of this dura also greatly facilitates control of the severe bleeding from the middle meningeal artery. Not infrequently control of this bleeding is best accomplished by immediately following the middle meningeal artery to the foramen spinosum. Ligation or cauterization of the trunk of this vessel is usually far easier and safer than attempting to control the numerous bleeding points from its many branches.

The problems associated with the intracranial portion of these tumors are those encountered in any series of brain tumors. The risk involved in removing combined intraorbital and intracranial growths is confined almost exclusively to the part of the tumor within the cranial chamber, and the group of cases described shows that, even with enormous growths, the danger is relatively slight.

Occasionally the internal carotid artery is surrounded by tumor, or at least attached to it. This complication occurred once in this series of cases. To injure the internal carotid artery or the middle cerebral artery would mean disaster and must be avoided at all hazards. Rather than invite hemiplegia and probably death from arterial thrombosis by shaving the tumor too closely, there is no choice but to leave a nest of cells on this vessel.

When there is some exophthalmos and a dural endothelioma has been completely removed from the middle or anterior fossa, should one open the orbit? The answer is dictated by the fact that the bone about the tumor is thickened because of tumor contained within it. Since the additional exposure of the orbit is simple and not time-consuming and adds practically nothing to the operative risk, the surgical possibilities should be completed in one stage. Moreover, a second stage is much more difficult and the possibilities of a complete cure are reduced.

Conclusion

The operation is offered not only for all combined intraorbital and intracranial tumors, but also for those that are restricted to the orbital cavity. As a matter of fact, it is rarely possible before the operation to be certain whether or not the tumor also lies within the cranial chamber, as so many of them do (roughly 75–80% in this series). Their co-existence should, therefore, be assumed by the law of probability.

For tumors confined to the orbit this operation offers a far better exposure than is possible by any other method. Deliberate, careful dissection of the tumor is possible only by this approach. There is, therefore, much less chance of injury to the extraocular muscles, their nerve supply, the optic nerve, and the ophthalmic vessels by this approach.

It offers the only hope of a permanent cure when the tumor is in both cavities, and for incurable cases it offers the maximum palliative result.

The operative risk—in safe hands—should be very low (4.1% in this series) both for tumors confined to the orbit and for those with intracranial extensions. Prior exenteration of the orbit, or removal of the eyeball, will prevent the utilization of this operation because the orbital tissues will be infected.

Comment: Ever since Dandy launched the operation of transcranial orbitotomy, the procedure has been embraced enthusiastically by the neuro-

346

surgeons, who maintain that unroofing the orbital cavity and resection of the bone covering the optic canal gives the clearest view of the orbital cavity and its contents and permits removal of the tumor without damage to intraorbital structures and without visible deformity and scar. With this technique the globe may be retained without damage except when an optic nerve tumor is close to the eyeball. Meningiomas of the sphenoidal ridge that invade the orbit and meningiomas of the optic nerve sheath that extend extraorbitally are now recognized as falling in the neurosurgeon's domain. Transfrontal orbitotomy is favored for the complete extirpation of gliomas of the optic nerve since they frequently involve the chiasm. Transcranial orbitotomy has also been used for encephaloceles, orbital foreign bodies, orbital abscess, and for decompression of the optic nerve in affected cases of Paget's disease, fibrous dysplasia of the skull and compression of the nerve by a sclerotic carotid artery. Ray favors also the intracranial approach for lesions of the frontal sinus that involve the orbit, such as osteomas or mucoceles, because of the cosmetic advantage over other types of operation. Stallard objects to transcranial orbitotomy because of its significant surgical mortality, stormy postoperative course and the incidence of meningitis, blepharoptosis and weakness of the superior rectus muscle. He maintains that most orbital conditions are satisfactorily handled by a modification of Krönlein's lateral orbitotomy. Naquin reported that after exhausting all diagnostic methods, such as radiography, angiography of both arteries and veins of the orbit, orbital pneumography and ultrasonic mapping, the size, location and character of the orbital tumor often remains still obscure. When a tumor is in the anterior third of the orbit, it should be removed through one of the anterior routes, the size and position of the tumor determining whether the most accessible approach is superior temporal, superior nasal, inferior orbital or lateral transconjunctival. Should the histopathologic report disclose malignancy, exenteration of the orbit is indicated, but only if no evidence of tumor metastasis elsewhere is found.

References

Ray, B. S. Intracranial operations for diseases of the orbit and adjacent structures. Am. J. Ophth., *54:* 581–591, October, 1962.
Stallard, H. B.: A plea for lateral orbitotomy. Brit. J. Ophth., *44:* 718, 1960.
Naquin, H.: Surgical treatment of exophthalmos. Tr. Am. Acad. Ophth. & Otol., *65:* 873–878, Nov.–Dec., 1961.

Biographical Note

Walter Edward Dandy (1885–1946) was born in Sedala, Missouri, 2 years after his parents emigrated from England. On graduation from the University of Missouri in 1907 he declined a Rhodes scholarship so as not to delay his medical training at Johns Hopkins Medical School. While a senior medical student he described in detail a 2 mm. human embryo, the youngest specimen in Prof. Mall's collection. After graduation he started a career of investigation, and at Cushing's direction began with the vascular and nervous connections of the pituitary gland. On leaving for Harvard, Cushing first invited Dandy to join him, then changed his mind, and thereafter the future relations between the two were strained. Dandy's first major research was on the cause of hydrocephalus. He found that nearly half of all brain tumors are in the brain stem or cerebellum in a location where they interfere with the circulation of cerebrospinal fluid and so give rise to hydrocephalus. He initiated the use of phenolsulfonphthalein for testing the patency of the aqueduct of Sylvius. In 1918, he introduced pneumo-ventriculography, the greatest single contribution ever made for the early diagnosis and precise localization of brain tumors. Dandy perfected the technique for total removal of acoustic nerve tumors, reducing the postoperative mortality from 70 to 10 per cent; and popularized the operation of intracranial section of the vestibular nerve for Ménière's disease. In 1922, the year that he became the neurosurgeon of Johns Hopkins Hospital, he devised an operation for the relief of internal hydrocephalus in infants and made his signal contribution to ophthalmology by inaugurating the transcranial approach for the removal of orbital tumors. In 1941 he reported intracranial extension of a primary orbital tumor in 80 per cent of 31 patients. Meningioma was the commonest tumor that involved both the intracranial cavity and the orbit. In 1927 and 1928 he removed the entire right hemisphere in 5 patients with an invasive brain tumor, all of whom exhibited no subsequent mental symptoms nor loss of memory. Though Cushing was America's pioneer neurosurgeon, Dandy had to an even greater extent the creative imagination, intuition, and persistence that is characteristic of genius.

Reference

Crowe, S. J.: *Halsted of Johns Hopkins: The Man and His Men.* Ch. V, pp. 85–111. Charles C Thomas, Springfield, Ill., 1957.

On Semi-decussation of the Optic Nerves

WILLIAM HYDE WOLLASTON, M.D., F.R.S.

London

ROYAL SOC. OF LONDON, PHILOSOPHICAL TRANS., 1824, *114* (1): 222–231

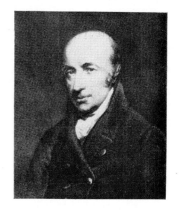

The subject of my inquiry relates solely to the course by which impressions from images perfectly formed are conveyed to the sensorium, and to that structure and distribution of the optic nerves on which the communication of these impressions depends.

Without pretending to detect by manual dexterity as an anatomist, the very delicate conformation of the nerves of vision, I have been led, by the casual observation of a few instances of diseased vision, to draw some inferences respecting the texture of that part which has been called the decussation of the optic nerves, upon which I feel myself warranted to speak with some confidence.

It is well know that in the human brain these nerves, after passing forward to a short distance from their origin in the thalami nervorum opticorum, unite together, and are, to appearance, completely incorporated; and that from this point of union proceed two nerves, one to the right, the other to the left, eye.

The term decussation was applied to this united portion, under the supposition that, though the fibers do intermix, they still continue onward in their original direction, and that those from the right side cross over wholly to supply the left eye, while the right eye is supplied entirely from fibers arising from the left thalamus.

In this opinion, anatomists have felt themselves confirmed by the result of their examination of other animals, and especially that of several species of fish, in which it is distinctly seen that the nerves do actually cross each other as a pair of separate cords, lying in contact at their crossing, but without any intermixture of their fibers.

In these cases it is most indisputably true, that the eye upon the right side of the animal does receive its optic nerve from the left side of the brain, while that of the left eye comes from the right side; but it is not a just inference to suppose the same continuity preserved in other animals, where such complete separation of the entire nerves is not found.

On the contrary, not only do I see reason, from a species of blindness which has happened to myself more than once, to conclude that a different distribution of nerves takes place in us, but I think my opinion supported by this evident difference of structure in fishes.

It is now more than 20 years since I was first affected with the peculiar state of vision, to which I allude, in consequence of violent exercise I had taken for two or three hours before. I suddenly found that I could see only half the face of a man I met; and it was the same with respect to every object I looked at. In attempting to read the name JOHNSON, over a door, I saw only "SON"; the beginning of the name being wholly obliterated to my view. In this instance the loss of sight was toward my left, and was the same whether I looked with the right eye or the left. This blindness was not so complete as to amount to absolute blackness, but was a shaded darkness without definite outline. The complaint was of short duration, and in about a quarter of an hour might be said to be wholly gone, having receded with a gradual motion from the center of vision obliquely upward to the left.

Since this defect arose from overfatigue, a cause common to many other nervous affections, I saw no reason to apprehend any return of it, and it passed away without need of remedy, without any further explanation, and without my drawing any useful inference from it.

It is now about 15 months since a similar affection occurred again, without my being able to assign any cause whatever or to connect it with any previous or subsequent indisposition. The blindness was first observed, as before, in looking at the face of a person, whose left eye was obliterated to my sight. My blindness was in this instance the reverse of the former, being to the right (instead of to the left) of the spot to which my eyes were directed; so that I have no reason to suppose it in any manner connected with the former affection.

The new punctum cecum was situated alike in both eyes, and at an angle of about three degrees from the center; for, when any object was viewed at the distance of about five yards, the point not seen was about 10 inches distant from the point actually looked at.

On this occasion the affection, after having lasted with little alteration for about 20 minutes, was removed suddenly and entirely by the excitement of agreeable news respecting the safe arrival of a friend from a very hazardous enterprise.

In reflecting upon this subject, a certain arrangement of the optic nerves has suggested itself to me, which appears to afford a very probable interpretation of a set of facts, which are not consistent with the generally received hypothesis of the decussation of the optic nerves.

Since the corresponding points of the two eyes sympathize in disease, their sympathy is evidently from structure and not from mere habit of feeling together, as might be inferred, if reference were had to the reception of ordinary impressions alone. Any two corresponding points must be supplied with a pair of filaments from the same nerve, and the seat of a disease in which similar parts of both eyes are affected must be considered as situated at a distance from the eyes at some place in the course of the nerves where these filaments are still united, and probably in one or the other thalamus nervorum opticorum.

It is plain that the cord, which comes finally to either eye under the name of optic nerve, must be regarded as consisting of two portions, one half from the right thalamus and the other from the left thalamus nervorum opticorum.

According to this supposition, decussation will take place only between the adjacent halves of the two nerves. That portion of nerve which proceeds from the right thalamus to the right side of the right eye, passes to its destination without interference; and in a similar manner the left thalamus will supply the left side of the left eye with one part of its fibers, while the remaining halves of both nerves, in passing over to the eyes of the opposite sides must intersect each other, either with or without intermixture of their fibers.

Now, if we consider rightly the facts discovered by comparative anatomy in fish, we shall find that the crossing of their entire nerves to the opposite eyes is in perfect conformity to this view of the arrangement of the human optic nerves. The relative position of the eyes to each other in the sturgeon is so exactly back to back, on opposite sides of the head, that they can hardly see the same object; they can have no points which generally receive the same impressions as we do; there are no corresponding points of vision requiring to be supplied with fibers from the same nerve. In this animal, an injury to the left thalamus might be expected to occasion entire blindness of the right eye alone, and want of perception of objects placed on that side. In ourselves, a similar injury to the left thalamus would occasion blindness (as before) to all objects situated to our right, owing to insensibility of the left half of the retina of both eyes.

A disorder that has occurred within my own knowledge in the case of a friend, seems fully to confirm this reasoning, as far as a single instance can be depended upon. After he had suffered severe pain, for some days, about the left temple and toward the back of the left eye, his vision became considerably impaired, attended with other symptoms indicating a slight compression on the brain.

It was not until after the lapse of three or four weeks that I saw him, and found that, in addition to other affections which need not here be enumerated, he labored under a defect of sight similar to my own, but more extensive, and it has unfortunately been far more permanent. In this case the blindness was at that time, and still is, entire, with reference to all objects situated to the right of his center of view. Fortunately, the field of his vision is sufficient for writing perfectly. He sees what he writes, and the pen with which he writes, but not the hand that moves the pen. This affection is, as far as can be observed, the same in both eyes, and consists in an insensibility of the retina on the left side of each eye. It seems most probable, that some effusion took place at the time of the original pain on that side of the head, and has left a permanent compression on the left thalamus. This partial blindness has now lasted so long without sensible amendment, as to make it very doubtful when my friend may recover the complete perception of objects on that side of him.

In reviewing the several phenomena that I have described, we find partial blindness occurring at the same time in both eyes. This sympathy from disease is readily explained, on the supposition that the parts which sympathize receive their nerves from the same source, while the opposite halves of the eyes, which are not at the same time similarly affected, are supplied from an opposite source; and the inference is immediate, that in common vision also the sympathy of corresponding points, which receive similar impressions from the same object, is dependent on the arrangement of nerves thus detected by disease.

We find, moreover, in the sturgeon (and it is the same in some other fish) whose eyes can scarcely see the same object at once and have no corresponding points which ordinarily sympathize, that the two eyes do not receive any nervous fibers from the same source; but one eye receives its nerve wholly from one side, and the other from the other side of the brain.

From the structure of these fish we learn distinctly, that the perception of objects toward one side is dependent on nerves derived from the opposite side of the brain; and in the last case of diseased vision above related, we find apparent injury to one side of the brain, followed by blindness toward the opposite side of the point to which both eyes are directed.

A series of evidence in such apparent harmony throughout, seems clearly to establish that distribution of nerves I have endeavored to describe, which may be called the semi-decussation of the optic nerves.

It may perhaps to some person appear surprising, that so many as three instances of a disorder which they presume to be rare, should have been witnessed by one individual; but I apprehend, on the contrary, this half-blindness to be far more common than is generally supposed; and I might with as much reason express surprise at its having so far escaped notice, were I not aware of how many facts commonly remain disregarded, merely for want of explanation. It is evident that I once, and for a long time, overlooked the inference that is to be drawn from this affection; and if the disorder had not happened to me a second time, I might never have reconsidered its cause.

Even since the preceding pages were written, I have met with two more cases of this disease. One of my friends has been habitually subject to it for sixteen or seventeen years, whenever his stomach is in any considerable degree deranged. In him the blindness has been invariably to the right of the center of vision, and, from want of due consideration, had been considered as temporary insensibility of the right eye; but he is now satisfied that this is not really the case, but that both eyes have been similarly affected with half-blindness. This symptom of his indigestion usually lasts about a quarter of an hour or twenty minutes, and then subsides, without leaving any permanent imperfection of sight.

I have not seen the subject of the fifth case, but I am informed that he has had many returns of this affection, generally attended with headache, and always lasting about twenty minutes, with very little variation.

Comment: Isaac Newton in the first edition of *Opticks* (1704) first formulated the hypothesis of semi-decussation. The hemianopsia accompanying the migraine to which Newton was subject very probably suggested the concept. In 1723, Vater and Heinicke (cited by Mackenzie) described several clinical cases of hemianopsia for which an explanation by Newton's hypothesis was offered. Chevalier Taylor also adopted this view and contributed a drawing clearly illustrating this assumption (*The Mechanism, or New Treatise of the Anatomy of the Globe of the Eye,* 1738). After Wollaston revived the theory, the idea of semi-decussation received immediate acceptance and was popularized by the physiologist, Johann Müller; but a half-century later the question became a controversial issue. Though Gudden apparently had confirmed its occurrence by serial sections of the chiasma, Michel held that his personal studies indicated that the

353

nerve fibers crossed completely. He argued that the semi-decussation theory could not account for binocular nasal hemianopsia on the basis of a single lesion and that only by assuming total decussation could all possible forms of hemianopsia be logically explained. Schoen countered that bi-nasal hemianopsia, if it did exist, was extremely rare. Other champions of semi-decussation were von Graefe, Hirschberg, Knapp, Mauthner and Hughlings Jackson; and this viewpoint became definitely established by the authoritative studies of Cajal and the accumulation of postmortem evi-dence. Three years after Wollaston's paper on hemianopsia he noted an immobility of the right pupil and numbness of the left arm. At his death the following year an autopsy revealed that a tumor as large as a hen's egg had invaded the right optic thalamus. Considering the size of the lesion it is surprising that his intellect remained unclouded to the last. The tumor was evidently sufficiently slow-growing to permit for some time an adjustment of the nerve structures.

Biographical Note

William Hyde Wollaston (1766–1828) was the second of 17 children. His grand-uncle was the eminent Dr. William Heberden. After study in Cam-bridge and London, he graduated in medicine in 1793 but failed to win success as a practitioner. On receiving a small legacy in 1800, he abandoned practice and zealously embarked on a career of independent investigation. From a process of purifying and welding platinum, he made $150,000 and incidentally discovered the elements, palladium and rhodium. His op-tical contributions include the determination of the refractive index by utilizing the critical angle, the discovery of the dark lines in the solar spec-trum and of ultraviolet activity. The most noteworthy of his numerous in-ventions were the reflecting goniometer for the measurement of crystals, the doublet used as the objective of the compound microscope, the camera lu-cida, the double-image prism, and meniscus lenses. Other investigations con-tributed to astronomy, acoustics, mechanics, mineralogy and botany. The present British imperial gallon was standardized at his suggestion to that containing 10 pounds of distilled water at 62°F. After learning the fatal nature of his illness, he bequeathed his wealth for the promotion of re-search and spent his last months in completing unfinished scientific papers and experiments.

References

Bell, J. M.: Chiasma. in *The American Encyclopedia of Ophthalmology*, 1914, *3:* 2039–2046.
Lebensohn, J. E.: Wollaston and hemianopsia. Am. J. Ophth., 1941, *24:* 1053–1056.

Four Cases of Spinal Myosis; with Remarks on the Action of Light on the Pupil

D. ARGYLL ROBERTSON, M.D.

Edinburgh, Scotland

EDINBURGH MEDICAL JOURNAL, *15:* 487–493 (DEC.) 1869

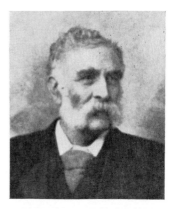

George Smith, age 51, tailor, applied to me for advice on account of dimness of sight. He had, moreover, occasional numbness in his legs, especially the right, with want of power, so that in walking he staggered, and had to use a stick. He could not stand steadily in the dark, but had to grasp at some object for support. He has noticed that objects appear darker than they used to, and that he requires more light while working than formerly sufficed. On examination, I found that while walking his gait was unsteady, and that he also exhibited considerable awkwardness in turning. On looking at the eyes, the drooping of the lids and the small size of the pupils at once attracted attention. The left palpebral aperture at the widest point measured only 3¾ lines, while the right measured 4 lines. Each pupil measured ¾ line in diameter; they were insensible to the influence of light, but contracted to ½ line during the act of accommodation for a near object. Under repeated instillations of a strong solution of sulphate of atropine, the right pupil became dilated to a little beyond medium size, so that it measured 2¾ lines in diameter, and was quite immobile. With the ophthalmoscope a slight degree of atrophy, with shallow cupping of the right optic nerve was discovered.

John Grey, age 35, a clerk, was admitted to the Royal Infirmary, complaining of weakness in his legs and right arm. He enjoyed good health until fifteen years ago, when he contracted syphilis. He has never had any eruption, nor sore throat. Nine years ago, he had an attack of hemiplegia, which affected the left side of the face and right side of the body. When nearly convalescent, he consulted Dr. Christison for convergent squint of the left eye. There is very marked contraction of

354

pupils. They each measure half a line in diameter, are insensible to light, but contract during the act of accommodation for near objects. There is no drooping of the eyelids. He walks with a peculiar straddling gait. There is partial anesthesia in the right iliac and inguinal regions. He does not complain of headache, but considers his memory affected. With either eye he is able to read fine print, and is able to distinguish colors perfectly. A drop of a strong solution of atropine was introduced into the left eye. The following day the left pupil measured two lines in diameter. With the ophthalmoscope a slight degree of cupping and lighter color of the optic disc, indicating a little atrophy of nerve substance, was discovered.

John Dann, age 43, iron-turner, was admitted to the Royal Infirmary complaining of a staggering and inability to walk, and dimness of sight. He observed, while washing his face, that, on shutting his eyes, he could not help falling forwards on to the basin. Dr. Balfour found that the skin of the trunk and extremities was insensible to pain. He complained of the sensation of a tight cord round his waist. On examining his eyes I found the left pupil more contracted than the right; the left measuring ¾ line, the right 1 line in diameter. There is a tendency to divergent strabismus of the left eye. Vision in the right eye is perfect, but with the left only moderate-sized print can be read. The pupils are insensible to light, while atropine only occasions medium dilatation (to 2 lines). On ophthalmoscopic examination both optic nerves were found considerably injected.

Robert Clerk, age 66, a clerk, was admitted complaining of general debility. His gait is unsteady. Both pupils are of the same size, and markedly contracted, measuring barely 1 line in diameter, and only partial dilatation (to 2½ lines) ensues on the application of a strong atropine solution. No alteration in the size of the pupil is observable under the influence of light, but when near objects are looked at contraction at once ensues. Vision is good, though not perfect in both eyes, and there is no color blindness. On ophthalmoscopic examination a slightly atrophic condition of the optic nerves was observable.

* * * * *

These four cases serve well to illustrate the connexion between certain eye symptoms and a diseased condition of the spinal cord. In all of them there was marked contraction of the pupil, which differed from myosis due to other causes, in that the pupil was insensible to light, but contracted still further during the act of accommodation for near objects, while strong solutions of atropine only induced a medium dilatation of the pupil. In three of the cases a slight degree of atrophy of the optic nerves existed, as was evinced by a shallow excavation and lighter color of the optic disc. In one, we observed a symptom which has been noticed occasionally in spinal disease—namely, a drooping of the upper lids. In none of the cases was there appreciable color-blindness. As regards the nature of the spinal lesion, in one case the characters of locomotor ataxy were well marked; in the others the form of spinal affection is doubtful.

To most of the eye-symptoms found in these cases I alluded at length in a previous communication (On an Interesting Series of Eye-Symptoms in a Case of Spinal Disease, with Remarks on the Action of Belladonna on the Iris. Edinburgh Med. J., *14:* 696–708 (Feb.) 1869). But I now desire to direct special attention to a very remarkable circumstance which I noticed in the case that formed the subject of my previous paper, and which I again observed in all the above cases, viz., that although the retina is quite sensitive, and the pupil contracts during the act of accommodation for near objects, yet an alteration in the amount of light admitted to the eye does not influence the size of the pupil. This cannot be explained by the supposition that the pupil is already so small as to be incapable of further contraction under light; because (in the healthy eye) a still further degree of contraction of the pupil may be effected by the use of the Calabar bean, and yet the pupil varies in size according to the intensity of the light. The only possible solution of the difficulty is to be found in the theory, that for contraction of the pupil under light it is necessary that the cilio-spinal nerves remain intact, and, as in these cases of myosis the cilio-spinal nerves are paralyzed, light does not influence the pupil. In all of them the retina was thoroughly sensitive to light, and in all of them the ciliary branches of the third nerve were healthy and active (as was shown by the further contraction of the pupil during the act of accommodation, which can only be referred to these nerves). But in all there were symptoms of spinal disease, and in all myosis due to paralysis of the cilio-spinal nerves. I am aware that a dilated immobile condition of the pupil has been found to follow division of the third pair in animals, and that in cases of complete paralysis of the third pair, the pupil is dilated usually and insensible to light. For a thorough solution of this question, further experiments and clinical observation are necessary.

Comment: All Robertson's cases were obviously syphilitic although syphilis of the central nervous system was not diagnosed in such cases till 1897. The typical Argyll Robertson pupil is most frequent in tabes (61 per cent) and dementia paralytica (50 per cent). When the treatment of these diseases with malaria is successful, recovery of the pupillary light reflex may occur. The essential characteristics of the Argyll Robertson pupil are inactivity to light, both directly and consensually, with unimpaired or increased contraction in accommodation and convergence and good visual acuity. Miosis is a prerequisite; the Argyll Robertson pupil does not lose its light reaction until the pupillary diameter is 2.5 mm. or less. If the pupil dilates with cocaine, it will constrict to light both directly and consensually. Accessory signs are irregularity and eccentricity of pupils, anisocoria and incomplete dilatation with atropine. The iris presents atrophy and depigmentation with thinning of the trabeculae and disappearance of the crypts. Pupils with only light rigidity have been noted in syphilis, mesencephalic tumors, lethargic encephalitis, herpes zoster ophthalmicus, disseminated sclerosis, diabetes and in lesions of the orbit involving the ciliary ganglion or its efferent path. In these conditions, as also in Adie's tonic pupils, the pupils are dilated. The site of the lesion that produces the bilateral or unilateral Argyll Robertson pupil is still unsettled. For many years the phenomenon was attributed to disease of the upper part of the cord, as originally suggested by Argyll Robertson, but later studies demonstrated that degeneration in this region does not necessarily occur. Langsworthy and Ortega, and recently Apter, proposed that the lesion involved the nerves within the iris. This is supported by the atrophy of the iris characteristic of syphilitic cases. According to Langsworthy and Ortega, a lesion to the blood vessels is primary. Following partial occlusion the intrinsic nerves of the iris become atrophied and weakened musculature results. As the accommodation reflex is more powerful than the light reflex, it would overcome the inertia of the weak sphincter pupillae. Apter found that the iris of every eye having an Argyll Robertson pupil was definitely abnormal; the crypts and collarette were obliterated, fine radial striations were seen and frequently the iris could be transilluminated. Using the biomicroscope she found unilateral Argyll Robertson pupils in 13 of 46 patients with neurosyphilis.

Reference

Apter, J. T.: The significance of the unilateral Argyll Robertson pupil. Am. J. Ophth., *38:* 34–43, 209–222, (July–Aug.) 1954.

Bibliographical Note

Douglas Argyll Robertson (1837–1909) was born in Edinburgh of a medical family. His father and two paternal uncles were distinguished surgeons. Robertson received his medical degree from St. Andrews College, Edinburgh in 1857 when Bowman and von Graefe were at the height of their fame. After studying with von Arlt in Prague and von Graefe in Berlin, he returned to Edinburgh to devote himself exclusively to ophthalmology. Robertson received an appointment to the Eye Dispensary of Edinburgh which his deceased father helped to found, and started a career of teaching ophthalmology at the University of Edinburgh to many generations of students. From 1867 to 1897 he also served as ophthalmic surgeon to the Edinburgh Royal Infirmary. In 1863 his paper, "On the Calabar bean as a new agent in ophthalmic medicine," created immediate interest in this first miotic. In 1869 and 1870 he directed attention to an eye finding in tabes—loss of the pupillary reaction to light while retaining that for accommodation. In regard to this, his friend Critchett remarked that it was far better to be an Argyll Robertson pupil than to have one. In 1876 he presented the first trephine operation for glaucoma. His total of over 50 papers, all marked by lucid language and orderly reasoning, covered also diphtheritic conjunctivitis, lupus of the eyelid, asteroid hyalitis, tenotomy of the superior rectus, ectropion surgery and subconjunctival Filaria Loa. In 1886 Robertson was elected president of the Royal College of Surgeons of Edinburgh, a post occupied by his father in 1848. In 1896 he was awarded an honorary LL.D. by the University of Edinburgh, and eventually was honored with every office of distinction in ophthalmology. He was in turn president of the Edinburgh Medico-Chirurgical Society (1896), of the Section on Ophthalmology of the British Medical Association (1898) and of the Ophthalmological Society of the United Kingdom (1893–95)—the first ophthalmic surgeon outside London to achieve this distinction. In 1894 he presided at the Edinburgh meeting of the International Congress of Ophthalmology. Robertson belonged to the German Ophthalmological Society and attended its meetings at Heidelberg; he was a Corresponding Fellow of the New York Academy of Medicine and an honorary member of the Neurological Society of New York.

Robertson had a handsome, striking appearance. His recreations were golf, shooting, archery, and fishing in all of which he excelled. His wife's favored ornament was a necklace formed of the numerous gold medals he had won at golf. Robertson loved travel and visited America in 1892 while touring the world. In recognition of his merit as an art connoisseur he was appointed a judge of the Royal Scottish Academy. He had a lively sense of humor and would exhort mothers to put the bread poultices in the child's stomach but never on the eye. When he retired in 1904 to make his home on the island of Jersey, his professional brethren presented him with his portrait painted by Sir George Reid. He died suddenly in India while paying a second visit to his friend, the Thakur of Gondal, escorting the latter's son and daughter, whose education had been intrusted to the Robertsons. His body was cremated at the burning ghat on the banks of the river Gondli. As a final tribute the Thakur himself kindled the funeral pyre.

Reference

Obituary. Ophthalmoscope, 7: 135–141, (Feb.) 1909.

The Importance in Clinical Diagnosis of Paralysis of Associated Movements of the Eyeballs, Especially of Upward and Downward Associated Movements

WILLIAM G. SPILLER, M.D.

Philadelphia, Pennsylvania

EXCERPTS FROM J. NERV. & MENT. DIS., *32:* 417–426, 497–530, 1905

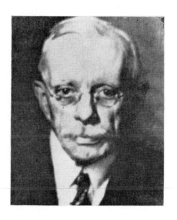

The disturbances of the upward or downward associated movements have been studied less than those of lateral associated movement. The former, though usually acquired, may be congenital. We have little anatomical or pathological evidence concerning the existence of a cortical center for upward or downward associated movements, but in reasoning from analogy we must assume that such a center or centers exist.

Parinaud pointed out that the downward movement in following a finger is a reflex act and better performed than a voluntary movement. The dissociation between the voluntary and reflex movements is not always hysterical. When the condition is hysterical, there is no inconvenience from the ocular disturbance, just as there is no inconvenience from the contraction of the visual fields and Parinaud has never seen a hysterical patient incline the head forward in order to make use of the superior part of the field of fixation.

All the pathological evidence that I have been able to obtain in cases of persistent palsy of associated upward or downward movement is indicative of a lesion near the aqueduct of Sylvius.

My first case is evidence that the nuclei of the superior rectus and inferior oblique muscles may be in the posterior part of the oculomotor nucleus, because there was paresis of upward associated movements and the nerve cells of the oculomotor nuclei were not diseased, but the posterior part of the nuclei was affected by pressure from the tumor in the pons, and the aqueduct of Sylvius was compressed. The paralysis of left associated lateral movement is explained by the almost complete destruction of the left half of the pons by a tubercle, and thereby involvement of the posterior longitudinal bundle. As downward movement was normal, this would seem to be evidence that the nucleus of the inferior rectus muscle must be in advance of those for the superior rectus and inferior oblique. It is probable therefore that a lesion of the nuclei of the inferior rectus muscles and of the fibers connecting them with the nuclei of the trochlear nerves would cause paralysis of downward movement.

It is striking that the paralysis of downward associated movement (necessitating the implication of two separate nuclei of ocular muscles) without paralysis of upward associated movement is exceedingly rare, far more so than is the isolated paralysis of upward associated movement.

I have studied 38 cases of paralysis of upward or downward associated movement reported in the literature, and 9 of my own. As a result of my study of these 47 cases,—

Paralysis of upward associated movement without paralysis or paresis of downward associated movement was found in 26 cases.

Paralysis of upward associated movement with paralysis or paresis of downward associated movement was found in 16 cases.

Paralysis of upward associated movement with impairment of lateral movement, often developing later, was found in 15 cases.

Paralysis of upward associated movement without impairment of lateral movement was found in 22 cases.

Paralysis of downward associated movement without paralysis of upward associated movement was found in 5 cases, but in none of my 9 cases.

The reaction of the iris was found to be impaired in 14 cases, and is said to have been normal in 4 cases. Convergence was impaired in 15 cases. Ptosis was found in 7 cases. Necropsy was obtained in 19 cases. In all of these cases except one parts about the aqueduct of Sylvius were implicated, and in that one a gumma was found in the cerebral peduncles. Tumor was found in 14 cases, a bullet wound in one case, a cyst in one case, hemorrhage in one case and an uncertain lesion in one case. Recovery or partial recovery occurred in 7 cases. Important symptoms other than ocular palsies were found in 41 cases.

As a result of my studies I believe that persistent paralysis of associated upward or downward movement indicates a lesion in the vicinity of the oculomotor nucleus. The paralysis of associated ocular muscles may be produced by inflammatory lesions or lesions of a similar character, as well as by tumor, and may disappear later in the course of the disease.

Comment: Paralysis of vertical movements is much more rare than paralysis of horizontal movements. The remarkable progress, since Spiller's investigations, in more precise localization of the areas involved in paralysis of vertical movements is well summarized by Duke-Elder (*Textbook of Ophthalmology*, Vol. IV, p. 4163): "It indicates with considerable exactitude a lesion (hemorrhagic, neoplastic or degenerative) in the upper peduncular region in front of the corpora quadrigemina and near the posterior commissure. In this region localized damage may cause loss of vertical movements, most usually of upward movements, and least frequently of downward movement alone. The supranuclear location of the lesion is proved if Bell's phenomenon is intact (i.e. if the eyes turn upwards when they are closed in sleep) and if vestibular reflexes can still be elicited when the head is flexed or extended. The center for upward movement is at a higher level than that for downward movement, since a lesion extending downward abolishes the former before the latter. With loss of elevation there is commonly a retraction of the upper lid and sometimes a disturbance of the pupillary reaction to light. On the other hand, a lesion in the lower half of the pons causes a palsy of downward deviation often associated with ptosis and paresis of convergence." The most common conditions leading to this type of palsy are neoplastic, such as tumors of the third ventricle, and vascular lesions in the midbrain. Small vascular lesions may clear up entirely. Since the supranuclear lesions which account for paralysis of voluntary vertical movements are situated in the vicinity of the afferent pupillomotor pathways, pupillary abnormalities are frequently associated. The pupillary changes may come before the paralysis of vertical movement.

References

Holmes, G.: Observations on ocular palsies. Brit. M. J., 2: 1165, 1931.
Lebensohn, J. E.: Parinauds syndrome: From obstetric trauma with recovery. Am. J. Ophth., 40: 738–740, 1955.

Biographical Note

William Gibson Spiller (1863–1940) was born in Baltimore, educated at a military academy near Philadelphia and graduated from the medical school of the University of Pennsylvania in 1892. He spent the next 4 years in postgraduate study under such masters as Edinger, Oppenheim, Dejerine and Gowers. He returned to Philadelphia to devote himself to neuropathologic research and did not engage in the private practice of neurology until 1910. In 1901 he headed the neurologic department of the Philadelphia Polyclinic Hospital; in 1902 he was appointed Professor of Nervous Diseases at the Women's Medical College; and in 1903 he became professor of neuropathology at the University of Pennsylvania. His presidential address to the American Neurological Association in 1905 on paralysis of vertical conjugate movements was published in the *Journal of Nervous and Mental Diseases* of which he was editor. In 1915 he succeeded Mills to the Chair of Neurology at the University of Pennsylvania and became one of the chiefs at the Philadelphia General Hospital. Spiller was the first to recognize the medullary syndrome resulting from occlusion of the anterior spinal artery and reported the first necropsy of a case having the anterior internuclear paralysis of Lhermitte. His papers on surgical intervention for trigeminal neuralgia led to the modern operation of retro-Gasserian neurectomy. His publications totalled almost 250. Among his major works was *The Eye and Nervous System* (1906), edited by him and W. C. Posey. In 1935 Spiller received the honorary degrees of D.Sc. from the University of Pennsylvania and LL.D. from Lafayette College. Other honors included corresponding membership in the neurologic societies of Paris, Vienna, Germany and Estonia. American neurology was cradled by Weir Mitchell, reached adolescence under Mills and attained maturity under Spiller and Sachs.

Reference

McConnell, J. W.: Obituary. Arch. Neurol. & Psychiat., *44:* 175–179, 1940.

Paratrigeminal Paralysis of
Oculo-pupillary Sympathetic

J. G. RAEDER, M.D.

Oslo, Norway

Brain, *47:* 149–158, May 1924

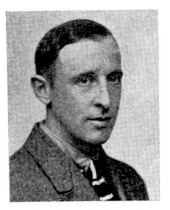

The syndrome of Horner has its name from a case of paralysis of the cervical sympathetic described by Horner in 1869, in which the clinical symptoms were ptosis, miosis, enophthalmos, and hypotonia of the right eye; also hyperemia and moistness of the skin of the same side of the face. Without going into details I shall briefly recapitulate the anatomy of these fibers. The oculo-pupillary fibers reach the base of the brain with the internal carotids, as the plexus caroticus internus. Some of these run as fine filaments to the Gasserian ganglion and join the first branch of the trigeminal nerve, others accompany the oculo-motor nerve. Those that join the trigeminal nerve innervate the dilator pupillae, while the filaments which join the oculo-motor nerves supply the involuntary superior and inferior palpebral muscles.

When the cervical trunk is injured all the symptoms are usually present; they are less complete when the lesion involves the spinal cord. I shall describe some cases of paralysis of the ocular sympathetic in which the lesions could be localized to a limited space, the situation of which justifies the designation "paratrigeminal" paralysis of the sympathetic.

Case 1. A laborer, aged 18, suffered from pains in the left eye, which later extended to the whole left side of the head, cheek, and teeth of the left upper jaw. There was no difference between the two sides of the face, and no change in perspiration. The left palpebral fissure was not so wide as the right. This diminution was due to a ptosis of the upper lid and to a slight elevation of the lower. The pupils were unequal, the right being 5 and the left 3 mm. in diameter. They reacted promptly to light, directly and consensually, accomodation and convergence. Both pupils reacted only slightly to painful stimuli. Intraocular pressure was

363

15.5 mm. of mercury in the right, 11 mm. in the left eye. The narrower fissure on the left side gave the impression of enophthalmos. Examination also revealed normal acuity and visual fields. The lower jaw deviated to the left when he opened his mouth. From time to time he complained of diplopia; we had the impression that there was a variable paresis of several muscles. The left sympathetic did not react to 1 per cent cocaine. There was therefore a sympathetic pupillary paresis. The radiating pains in the left trigeminal area pointed to disease at the base of the skull. If this lay in such a position as to involve the sympathetic fibers from the internal carotid plexus to the third and fifth cranial nerves, all the symptoms could be explained by a single lesion. No hyperemia of the skin or disturbance of sweat secretion on the face may be explained by the fibers subserving these functions leaving the sympathetic trunk lower down. The patient grew worse and died. Postmortem examination revealed a grayish tumor of firm consistency on the left side. Medially it reached the hypophysis, laterally the Gasserian ganglion. The oculo-motor nerve extended over the tumor, the abducens was displaced laterally. The trochlear nerve seemed to lie underneath the tumor. The growth covered the internal carotid artery. The tumor was regarded as an endothelioma.

Epicrisis. Paresis of the pterygoid muscles, radiating pains in the face and epiphora, indicated a lesion of the trigeminal nerve in addition to paralysis of the sympathetic. The diplopia was due to infiltration of the abducens, trochlear and oculo-motor nerves where they all lie fairly close together.

Case 2. A man aged 65 developed an inward squint of the right eye six months ago. At the same time he noticed that the right eyelid had fallen a little. He suffered with neuralgic pains round the right eye and right part of the forehead, epiphora and headache. The right eye was converged and could not be moved outwards; its downward movement was also defective. The right palpebral fissure was smaller than the left. The pupils were unequal, the right being smaller than the left. An affection of the sympathetic was confirmed by instillation of 1 per cent cocaine. There was also a slight reduction of tactile sensibility in the area of the upper branch of the right trigeminal nerve. Perspiration and the vasomotor state were the same on both sides.

Epicrisis. Paresis of the right fourth and sixth cranial nerves was associated with epiphora, neuralgic pains, and reduced tactile sensibility in the area of the first branch of the trigeminal nerve. The lesion must have lain in the same position as in the first case.

Case 3. A man aged 48 was run over by a motor car. An incomplete syndrome of Horner was found, probably due to a fracture of the base of the skull through the medial part of the left middle fossa. There was ptosis and miosis on the left side, hypesthesia of the left side of the face, and a paracentral temporal scotoma in the left eye. Here the optic nerve, which is situated very close to the region in which we assumed the lesions in the other cases to lie, was involved.

Case 4. A man aged 28. Trigeminal neuralgia on left side. The pain was limited to the distribution of the frontal and supraorbital nerves. There was a definite sympathetic ptosis on the same side. The pronounced inequality that followed the instillation of 1 per cent cocaine indicates a paresis of the sympathetic fibers. This case resembles the affection of the sympathetic by herpes zoster ophthalmicus described by Bing.

Case 5. A laborer, aged 48, was injured by a runaway horse. He was hit in front of the left ear, and was unconscious for several hours. The hearing of his left ear was somewhat reduced, the left side of his face was paretic and anesthetic, and the sight of his left eye was affected. On examination, no ptosis, lagophthalmos, or enophthalmos was observed. The left pupil was smaller than the right in all degrees of illumination and after instillation of 1 per cent cocaine. The left optic disc appeared pale. Vision was reduced to counting fingers at 75 cm., and the field of vision was contracted. There was a left-sided motor trigeminal paresis, the lower jaw deviating to the left. Sensation was diminished in the areas of all three branches of the left trigeminal nerve. No vasomotor disturbances were observed in the face and there was no hypotonia of the eye. The disturbances were probably due to a fracture of the base of the skull through the left middle fossa. In addition to a lesion of the second and fifth cranial nerves, there was a paralysis of the sympathetic which involved only the fibers to the dilator. It must be assumed that the lesion lay in front of the anastomosis between the carotid plexus and the oculomotor nerve, so that the sympathetic fibers to the involuntary palpebral muscle were not injured.

A number of cases of trigeminal neuralgia have been described in which there was also homolateral miosis. I submit that the majority of these cases were actually due to paratrigeminal lesions. The anatomical lesion responsible may be assumed to have more or less the same localization as the tumor found in Case 1.

Comment: Raeder described his first case of the paratrigeminal syndrome in 1918 (Norsk. mag. laegevid., *79:* 999–1015, Sept., 1918). The publication excited extreme interest, since it presented a distinct intracranial localization in which the lesion produced an incomplete Horner's syndrome with involvement of one or more cranial nerves. Anhydrosis was absent, since the sympathetic sudomotor fibers of the face are associated with the external carotid artery and its branches, and not with the internal carotid. Bedrossian reported, in 1952, an apparent case of Raeder's syndrome in which the patient had severe pain and somewhat blurred vision in the left eye for 10 days. Instillation of cocaine dilated the right pupil but not the left, and the instillation of epinephrine (1:1000) dilated the left pupil but not the right. On the following day the patient had pain over the left side of his upper jaw and the dentist extracted an abscessed left upper lateral incisor, after which all symptoms rapidly subsided. Klingon and Smith also encountered a temporary Raeder syndrome that was produced by the inflammatory extension of a right frontomaxillary sinusitis. In their case, the right eye exhibited ptosis, miosis, and enophthalmos, and the sensation of the right cornea was diminished. It is noteworthy that in both cases anhydrosis was present, and was demonstrated in the last patient by the starch-iodine sweat test, whereas in the typical Raeder syndrome anhydrosis is absent. Nevertheless, when Raeder's syndrome is suspected, confirmation by heroic measures such as arteriography and air study should be delayed until the diagnosis is supported by a progression of signs and symptoms.

References

Bedrossian, E. H.: Raeder's syndrome. A. M. A. Arch. Ophth., *48:* 620–623, 1952.
Klingon, G. H., and Smith, S. M.: Raeder paratrigeminal syndrome. Neurology, *6:* 750–753, 1956.

Biographical Note

Johan Georg Raeder (1889–1956), the son of a headmaster, was born in Oslo, Norway. On receiving his medical qualification in 1915, he embarked forthwith for Angola as ship surgeon on a whaling vessel. He fell in love with Africa and it was henceforth his favorite vacation area. In later years he revisited his hunting grounds with a camera and published an illustrated book of his experiences. After his return from his first voyage, Raeder became attached to various eye infirmaries in Oslo and from 1920 to 1925 taught physiologic optics at the University. In 1926 he was appointed ophthalmologist to the Ullevaal Hospital. His assistant in private practice was for many years Dr. Arne Mohn. Raeder was always a zealous innovator. In 1924 he achieved his medical doctorate in ophthalmology with a thesis on the crystalline lens which he studied by an original method. In 1927 he contributed an article with original ideas on the surgical treatment of glaucoma. At home, foil fencing was his hobby and he was an ardent member of the Oslo Fencing Society. He retired because of chronic nephritis, and after a lingering illness died of uremia.

Reference

Keyser, G. W., Oslo, Norway: Personal communication.

Sleep as a Problem of Localization

CONSTANTIN VON ECONOMO, M.D.

Vienna, Austria

J. NERV. & MENT. DIS., 1930, *71:* 249–259

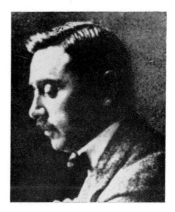

The Viennese ophthalmologist, Mauthner, (Wien. Klin. Wochnschr., *3:* 445, 1890) assumed on the basis of Wernicke's description of encephalitis hemorrhagica superior in drinkers associated with sleep and paralysis of ocular muscles that this interruption of conduction takes place in the region of the aqueduct in the cap of the peduncular region in the interbrain. He thought, then, that a physiological recurring swelling "fatigue edema" of these parts of the brainstem blocked the conduction of the nerve fibers. In a somewhat more complicated manner the interruption was explained by Veronese and Troemner who assumed that the thalamus opticus was the point where the blockade of activity took place.

But even the very promoters of these theories themselves realized that they were not sufficient to explain the sleep mechanism which seemed much more complicated. Purkinje, for instance, who was the first to conceive the idea that the congestion of stem ganglia squeezing the mass of fibers of the corona radiata interrupts conduction, claims in order to explain the periodic return of that congestion that the blood has a chemical action during sleep that provokes that swelling and that it again changes and stimulates the nervous system during the waking state.

We must acknowledge that the chemical theories mentioned, especially that of Weichhardt, Piéron and the hormonal theory of Mingazzini are able to satisfy our desire for seeing cause and effect more than all the others mentioned. And in fact, most of the scientists, physiologists as well as pathologists, were thoroughly contented with these explanations of sleep.

So stood the facts when two years later the appearance of lethargic encephalitis, which I first described in 1916–17, refuted all these state-

368

ments however well founded they appeared. The lethargic epidemic encephalitis shows in its most ordinary somnolent-ophthalmoplegic form, outside of disturbances of the eye muscles, as the most striking symptom, a sopor of different degree varying from simple somnolence to the deepest sopor in which the patients may sleep for weeks and months but from which in the majority of cases, it is possible to arouse them. The disease is produced by an inflammation of the central grey matter localized in the main in the cap of the interbrain at its junction with the thalamus. The inflammation may spread frontally and caudally to other parts of the nervous system and produce other symptoms. So it could be shown later that those cases of encephalitis which began with choreatic unrest presented at the beginning a striking and tormenting insomnia. The combinations chorea and insomnia on the one hand, eye muscle disturbances and sleep on the other hand, and our knowledge that many choreiform diseases originate in the region of the stem ganglia, leads to the assumption that the inflammation in cases associated with insomnia, is localized anteriorly in the lateral wall of the third ventricle, near the corpus striatum while it is localized in cases showing disturbances of ocular muscles with sopor in the posterior wall of the third ventricle near the nuclei of the oculomotorius in the cap of the interbrain.

The lethargic encephalitis produces, furthermore, outside of insomnia and sopor, a number of other disturbances of sleep, for instance, the inversion of sleep *i.e.,* the reversal of the periodicity of sleeping and waking, patients sleeping in the day time and being awake at night. Another very frequent sleep disturbance in encephalitis is what I call the dissociation of cerebral and body sleep and observed in a series of akinetic cases, patients being in day time mentally wideawake while their bodies were akinetic and drowsy as in sleep; at night these patients are again mentally asleep while their bodies are restless, which circumstance produces states of somnambulism. It was supposed by many investigators that it might be the toxic effect of lethargic encephalitis being an infectious disease, that was the reason for the sleep symptoms. But I called attention to the fact that quite a number of other diseases affecting the same region of the nervous system, as lethargic encephalitis does, namely, Wernicke's disease, Gayet's disease, then tumors of the infundibular region present outside of disturbances of the eye muscles, also sopor. Some recent findings in cases of softening (in hemorrhages) of this region have shown the same symptomatology. The consideration that diseases of such different nature can always be productive of sleep if they occur in this region of the nervous system, proves the correctness of the statement that not the individuality of the disease as such, but its localization at this very definite area of the nervous system is decisive for the occurrence of sleep. Inasmuch as furthermore in lethargic encephalitis sleep is disturbed in such various ways as sopor, insomnia, inversion of sleep, dissociation of sleep, etc., we have additional proof that we must consider this region of grey matter as the site from which sleep can be primarily and directly influenced. This area is therefore selective for the function of sleep and as in more than 85 per cent of the cases of encephalitis there occur some troubles of the sleep function, we must suppose that the virus of encephalitis has a special affinity to these accumulations of grey matter which are of special importance for the sleep and which I designate as the "center for regulation of sleep."

We must insist on the anatomical fact that the center for regulation of sleep is in the immediate vicinity of the other important vegetative centers located in the infundibular region and we can suppose that it forms with them a larger physiological entity but that it is, anyhow, to be distinctly separated from the other vegetative centers by its localization as well as by its chemical affinity as its affinity to the virus of encephalitis proves, because in the acute stage of that disease we generally do not find other disturbances of the vegetative nervous system.

Outside of the effects of cerebral functions, the center of sleep regulation certainly exerts a regulating influence as previously mentioned, on the other vegetative and animal components of sleep which we might call "body sleep" for instance the change of respiration, perspiration, metabolism, etc. That influence is effected directly on the neighboring vegetative centers as for instance the centers of temperature, for sugar and calcium content of the blood, for regulation of the water metabolism, etc., which all change during sleep and the centers of which are located in the subthalamic region and in the wall of the third ventricle.

We may, then, assume that the localized mechanism we postulate for the supervision of sleep is really existing and we must look out how best we can localize it. Our experience with cases of lethargic encephalitis and other infundibular processes shows that sopor may occur in these diseases as an isolated symptom but that it appears principally associated with paralysis of eye muscles, especially with ptosis. That corresponds to the most frontal part of the nucleus oculomotorius, so we must place the posterior border of the center for sleep regulation immediately in front of the nuclei of the eye muscles in the grey junction of interbrain and thalamus where the aqueduct of Sylvius opens into the third ventricle.

The anterior part of that center may be located further frontally in the grey walls of the third ventricle near the caput of the corpus caudatum, as we find the symptom of insomnia combined with choreatic disturbances. Pathological-anatomical examination of encephalitis material has not resulted in a more exact localization but I am under the impression that we have to do not so much with a narrowly circumscribed grey nucleus but with a mass of grey substance spreading over the posterior and lateral walls of the third ventricle and reaching laterally also into the hypothalamus. The different parts of that grey matter act in a sort of balancing way. I arrive at this conclusion on account of the multiplicity of sleep disturbances observed in the course of encephalitis.

The problem of more exact localization could only be solved in a conclusive way by physiological experiments. Different attempts in this direction have been made. If these results are verified in the future, irrefutable proof is furnished for the correctness of our conception of a center for the supervision of sleep situated at the junction of the thalamus and the interbrain from which sleep is actively initiated. It is therefore manifest by all these recent studies, that there is an apparatus which controls the general periodic alternation of sleeping and waking, the constellation of our organism similar to high and low tide and similar to other vegetative function centers of the central nervous system.

As we have seen not only lethargic encephalitis but also other diseases of that region in the diencephalon may produce sleep disturbances.

Comment: On May 30, 1890, the Viennese ophthalmologist, Ludwig Mauthner, announced in a brief communication to the Vienna Medical Society an original conception of the mechanism of sleep. Mauthner observed that all chronic forms of sleeping sickness have as a complication ptosis and ocular muscle paralysis and reveal on autopsy engorgement of the walls of the third ventricle and the sylvian aqueduct. Hence he conceived that physiological sleep depends on a cyclic interruption of conduction between the periventricular gray matter and the cortex. He suggested that in drowsiness the drooping of the lids and diplopia indicated that the innervational disturbance that produces sleep extends to the adjacent oculomotor nuclei. Mauthner's notion was ignored for a quarter of a century. As late as 1914, Dejerine, who held the chair of neurology at Paris, asserted with finality that sleep cannot be localized. But in 1916, Economo, after exhaustive study of the pathology in lethargic encephalitis and other forms of epidemic encephalitis, revived the idea of a sleep regulation center, which has been convincingly demonstrated since experimentally. Kleitman, in his monograph, *Sleep and Wakefulness,* agreed with Mauthner in conceiving sleep as a functional break between the cortex and the lower centers. The positive Babinski sign in sleep supports this concept. The diurnal periodicity of sleep arises from the diurnal variations of afferent impulses to the hypothalamic center. The highest temperature of the body, the best performance rate, including visual reaction time and the lowest fatigability are reached in the afternoon. Physiologic sleep stems from an interrelated sequence of muscular fatigue and depression of sympathetic and cortical activity. There are no afferent sympathetic fibers; the sympathetic hypothalamic center is excited wholly by somatic stimuli. The excitation of the hypothalamus, in turn, is the indispensable substratum of cortical activity.

In prolonged vigil, the chief complaints are ocular. Pain in the eyes with itching, burning, dryness and grittiness become increasingly troublesome and are exaggerated by any attempt to read. Edema of the lids and dark circles under the eyes become evident; convergence fails, fixation becomes unsteady and by the fourth day a manifest exotropia of 4 to 5 prism diopters can be measured. All the abnormal ocular findings of prolonged vigil disappear after adequate sleep. Sleep begins with a spastic closure of the lids. A flaccid closure follows, the folds of the lids smooth out and muscular twitchings cease. With the closing of the lids the eyeballs assume their position of rest (Bell's phenomenon). In deep sleep disjunctive movements may occur in the adult, reminiscent of the ocular performance in the first few weeks of life. The pupil constricts, the degree depending on the depth of sleep. On awakening the pupils instantly dilate even though the sleeper is aroused by illumination. The ocular concomitants of sleep are now readily explained. On account of the depression of the sympathetic nerves the deep layer of the levator muscle loses tone, lacrimation ceases, vasomotor tone lessens and vasodilation occurs exciting the production of mucus with the accompanying sensations of grittiness and veiled vision. The extreme miosis of deep sleep, like the positive Babinski sign then present, results from an absence of inhibitory cortical control over the lower motor centers.

Reference

Lebensohn, J. E.: The eye and sleep. Arch. Ophth., *25:* 401–411, 1941.

Biographical Notes

LUDWIG MAUTHNER

Ludwig Mauthner (1840–1894) was born in Prague of Jewish parents and attended the University of Vienna. At the age of 18 he presented his first contribution, "The Structure of the Spinal Cord of the Lower Vertebrates." After graduating medicine at 21, he trained in ophthalmology under the discerning Eduard von Jaeger, who gave him a free hand, saying "I owe it to ophthalmology—for he is a genius." In 1868, at the age of 28, he published a comprehensive text on ophthalmology, with 468 plates and a full bibliography. In the following year Mauthner was called to the chair of ophthalmology at the newly created medical school at Innsbruck. During his incumbency he published an exhaustive work on the optical errors of the eye and edited the German edition of Knapp's *Archives of Ophthalmology and Otology*. After 8 years in this irksome post he resigned and returned to Vienna, where he achieved fame as a lecturer and published a series of ophthalmic monographs. In 1894 he was selected for the chair of ophthalmology at Vienna. On October 19, his nomination was announced; on the following night he died. On March 19, 1899, his friend Schnabel spoke at the unveiling of a memorial bust placed in the arcade of the Vienna University.

Reference

Hirschberg, J.: Obituary. Am. J. Ophth., *11:* 386–388, 1894.

CONSTANTIN VON ECONOMO

Constantin von Economo (1876–1931) was born of Greek parents in Romania, but was educated in Trieste where his family moved the year after his birth. At the age of 14 the reading of Lombroso's *Genius and Insanity* so impressed him that he decided to study medicine. While still an undergraduate at the Vienna Medical School he completed a paper on the avian hypophysis. After graduating medicine in 1901 he studied neurology and psychiatry in Paris, Strassburg and Munich. In 1906 he returned to Vienna as assistant at the psychiatric clinic of Wagner von Jauregg. An enthusiastic amateur aviator, he served during World War I as a pilot on the South Tyrol front until he was ordered back to his medical duties at the University. He then began his outstanding studies on encephalitis lethargica and the nature of sleep for which he is best known. In 1920 he married a daughter of an Austrian general who later cooperated with von Jauregg in writing his biography. In 1925 he published his great atlas on the cytoarchitecture of the adult human cerebral cortex. On the retirement of von Jauregg he was urged to take over the chair of psychiatry but declined since he preferred to pursue research unhampered by administrative duties. Economo possessed independent means, traveled extensively and had a wide range of interests.

Reference

J. von Wagner-Jauregg: Baron Constantin von Economo. His life and work. English translation by R. Spillman. Free Press, Burlington, Vt., 1937.

Pseudo-Argyll Robertson Pupils with Absent Tendon Reflexes

W. J. ADIE, M.D.

London, England

BRIT. M. J., 1931, *1*: 928–930

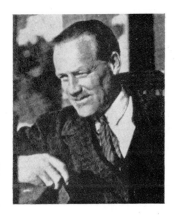

I wish to draw attention to a benign symptomless disorder characterized by pupils which react on accommodation but not to light, and by absent tendon reflexes.

Five of the six cases I am about to describe came under my notice in the course of a few weeks; the condition therefore cannot be very rare. Though harmless in itself it merits recognition because it is often mistaken for a manifestation of syphilis of the nervous system, with unfortunate consequences for the patients and their families.

Case I. A woman aged 36 was admitted to the Hospital for Tropical Diseases under the care of Dr. G. Carmichael Low for an "overhaul" on her return from abroad. Physical examination and routine laboratory tests revealed no evidence of disease apart from the neurologic signs that concern us here. There was nothing in the family or personal history to explain these signs. Ten years ago she noticed that her pupils were unequal. On examination I found pupils of moderate size, the right just larger than the left, which was slightly oval; neither reacted to light, direct or consensual; both contracted fully on convergence, but the movement was remarkably slow; after the effort to converge was relaxed they remained small for several seconds, then dilated very gradually to their original size. All the tendon reflexes in the upper and lower limbs were completely abolished. There were no other signs of organic nervous disease. I knew that this myotonic pupillary reaction had nothing to do with syphilis, but had never seen or heard of it in association with absent tendon reflexes. I reported as follows: "A most unusual case; I prefer not to make a diagnosis; the condition is benign, and should not prevent her from returning to her work abroad." After her

374

discharge, Dr. Low kindly allowed me to consult the hospital notes, and I found that Wassermann's test had been done on the blood and cerebrospinal fluid with negative results.

Case II. A woman aged 23 attended hospital because her brother, an optician, had found that she had Argyll Robertson pupils. She was admitted to the National Hospital for investigation. She knew "what they thought," and was greatly distressed. With the first case in mind I promised her that she should leave the hospital with the stigma removed. Apart from the special signs, nothing of importance was discovered in the course of a thorough routine investigation. The following observations were made: the pupils were unequal, right 3½ mm., left 3 mm.; the right was irregularly oval with the long axis vertical, the left regularly oval with the long axis horizontal. The reaction to light was completely absent in both; the reaction on convergence was present in both, but was abnormal; the contraction was delayed and proceeded slowly until the pupils reached pinpoint size. When the effort to converge was relaxed they dilated very slowly to their original size. The knee and ankle jerks were completely absent. These observations were confirmed repeatedly by myself and my colleagues. The Wassermann reaction was negative in the blood and cerebrospinal fluid. The report on the fluid was as follows: clear, colorless; no cells seen; total protein 0.035 per cent; Nonne-Apelt and Pandy reactions negative; Lange's colloidal gold test, no change (Dr. J. G. Greenfield).

Case III. A young man now aged 32 was brought to me 12 years ago by his sister, a medical student, who discovered that he had Argyll Robertson pupils. I found that his knee jerks were absent, and thought that he was a case of congenital tabes. He came to see me recently about another matter, and I went into his family and personal history and made a complete physical examination. Nothing apart from the neurologic signs suggested syphilis, congenital or acquired. His general health was good. The pupils were moderate in size and unequal, right larger than left. The right was totally inactive to light, the left reacted very feebly. On convergence both pupils contracted very slowly to pinhead size, then dilated still more slowly when he looked into the distance. He had noticed himself that the pupils varied in size from time to time. All the tendon reflexes in the upper and lower limbs were absent. There were no other neurologic signs. He has submitted to several tests of the blood and cerebrospinal fluid, all with negative results.

Case IV. A woman aged 45 attended the Royar London Ophthalmic Hospital for glasses and was referred to me by Mr. Foster Moore, who had noticed the abnormal pupils. There was nothing worthy of note in the family or personal history. Her general physical condition was good. Vision improved to 6/9 right, 6/18 left; no optic atrophy (Mr. Foster

Moore). The pupils were unequal; right 3 mm., left 2½ mm. The left pupil did not react to light; on convergence it contracted slowly but fully, and maintained its smaller size long after convergence had ceased; it then dilated very gradually. The right pupil contracted feebly to light, slightly better on convergence; the contraction was not slow or unduly maintained. The knee jerks were easily obtained and equal, but the ankle jerks were completely absent. The Wassermann reaction in the blood was negative. The cerobrospinal fluid has not yet been examined.

Case V. A girl aged 17 was referred to me by Mr. Foster Moore and admitted to the National Hospital for investigation. She noticed about two years ago that her pupils were unequal, and that the left pupil varied in size from time to time. Four months ago the left pupil became permanently large; since then she has not been able to use it for close work. Otherwise she has always been in perfect health. Examination revealed no other signs except the following: The pupils were unequal; right 2½ mm., left 8 mm. They were both inactive to light; on convergence the right pupil contracted slowly to pinpoint size, and when convergence ceased it again dilated very slowly. The left did not contract on convergence. The knee jerks were brisk. For a patient of her age and compared with the active knee jerks, the ankle jerks were certainly abnormally sluggish. The Wassermann reaction was negative in the blood and cerebrospinal fluid. Report on the cerebrospinal fluid: clear, colorless, 1 cell per cu. mm.; total protein 0.03 per cent.; Nonne-Apelt and Pandy reactions negative; Lange's colloidal gold reaction 0001100000 (Dr. J. G. Greenfield).

Case VI. In an article on the myotonic pupil in Wilbrand and Saenger's Neurologie des Auges, I found a reference to a case described by Gehrcke in which eye signs like those in my cases were found in a patient with "imperfect stationary tabes." The following is an extract of the case history: A woman aged 45; right pupil inactive to light, very slow contraction and relaxation on convergence; ankle jerks absent. There were no other signs of organic nervous disease. The family history was not given. The Wassermann reaction was negative in the blood and cerebrospinal fluid. The Nonne-Apelt, Weichbrodt, and Pandy reactions were all negative; no increase of cells; pressure normal. Nevertheless, because the ankle jerks were absent the diagnosis of tabes was made. This is the only case resembling my own that I have been able to find in the literature. I have not yet completed my search. (See note at end.)

Commentary

It is not surprising that all of these patients with "Argyll Robertson pupils" and absent tendon reflexes were thought to be suffering from syphilis of the nervous system, congenital or acquired. The correct diagnosis can be made with certainty by closely observing the contraction of the pupil during the act of accommodation for near objects. The true Argyll Robertson pupil reacts promptly and fully, often excessively, on convergence, and dilates again as soon as the effort to converge the visual axes is relaxed. In these cases the pupils show the so-called myotonic reaction; they do not respond to light; they contract very slowly through a wide range during a sustained effort to converge; often remain small long after the efforts ends, and when they dilate again, do so slowly. They differ in other ways from the true Argyll Robertson pupil, but the above features are sufficient to distinguish them. This myotonic reaction is well known to ophthalmologists, and it has been firmly established that syphilis plays no part in its production. Mr. Foster Moore has described seven cases under the title "nonluetic Argyll Robertson pupil," and has told me of several others he has seen. The characteristics of his cases are, he says, the complete or substantially complete inaction of the pupil to the light stimulus, the leisurely manner in which it contracts with convergence, and in which it again dilates after relaxation of convergence; the frequency with which it is unilateral; the integrity of accommodation; the absence of syphilis; the presence of knee jerks, and the absence of signs of any nervous disease even after many years.

It seems to me more than probable that some of his cases with nonluetic Argyll Robertson pupils but normal tendon reflexes are examples of a milder form of the same benign disorder that I have described here. I think, too, that my cases are related to those described by Mr. Gayer Morgan and Dr. C. P. Symonds under the titles "A series of cases with rapid onset of unequal pupils and failure of accommodation: a *forme fruste* of encephalitis lethargica," and "Internal ophthalmoplegia with absent tendon reflexes." In their cases the defect was most often unilateral, the affected pupil was dilated, and reacted not at all or incompletely both to light and on convergence; further, accommodation was partially paralyzed, so that visual symptoms were produced. In some of their cases the tendon reflexes were diminished or lost.

My fifth patient seems to me to provide evidence that links the three groups. In one eye her pupil was dilated and fixed, with paralysis of accommodation, as in the cases described by Mr. Morgan and Dr. Symonds; in the other eye accommodation was normal, the light reflex was absent, and the reaction on convergence was myotonic as in the nonluetic Argyll Robertson pupils of Mr. Foster Moore. My fourth case also showed a myotonic pupil on one side and a partially fixed pupil on the other. I have reason to believe that a large fixed pupil is sometimes the forerunner of a myotonic pupil. These and other more academic aspects of the subject I hope to deal with at another time. My object now is to make it known that pupils conforming to the prevailing loose definition of an Argyll Robertson pupil, and easily mistaken for the true Argyll Robertson sign, may be found associated with loss of tendon reflexes in patients with a benign disorder that has nothing to do with syphilis whatsoever.

Note. After this was written, Mr. Foster Moore kindly allowed me to read the typescript of his paper on the nonluetic Argyll Robertson pupil, which he read at the recent Ophthalmological Congress. In one of his 15 patients with this abnormal reaction of the pupil, the knee jerks were absent; in another they were obtained with reinforcement only.

Comment: The myotonic pupillary reaction had been previously described independently by Saenger and Strasburger in 1902. Nonne then observed the association with absent knee and ankle jerks. Adie's first paper on the subject in the British Medical Journal was followed by two additional contributions the following year (Brain, 1932, *55:* 98; Brit. J. Ophth., 1932, *16:* 449) in which he emphasized the atypical forms of the malady and its widespread incidence. The importance of the Adie syndrome, which is essentially benign, rests chiefly in its differential diagnosis from the Argyll Robertson pupil and tabes. The Adie pupil occurs predominantly in females, and is unilateral in 80 per cent of cases. The affected pupil is relatively dilated and its response to a light stimulus (either direct or consensual) and to convergence is so excessively slow as hardly to be noticeable except after dark adaptation, though the fellow pupil reacts normally. The condition is most common in the third decade, is noted suddenly and is permanent. The reactions to atropine, homatropine, cocaine, epinephrine, eserine and pilocarpine are normal though a relative difference in the size of the pupils continues. In contradistinction, the Argyll Robertson pupil affects males predominantly, and is bilateral in 90 per cent of cases; the pupils react readily to convergence and mydriatics produce a slow, incomplete response. Scheie noted that while the instillation of methacholine chloride (mecholyl) in 2.5 per cent concentration does not affect the normal pupil, it produces a prompt constriction of the myotonic pupil. This diagnostic test would seem to place the site of the lesion at the ciliary ganglion or postganglionic fibers. In support of this view Weekers reported four cases in which the retrobulbar injection of ethyl alcohol caused a permanent myotonic pupil, which constricted promptly to stable derivatives of acetylcholine such as mecholyl but not to cholinesterase inhibitors (eserine, isoflurophosphate). Much clinical evidence, however, suggests also an involvement of the diencephalon and its connections.

Reference

Scheie, N. G.: Site of disturbance of Adie's syndrome. Arch. Ophth., 1940, *24:* 225.

Biographical Note

William John Adie (1886–1935) was born in Geelong, Australia, and qualified in medicine at Edinburgh University. In World War I he was cited for gallantry in the field and during the initial gas attacks improvised a urine-dampened mask. After the war he rejoined the neurologic staff of the National Hospital and was appointed physician to the Royal London Ophthalmic Hospital. While at the latter institution Adie wrote on the syndrome of tonic pupils and absent tendon and periosteal reflexes. He was the first to describe the syndrome in detail and to delineate complete and incomplete forms. His other principal contributions were on dystrophia myotonica and narcolepsy. His clinical acumen and teaching ability were noteworthy. In his last years while convalescing from coronary thrombosis at Majorca, he became increasingly engrossed in his hobby of ornithology and bird watching.

Reference

Jelliffe, S. E.: Obituary. J. Nerv. & Ment. Dis., 1935, *81:* 726.

Part Thirteen

Comparative Ophthalmology

The Evolution of the Eye

CHARLES DARWIN

Down, England

EXCERPT FROM *The Origin of Species,* CH. VI, ED. 1, 1859

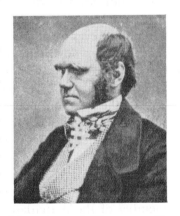

To suppose that the eye with all its inimitable contrivances for adjusting the focus to different distances, for admitting different amounts of light, and for the correction of spherical and chromatic aberration, could have been formed by natural selection, seems, I freely confess, absurd in the highest degree. When it was first said that the sun stood still and the world turned round, the common sense of mankind declared the doctrine false; but the old saying of Vox populi, vox Dei, as every philosopher knows, cannot be trusted in science. Reason tells me, that if numerous gradations from a simple and imperfect eye to one complex and perfect can be shown to exist, each grade being useful to its possessor, as is certainly the case; if further, the eye ever varies and the variations be inherited as is likewise certainly the case; and if such variations should be useful to any animal under changing conditions of life, then the difficulty of believing that a perfect and complex eye could be formed by natural selection, though insuperable by our imagination, should not be considered as subversive of the theory. How a nerve comes to be sensitive to light, hardly concerns us more than how life itself originated; but I may remark that, as some of the lowest organisms, in which nerves cannot be detected, are capable of perceiving light, it does not seem impossible that certain sensitive elements in their sarcode should become aggregated and developed into nerves, endowed with this special sensibility.

In searching for the gradations through which an organ in any species has been perfected, we ought to look exclusively to its lineal progenitors; but this is scarcely ever possible, and we are forced to look to other species and genera of the same group, that is to the collateral descendants from the same parent-form, in order to see what gradations are possible, and for the chance of some gradations having been transmitted in an unaltered or little altered condition. But the state of the same organ in distinct classes may incidentally throw light on the steps by which it has been perfected.

The simplest organ which can be called an eye consists of an optic nerve, surrounded by pigment-cells and covered by translucent skin, but without any lens or other refractive body.

In the great class of the Articulata, we may start from an optic nerve simply coated with pigment, the latter sometimes forming a sort of pupil, but destitute of a lens or other optical contrivance. With insects it is now known that the numerous facets on the cornea of the great compound eyes form true lenses, and that the cones include curiously modified nervous filaments.

When we reflect on these facts, here given much too briefly, with respect to the wide, diversified, and graduated range of structure in the eyes of the lower animals; and when we bear in mind how small the number of all livings forms must be in comparison with those which have become extinct, the difficulty ceases to be very great in believing that natural selection may have converted the simple apparatus of an optic nerve, coated with pigment and invested by transparent membranae, into an optical instrument as perfect as is possessed by any member of the Articulate class.

He who will go thus far, ought not to hesitate to go one step further, if he finds on finishing this volume that large bodies of facts, otherwise inexplicable, can be explained by the theory of modification through natural selection; he ought to admit that a structure even as perfect as an eagle's eye might thus be formed, although in this case he does not know the transitional states. It has been objected that in order to modify the eye and still preserve it as a perfect instrument, many changes would have to be effected simultaneously, which, it is assumed, could not be done through natural selection; but as I have attempted to show in my work on the variation of domestic animals, it is not necessary to suppose that the modifications were all simultaneous, if they were extremely slight and gradual. Different kinds of modifications would, also, serve for the same general purpose: as Mr. Wallace has remarked, "If a lens has too short or too long a focus, it may be amended either by an alteration of curvature, or an alteration of density; if the curvature be irregular, and the rays do not converge to a point, then any increased regularity of curvature will be an improvement. So the contraction of the iris and the muscular movements of the eye are neither of them essential to vision, but only improvements which might have been added and perfected at any stage of the construction of the instrument." Within the highest division of the animal kingdom, namely, the Vertebrata, we can start from an eye so simple, that it consists, as in the lancelet, of a little sack of transparent skin, furnished with a nerve and lined with pigment, but destitute of any other apparatus. In fishes and reptiles, as Owen has remarked, "the range of gradations of dioptric structures is very great." It is a significant fact that even in man, according to the high authority of Virchow, the beautiful crystalline lens is formed in the embryo by an accumulation of epidermic cells, lying in a sack-like fold of the skin; and the vitreous body is formed from embryonic sub-cutaneous tissue. To arrive, however, at a just conclusion regarding the formation of the eye, with all its marvellous yet not absolutely perfect characters, it is indispensable that the reason should conquer the imagination; but I have felt the difficulty far too keenly to be surprised at others hesitating to extend the principle of natural selection to so startling a length.

It is scarcely possible to avoid comparing the eye with a telescope. We know that this instrument has been perfected by the long-continued efforts of the highest human intellects; and we naturally infer that the eye has been formed by a somewhat analogous process. But may not this inference be presumptuous? Have we any right to assume that the Creator works by intellectual powers like those of man? If we must compare the eye to an optical instrument, we ought in imagination to take a thick layer of transparent tissue, with spaces filled with fluid, and with a nerve sensitive to light beneath, and then suppose every part of this layer to be continually changing slowly in density, so as to separate into layers of different densities and thicknesses, placed at different distances from each other, and with the surfaces of each layer slowly changing in form. Further we must suppose that there is a power, represented by natural selection or the survival of the fittest, always intently watching each slight alteration in the transparent layers; and carefully preserving each which, under varied circumstances, in any way or in any degree, tends to produce a distincter image. We must suppose each new state of the instrument to be multiplied by the million; each to be preserved until a better one is produced, and then the old ones to be all destroyed. In living bodies, variation will cause the slight alterations, generation will multiply them almost infinitely, and natural selection will pick out with unerring skill each improvement. Let this process go on for millions of years; and during each year on millions of individuals of many kinds; and may we not believe that a living optical instrument might thus be formed as superior to one of glass, as the works of the Creator are to those of man?

Comment: Darwin stressed that vision resulted from a continuous adaptive response to light and that any favorable mutation, however subtle and minute, gave its possessor a better chance for surviving the challenges of environment. The evolution of sight is no more wondrous than that of flight which progressed from gliding to annual distant migrations.

The simplest protozoa exhibits a surface photosensitivity that steers the organism to its optimum environment. In the ameba this is attributed to a change in viscosity of its outer layer. The photomotor response increased in efficiency with the successive evolution of specialized light-sensitive cells in the anterior part of the organism, the addition of insulating and sensitizing pigments and of focusing devices to concentrate the light. In both plant and animal kingdoms the light-sensitizing pigment is derived from carotenoids. The derivative vitamin A systems, essential for image formation, are similar in eyes as widely diverse as those of man and the octopus.

In invertebrates, the retina, derived from the surface ectoderm, is connected secondarily to the nervous system. In vertebrates, however, the eyes arise from the neuroectoderm and a multi-layered retina assumes the function of the invertebrate optic ganglion. Though the vertebrate retina is always inverted and the invertebrate retina is usually erect, inverted retinas are seen in six of the spider's eight eyes and in the eyes of the scallop.

Ray Lankester (1880) suggested that the original pre-vertebrate eye was buried in the central nervous system as in the larval sea-squirt, a protochordate. He assumed that light traversed the transparent body and that as the body became more opaque with the progress of evolution, the eye travelled gradually to the surface. The transparent media of the eye retain the primitive transparency. The cornea, for example, resembles the integument of Amphioxus.

The neural tube had to come into being before the vertebrate retina could evolve. A suggestion of its incipiency is the median infundibular organ of Amphioxus, considered by Walls to be derived from photosensory ependyma. The rods and cones have been traced to the flagellae of ependymal cells, a conception that brings them in line with sensory hair cells in general. The course of evolution intimates that the cones are the older form since diurnality was the primitive status of Vertebrates. The lens, as shown by experimental embryology, is a secondary structure called forth by a chemotactic response to the developing optic cup. The semisold vitreous first served to prop the lens in place, as the eye of the lamprey demonstrates. Diverse methods of effecting accommodation are illustrated in the fish, bird, horse and man. The fibrous and vascular coats of the eye are probably modifications of the meningeal envelops—dura mater and pia arachnoid respectively.

The pupil, fixed in lampreys and fishes, attains maximum motility in mammals. The rapid equalizing device of an active iris displaced the photo-mechanical changes of pigment migration used by the retinas of primitive forms. With evolution the acuity requirements steadily increase. Consequently in man the posterior segment becomes larger so that the visual cells are more numerous per angular unit of image, and the lens becomes flatter to be adapted for the greater focal distance. In the rabbit the depth of the vitreous chamber is less than the anterior-posterior diameter of the lens; in man it is about three times as great.

The ancestral vertebrates had a third eye, directed upwards. In fossil ostracoderms, a socket for this eye is universally present, although much smaller than those for the paired eyes. Despite loss of function, the third eye persists, transformed into the pineal body.

The vexing problems of the ancestry of the Vertebrates and of the Primates have been clarified. The best clues to chordate origins are found in the Echinoderms. Their larvae, which exhibit bilateral symmetry, resemble the larval forms of proto-chordates; and unlike other invertebrates, the Echinoderms use creatine phosphate instead of arginine phosphate to spark the energy release for muscle activity. The earliest phase in the evolution of the Primates is represented approximately by the tree-shrew. In contrast to the true shrews, which are properly classified as Insectivores, the tree-shrew has a high visual development, stimulated undoubtedly by its arboreal life.

An outstanding feature of the evolution of the Primates is the progressive elaboration of the sense of vision. In the higher Primates the orbital apertures become directed forwards and stereoscopic vision is developed as a distinctive acquisition. The most marked trend in the evolution of man has been the special development of the brain. "Human vision is the product of a complex brain teamed with a relatively simple eye" (Walls).

Reference

Duke-Elder, S.: *The Eye in Evolution*. C. V. Mosby Co., St. Louis, 1958.

Biographical Note

Charles Robert Darwin (1809–1882) was born on the same day as Abraham Lincoln, February 12, 1809. His father, a physician, had planned for Charles to follow his profession, but young Darwin found the medical teaching at Edinburgh uninspiring. Starting anew at Christ's College, Cambridge, he took his degree in 1831. Early in youth his scientific bent was stimulated by reading *The Natural History of Selborne* by Gilbert White—a classic in its field. At both Edinburgh and Cambridge he gained the friendship of the scientists there and worked with them at off hours. He spent the vacation after his commencement with Prof. Sedgwick, studying the geology of North Wales. On his return home he found a letter from Prof. Peacock of Cambridge inviting him to be the naturalist on H. M. S. Beagle in its surveying cruise around the world. When he left, on December 27, 1831, Darwin was 22 years old. He returned 5 years later with the finest collection of animals, plants and rocks ever assembled. At Galapagos, Darwin found seven distinct species of finches in the separate islands which he proved were all derived from a single species on the South American mainland. Though

384

this and much other evidence convinced Darwin of the fact of evolution, the mechanism of evolution baffled him until in October 1838 he read Malthus on *Population* when the idea of natural selection flashed upon him. In 1839 he married his cousin, Emma Wedgwood, and in 1842 he finally published the journal of his voyage. In June 1858, A. R. Wallace, then in the Moluccas, sent Darwin a manuscript in which the theory of evolution and natural selection was independently developed. Darwin and Wallace presented their papers jointly before the Linnaean Society on July 1, 1958. Darwin's formal work *On the Origin of Species* was published on November 24, 1859, and the entire edition of 1250 copies was exhausted on the day of issue. During his last 40 years Darwin published 17 books, including the famous *Descent of Man* (1871). He is buried in Westminster Abbey; his home at Down, 20 miles from London, is now a museum.

References

Sears, P. B.: *Charles Darwin*. New York, Scribner's Sons, 1950.
Eiseley, L.: *Darwin's Century*. New York, Doubleday, 1958.

Ophthalmoscopy of the Fundus in Living Birds

CASEY ALBERT WOOD, M.D.

Chicago, Illinois

The Fundus Oculi of Birds, pp. 33–48. Lakeside Press, Chicago, 1917

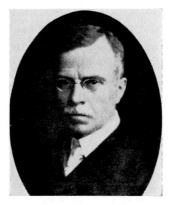

For a proper exploration of the vertebrate fundus it is highly desirable that the pupil be widely dilated. This is accomplished in Man and other Mammals by such mydriatics as atropin, homatropin, euphthalmin, etc., which bring about an enlarged pupil mainly by inhibiting the action of the non-striated sphincter muscle fibres of the iris In birds, however, these agents have little *direct* effect on the striated, voluntary, sphincter musculature of the iris; hence they are of little value in an ophthalmoscopic examination. One is obliged, therefore, to resort to such agents as galvanism, nicotine, strophanthin, curare, stipticin, etc., and to such drugs as render the bird unconscious without actually killing it.

In collecting the heads of birds for macroscopical and histological studies the writer found that satisfactory ophthalmoscopic view of the fundi can be had a few minutes before and after the death of the specimen, during which period the pupil not only dilates *ad maximum* but the bird does not use his third eyelid. Many of the appended reports were gathered in this way.

Owing to the peculiar arrangement of their lacrimal apparatus fluids instilled into the eye (conjunctical sac) of Birds run immediately into the throat and gullet, there to be absorbed and to produce precisely the same systemic effects as if they were poured directly down the throat of the animal. Great care should be used, therefore, in using eye drops for their expected effects upon the visual apparatus; if poisonous for the bird they may cause his death in short order. Some of the so-called mydriatics recommended for an examination of the ocular interior of the bird act as systemic intoxicants and not specifically upon the iris muscles, as is the case with the mammalian eye.

385

One per cent solution of nicotine brings about a dilation of the avian pupil that persists for several hours, and is probably the best agent one can use for the purpose. Experience has proved that the self-luminous, electric ophthalmoscope is the best instrument for exploring the avian fundus. Examinations by the erect image will be found the most satisfactory method, although, as in viewing the human fundus, it is advisable to use the indirect plan at the outset. The self-luminous ophthalmoscope is quite satisfactory for both purposes.

In making an examination of the avian fundus it must be remembered that it is *wild species* that present invariable ophthalmoscopic pictures. It will be found that after two or three generations of inbreeding, confinement and domestications, changes occur in the ocular apparatus coincident with variations in other parts of the organism.

The facility with which the ophthalmoscope can be used depends upon the conduct of the bird under examination. For instance, it is important that the macular region be carefully explored and it can generally be seen, but throwing the light on this very sensitive area often makes the animal restless and the greatest gentleness should be observed to keep it quiet if a complete examination is to be made. Most specimens, not excepting the Eagles, Hawks, Vultures and other large birds can be hypnotized and so quieted for the period of an ophthalmoscopic examination. To this end the assistant must, at first, quietly but firmly hold the mandibles with one gloved hand, the other pressing claws and wings against his chest. In a few minutes the bird ceases to struggle; the assistant's grasp of the bird is then slowly relaxed; the bird relaxes its muscles, no longer resists the attempt to examine it and the head can usually be turned in any desired direction to suit the observer.

There is sometimes difficulty in seeing the fundus of the bird because of frequent winking of the bird's nictitating membrane (rarely through shutting of the true lids) and because of occasional contractions of the pupil (unless it is artificially dilated) but these difficulties are, with time and patience, overcome—and almost always without damage to the bird, the observer or his assistant. Some birds, Cormorants, for instance, resist attempts to quiet them and become wild and restless when the light from the ophthalmoscope falls on the macular region; others, like the Raven, remain quiet for irregular periods during the examination but intelligently await an opportunity to use bill and claw on the captor.

As an extended study of the eyes of living birds is not without its dangers, both the student and his assistant should wear leather gloves during the ophthalmoscopic examination and should especially be on guard against facial bites, stabs and scratches—from the mandibles and talons of Raptores and Parrots in particular. In addition to these accidents, one of the writer's assistants was severely bitten by a European Raven, another was badly kicked by an Ostrich, while the writer himself barely escaped the loss of an eye from a stab on the margin of the orbit inflicted by the pointed beak of a little White Heron.

Reference is elsewhere made to the possibility of quieting or even hypnotizing birds for the purpose of making an ophthalmoscopic examination. In some cases flashing the light of the ophthalmoscope into the animal's eyes produces a quieting effect. The writer examined, in 1912, a young, adult ostrich, six feet high, healthy and very vigorous. The bird resisted capture and was thrown only after a struggle. A keeper sat on his prostrate body; another held his head and neck. After the light of a self-luminous skiascope had played over his dilated pupils in a darkened room for about five minutes he acted as if he were in a trance; he remained in the prone position without being held and a complete examination of his pupil reflexes, static refraction, fundus appearances, etc., was made without difficulty. Finally, after about twenty minutes or a half an hour (when this inquiry was completed) the bird refused to move or rise—and had to be pushed to his feet—after which he became his lively self again.

The small pupils of Wrens, Nuthatches, the smaller Warblers, Hummingbirds, etc., even when fully dilated, make it extremely difficult to view the fundus during the life of the bird and tax the perseverance of the observer to the utmost. It is, perhaps well not to attempt such tasks until the ophthalmoscopist has had a year or two of experience. Annoying, also, are the fugitive reflections and "shot-silk" colors that play over the retinal areas in some birds, but even these fail to obscure the fundus picture after some months of practice.

The task of *picturing the avian background for the purpose of conveying an intelligent idea of its appearance* is a serious one. The ophthalmologist may be a good observer but a poor artist; conversely, an expert in the use of brush and pencil may not be sufficiently conversant with normal and pathological, human and comparative ophthalmoscopy and ophthalmology to enable him to make an intelligent use of his artistic talents. These difficulties have been, in this research, largely met by an arrangement with Mr. Arthur Head, the well-known London artist, who for some twenty years past has been painting both human and animal fundi for confreres here and abroad. This artist and the writer have together examined and discussed in the Gardens of the London Zoological Society the ophthalmoscopic appearance of several hundred avian and other eyes.

The Avian Eyeground in General. The average eyeground or fundus oculi of most day birds resembles, as much as anything, the texture of the so-called "scotch mixtures" in smooth finished cloth—usually light brown, gray, gray-blue, blue mixed with striate rays, or fine concentric marking of lighter gray or white. Scattered over this background are numerous yellowish, yellow-white, brown or gray points of pigment. Although this matter has not been satisfactorily determined yet these punctate deposits are, in part at least, the colored oil droplets.

The Pecten and Optic Disc

Viewed ophthalmoscopically the avian pecten exhibits three fairly definite varieties which may be classified as follows:

1. *Those pectens whose mass uniformly springs from and equally covers the optic disc.* Such pectinate bodies do not extend into the vitreous cavity farther than the length of the widest segment, and they are sessile on the face of the papilla. This method of arranging the pectinate tissues makes provision for a blood reservoir large enough to supply nutritional needs but so placed that it does not materially obstruct visual or light rays. Such a disposition and configuration of the fundal organs meet the needs of many species, among them Eagles and Owls, who require very acute vision.

2. *Some pectens, while they originate from the whole surface of the optic disc, immediately slope away from the visual axis,* approach the bulbar wall and terminate without projecting far into the vitreous. In this type there is generally a disc-length or more between the free terminal of the pecten and the posterior surface of the crystalline lens.

3. This class includes those pectens (usually of slender proportions) that arise from the whole surface of the optic papilla and, then, either curve towards and follow the concave wall of the eyeball or they proceed in a straighter line until they touch (or nearly reach) the posterior surface of the lens, generally near its equator. In most instances there is less than a disc length between the pecten terminal and the lens capsule.

There are many species whose pectens occupy a position intermediate between Class 2 and Class 3. In some instances they radiate from the nerve-head as whitish, thread-like rays, in such a fashion as to cover the whole of a wide area about the optic entrance.

Comment: The eyeball of a bird is unusually large in proportion to its body. The eyelids although similar to those of man, have minute feathers for cilia. The nictitating membrane, which reaches its highest development in birds, cleanses the cornea and when necessary protects the eye from injury and intense sunlight. The lacrimal gland of Harder placed beneath this third eyelid functions simultaneously with it. The avian sclera is distinctive in having overlapping bony plates in its anterior segment. The deep anterior chamber permits significant anterior-posterior movements of the crystalline lens. The canal of Schlemm is remarkably capacious. Accommodation in birds is a more complex performance than in man. It is effected chiefly by the circular striated muscle of Crampton, an intraocular band that encircles the eye about the equator. With its contraction the crystalline lens is pushed into the anterior chamber and the cornea becomes more convex. At the same time the pectinate body fills with blood and occupies the space vacated by the lens. The erectile pecten is invariably a part of the avian eye. It projects into the vitreous from the optic disk to nearly the posterior aspect of the lens. It is found in the nasal half of the vitreous and hence does not interfere with the passage of light to the fovea. The hyaloid artery in the human fetus may be considered a vestigial pecten. The bird is able to make the adjustment "from a telescope to a microscope" in a fraction of a second, to see small objects a quarter-mile away and to pick seeds from the ground that would require a magnifier to distinguish them from the surrounding dust. The pecten probably takes the place of retinal vessels which are wanting in the avian fundus. Some species have two macular regions plainly differentiated. In the divergent eyes of eagles, hawks, and vultures, the double macula may permit monocular stereoscopic eyesight.

Although d- tubocurarine chloride (0.25 per cent) in a simple aqueous solution does not dilate the avian pupil appreciably, it is an excellent mydriatic in a solution of 1:4000 benzalkonium chloride; or in an oil suspension. Gallamine triethiodide (0.2 per cent) in 1:4000 benzalkonium is also a good mydriatic, but somewhat less effective. The reduction of surface tension with benzalkonium chloride, a cationic detergent, helps curare penetrate the corneal epithelium. When in an oil suspension, curare passes into the cornea because it is much more soluble in water than in lipid. Wood, in experimenting on English sparrows, found nicotine, 1 per cent, an effective mydriatic. However, its instillation in the eyes of pigeons causes only intense miosis and severe systemic intoxication.

References

C. A. Wood: The eyes of birds. In *The American Encyclopedia of Ophthalmology*, Vol. 2, pp. 979–999. Cleveland Press, Chicago, 1913.

H. S. Campbell and J. L. Smith: The pharmacology of the pigeon pupil. Arch. Ophth., *67:* 501–504, April, 1962.

Biographical Note

Casey Albert Wood (1856–1942) was born in Canada and was one of Osler's first pupils at the McGill University in Montreal, in which city he was later engaged for several years in general practice. In 1882 he returned from his studies in ophthalmology abroad and settled in Chicago where he rapidly developed an extensive practice. In 1904 he was appointed to the chair of ophthalmology at the University of Illinois. Always an indefatigable worker, he helped to found the present *American Journal of Ophthalmology*. His most important personal contributions were on toxic amblyopia (1896), *A System of Ophthalmic Therapeutics* (1909), *A System of Ophthalmic Operations* (1911), and *The Fundus Oculi of Birds* (1917). He edited besides the monumental *American Encyclopedia of Ophthalmology;* translated *De Oculis of Benevenuto Grassus* (1929) and the *Tadhkirat of Ala ibn Isa* (1936); and compiled *An Introduction to the Literature of*

Vertebrate Zoology (1931). After service in World War I, from which he was discharged with the rank of colonel, he did not return to private practice but devoted himself to world travel, writing, and the study of birds. His interest in birds dated from youth and was enthusiastically shared by his wife. McGill University had honored him with an LL.D. in 1922, and to this university he donated his extraordinary collection of ophthalmologic books, periodicals, and instruments, as well as his extensive library of ornithologic works.

Reference

Chance, B.: Obituary. Am. J. Ophth., *25:* 607–611, May, 1942.

Vision in the Evolution of Man

G. ELLIOT SMITH, M.D.

London, England

EXCERPTS FROM *The Evolution of Man*, OXFORD UNIVERSITY PRESS
LONDON, 1927

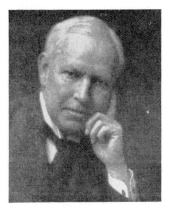

The ability to learn by experience necessarily implies the development, somewhere
in the brain, of a something that can act not
only as a receptive organ for impressions
of the senses and a means for enabling their
influence to find expression in modifying
behaviour, but also serve in a sense as a
recording apparatus for storing such impressions, so that they may be revived in
memory at some future time in association
with other impressions received simultaneously, the state of conscious-
ness they evoked, and the response they called forth.

Such an organ of associative memory is actually found in the brain
of mammals. It is the cortical area for the exact designation of which
I invented the term "neopallium." Into it pathways lead from all the
sense organs; and each of its territories that receives a definite kind of
stimulus, visual, acoustic, tactile, or any other, is linked by the most
intimate bonds with all the others.

Towards the close of the Cretaceous Period some small arboreal
Shrew-like creature took another step in advance, which was fraught
with the most far-reaching consequences. For it marked the birth of the
Primates and the definite branching off from the other mammals of the
line of Man's ancestry.

This change was associated with an enormous development of the
visual cortex in the neopallium, which not only increased in extent so
as far to exceed that of the Lemurs, but also became more highly specialized in structure. Thus, in *Tarsius,* vision entirely usurped the controlling place once occupied by smell; but the significance of this
change is not to be measured merely as the substitution of one sense for
another. The visual area of cortex, unlike the olfactory, is part of the
neopallium; and when its importance thus became enhanced the whole

391

of the neopallium felt the influence of the changed conditions. The sense of touch also shared in the effects, for tactile impressions and the related kinaesthetic sensibility, the importance of which to an agile tree-living animal is obvious, assist vision n the conscious appreciation of the nature and the various properties of the things seen, and in learning to perform agile actions which are guided by vision.

Increased reliance upon the guidance of the sense of sight awakened in the creature the curiosity to examine the objects around it with closer minuteness and supplied guidance to the hands in executing more precise and more skilled movements than the Tree Shrew attempts. Such habits not only promoted the development of the motor cortex itself, and cultivated the discriminative powers of the tactile and kinaesthetic senses, but they linked up their cortical areas in bonds of more intimate association with the visual cortex.

The process of devising the complex machinery for controlling skilled movements leads to the progressive development of the prefrontal territory, the size of which becomes a distinctive feature of the Primates, and in particular of Monkeys, Apes, and Men. In the lower mammals stimulation of the diminutive prefrontal area provokes movements of the head and the eyes (or at first only of the eye of the opposite side of the body). When a true Monkey evolves from a Tarsioid and the prefrontal territory suddenly attains a noteworthy increase in extent, electrical stimulation of this area produces a wide range of closely co-ordinated movements of the two eyes. These conjugate movements, and in particular the acts of convergence, are the necessary preliminaries for fixing the visual attention upon an object to be studied. Moreover, they are obviously also an essential part of the process involved in guiding the hands to learn to perform skillful actions. The prefrontal area is thus intimately concerned not only with the acquisition of skill, but also with controlling the automatic movements of the eyes, which are an essential part of the process of fixing the gaze and concentrating the attention upon some object. The purpose of such a psychological process is to make further observations or to extend the range of thought. The prefrontal area is thus a necessary part of the apparatus concerned with the process of learning and thinking. Such an organ co-ordinated the activities of the whole neopallium so as the more efficiently to regulate the various centres controlling the muscles of the whole body. In this way not only is the guidance of all the senses secured, but the way opened for all the muscles of the body to act harmoniously so as to permit the concentration of their action for the performance of delicate and finely adjusted movement.

But the cortical developments adumbrated in the last paragraphs could not take place until the range of conjugate movements of the eyes was considerably extended. This did not happen in *Tarsius:* but when some Eocene Tarsioid acquired the ability to move its two eyes in any direction in intimate correlation the one with the other a new impulse was given to cortical development and true Monkeys came into being. The essential factor in this profound transformation was the evolution in the prefrontal area of the mechanism for making possible a wider range of conjugate movements of the eyes.

In the vast majority of living animals behaviour is dominated either by smell or vision. Of these smell is the more primitive and fundamental factor. The cerebral cortex was evolved from the part of the brain which originally was little more than the receptive centre for impressions of smell and the instrument for enabling the sense of smell to influence the animal's behaviour. Unlike all the other sensory tracts, those which convey impulses from the olfactory organ reach the cerebral cortex directly—that is, without passing through the thalamus. From a psychological point of view, therefore, the sense of smell occupies a unique and distinctive position. It represents the germ of all the higher psychical powers, or, perhaps it would be more accurate to say, the cement that binds together the elements out of which the powers of the cerebral cortex, as the repository of the impressions of past experiences, the organ of discrimination and appreciation of space and time, are developed.

But the sense of smell conveys only the vaguest indications of spatial relations. An animal attracted by the scent circles around it until it comes within visual range of its quarry: then the eyes convey more precise information as to its position in space and as to its movements. Such visual information is almost entirely devoid of affective tone, of psychological meaning, which it acquires secondarily from the sense of smell.

I have emphasized this fundamental relationship of vision to smell because it is essential for the proper understanding of the respective roles of these dominant senses. Moreover, Sir Charles Sherrington, to whose pioneer work we are indebted for a definition of these problems, has not given adequate recognition to the dependence of vision upon smell for the acquistion of the meaning of vital experience.

In the whole history of living animals, both invertebrate and vertebrate, there has been a constant rivalry between smell and vision for dominance. Behaviour in the primitive members of every group is controlled pre-eminently by smell, and invariably in the more efficient members of such groups vision has usurped the control, as in the teleostean fishes, in birds, and the highest mammals. But in all vertebrate classes excepting mammals visual dominance is attained only at the expense of a precocious specialization of the brain that is fatal to progress, or, at any rate, to the kind of advancement that leads towards the attainment of the human type of intelligence. In the brain of the primitive vertebrate the cerebral hemisphere is essentially the receptive instrument for olfactory impulses, whereas visual impulses are received mainly by the midbrain. Hence a precocious increase of the influence of vision involves a development of the mid-brain at the expense of the fore-brain, and in that sense is fatal to the evolution of the brain in the direction of the enhancement of the functions of the cerebral cortex.

It is only in mammals in which vision, so to speak, has secured representation in the cerebral cortex that fuller reliance on this sense does not involve an impairment of the influence of the cerebral cortex. In mammals, in fact, the cultivation of vision acts as the most powerful stimulus to the growth and elaboration of the cerebral cortex and the progressive development of its psychological possibilities, because the receptive centre for impulses from the eyes is in the neopallium.

I have already referred to the fact that the adoption of vision as the dominant sense enhanced the functional importance of the neopallium, the dominant part of the nervous system, and, in fact, of the whole organism. It has been shown by Professor Magnus of Utrecht that with the enhanced importance of vision the eyes come to play a significant part in regulating posture and muscle tone. This assumption by the cerebral cortex of automatic functions hitherto controlled mainly by lower centres brings the regulation of posture into closer relationship with the functions of the neopallium. Such a development becomes a factor of fundamental importance in establishing the erect attitude.

Of the large series of supposed distinctive features of the human brain that have been extensively cited during the last half-century I shall refer here only to one directly relevant to the serious argument which I must now set forth, based upon the further investigation of the area surrounding the sulcus which Huxley labelled "calcarine."

The identification of this furrow was established by the study of the distribution of the cortical territory that in 1904, I called the *area striata* (in reference to its most obtrusive feature, the stria of Gennari), in front of which the *sulcus lunatus* is situated. This led to the measurement of the extent of the area striata, in which the optic radiations ends; and the discovery that the visual receptive territory is just as extensive in the brains of many Monkeys, even small Macaques, as it is in those of men. In other words, in proportion to the size of the brain the area of cortex concerned with vision is relatively enormous in the lowlier Primates. This investigation led to the realization of the important part played by the early cultivation of vision as the dominant sense in Man's ancestors, and pointed to the necessity for a detailed study of how and why this particular trend in evolution should have led to results of such vast significance as the emergence of the human mind.

Man has evolved as the result of the continuous exploitation throughout the Tertiary Period of the vast possibilities which the reliance upon vision as the guiding sense created for a mammal that had not lost the plasticity of its hands by too early specialization. Under the guidance of vision the hands were able to acquire skill in action and incidentally to become the instruments of an increasingly sensitive tactile discrimination, which again reacted upon the motor mechanisms and made possible the attainment of yet higher degrees of muscular skill. But this in turn reacted upon the control of ocular movements and prepared the way for the acquisition of stereoscopic vision and a fuller understanding of the world and the nature of the things and activities in it. For the cultivation of manual dexterity was effected by means of the development of certain cortical mechanisms; and the facility in the performance of skilled movements once acquired was not a monopoly of the hands but was at the service of all muscles. Skilful use of the hands was impossible without the appropriate posturing of the whole body. High co-ordination of hand movements and high co-ordination of movements of the muscles of the whole body must go together. The sudden extension of the range of conjugate movements of the eyes and the attainment of more precise and effective convergence were results that accrued from this fuller cultivation of muscular skill. They were brought about as the result of the expansion of the prefrontal cortex, which provided the controlling instrument, and also by the building up in the mid-brain of the mechanism for automatically regulating the complex co-ordination necessary to move the two eyes in association in any direction. The attainment of stereoscopic vision enormously enhanced the value of the information acquired by the eyes.

Man studies the actions and facial movements of his fellows and from them learns to interpret their sentiments and intentions—in particular their attitude towards himself. Not only does he acquire such information by means of his own eyes, but in addition the eyes of his fellows themselves afford the most illuminating signals of their owner's thoughts once he has learned to detect the subtle changes that occur in them. Just as the fixing of his own gaze implies the concentration of his attention upon some definite object, so he—as it were instinctively—interprets the immediate interests of his fellow men and women by appreciating the object or point in space towards which the visual axes of the individual he is watching are directed. When he "looks another man in the face" this involves a mutual inquiry and a frank communication of feeling and knowledge one to the other. Such ocular signalling

is the most eloquent form of intercommunication between the sexes—
as the slang expressions in every language reveal. Vision is obviously of
vast significance as an instrument of sexual selection in mankind. The
appreciation of beauty of form and colour, as well as the charm of posture and movement, is rendered possible by Man's distinctive powers of
vision. But vision has not only become the dominant influence in sexual
choice, but its potency has become so enhanced in Man as to override
all those conditions that in other living creatures restrict pairing to
certain seasons when the sexual glands reveal their distinctive activities
and scent glands excite the sexual appetite and almost automatically
impel a pair to mate. But when vision acquired its domination over
behaviour the factors that determine sexual discrimination and attraction were brought more definitely under the influence of the cerebral
cortex (the neopallium). With the superseding of smell by vision the
special scent glands that play so large a part in sexual excitation in some
animals disappeared, and in certain Monkeys nature replaced them by
brilliant colours as a sexual allurement. But in the highest Primates
these grosser forms of visual attraction were sublimated, and aesthetic
appreciation became the obtrusive factor in the conscious choice of
mates, and sexual intercourse was no longer restricted to definite
seasons. When due recognition is given to the unquestionable fact that
sexual selection in mankind is essentially determined by visual discrimination, the further problem arises as to what extent the profound transformations of Man's bodily form—the shape and proportions of the limbs, the erect attitude, the loss of hair on trunk and
limbs, the modelling of the female form by localized developments of
fat—are affected by such selection.

In his Croonian Lecture to the Royal Society in 1925 Professor Magnus called attention to the fact that in Monkeys (and certain other
mammals in which vision plays an important part in guiding movements) the eyes begin to assume the function of regulating posture and
muscle-tone—what Magnus calls the optical righting reflexes develop.
This involved the action of the cerebral cortex, whereas the more primitive nervous mechanisms for controlling posture are sub-cortical, in
other words are placed in the brain-stem. The increasing influence of
vision as the guiding sense added to the significance of the cortex as a
posture-regulating instrument. This was an important factor in the
development of the erect attitude in Man, which is maintained by conscious activity and is not an automatic posture to the same extent as
that of four-footed animals is. The erect attitude was not the cause, as so
many writers have assumed, of Man's intellectual pre-eminence. If it
liberated the hands from the function of locomotion and so enabled
them to attain higher possibilities of skilled action and tactile discrimi-

nation, it must not be forgotten that the erect attitude itself was made possible by the higher development of the brain, which not only conferred these aptitudes on the hands, but also created new conditions for the regulation of posture and a closer correlation between the functions of releasing muscle-tone and initiating a skilled movement.

The parietal area is the chief instrument whereby this intimate correlation of visual and tactile experience is acquired. The hand becomes the sense organ for this enormously enhanced aptitude for tactile discrimination, whereby the nature of things is so largely estimated and their meaning and identity established. The area concerned with these functions derives its power of spatial reference mainly from its connexion with the visual cortex.

The transference of the visual sensorium to the neopallium created the possibility for more intimate correlation of visual experience with that acquired by touch, hearing, smell, &c.; but in addition it conferred visual guidance on the limbs in the process of learning new modes of action.

But the mere process of learning gives him knowledge and understanding, appreciation of form and beauty, and the powers we significantly call insight, foresight, and the wider vision.

Comment: In fishes the roof of the midbrain (tectum) is expanded to form the bigeminal optic lobes, and in amphibians this becomes the corpora quadrigemina. As evolution proceeded the photostatic aspects of vision were retained in the tectum but the epicritic visual functions were transferred in an ever increasing degree to the cortex through the thalamic relay station. The thalamic nuclei control the lower centers and are themselves controlled by the cortical centers. In the Primates the lateral geniculate body of the thalamus is represented almost entirely by the dorsal nucleus—of laminated structure and point-to-point retinal representation—in which 75 per cent of the optic fibers terminate. The primitive ventral nucleus declines in importance as the visual system progresses from a tectal to a cortical orientation and only retains photostatic functions. In the higher vertebrates the paleocortex based upon the sense of smell is gradually superseded by the neocortex built around the sense of vision. "Only in man does ablation of the occipital cortex lead to permanent blindness with complete loss of all sensations of light. In him the only sub-cortical activity is pupillary, and in him alone is vision in its entirety a cortical function." (Duke-Elder).

Reference

Duke-Elder, S.: *System of Ophthalmology*, Vol. I.: *The Eye in Evolution*, pp. 531–537. C. V. Mosby Co., St. Louis, 1958.

Biographical Note

Sir Grafton Elliot Smith (1871–1937) was born at Grafton, New South Wales, and graduated from the University of Sydney Medical School in 1892. After completing his doctoral thesis on the histology of the cerebrum in nonplacental mammals, he obtained a travelling fellowship and continued his researches at Cambridge University where he was stimulated by contacts with Gaskell, Horsley, Langley and Mott. In his brilliant career, Smith occupied the chair of anatomy successively at Cairo (1900–1909), at Manchester (1909–1919) and at the University College, London (1919–1936). From an intensive investigation of ancient Egyptian life, mummies and paleopathology, he contributed several important books that demonstrated convincingly the Egyptian origin of Western culture: *The Migration of Early Culture,* 1915; *The Ancient Egyptians and the Origin of Civilization,* 1923; *Egyptian Mummies,* 1924; *Human History,* 1929. On finding in a mummy advanced calcific arteriosclerosis of the heart, he recalled the Biblical passage, "And the Lord hardened the heart of Pharaoh." In England he continued his studies on ethnology, anthropology and the evolution of the brain. In 1919 he delivered the Croonian Lectures on the cerebral cortex. His comparative analyses of the fissural pattern of the brain laid the basis for interpreting homologies of cerebral configuration. He showed that phylogenetic changes in the surface topography of the brain were due to subcortical and cortical factors that influenced the elaboration of the convolutions of the pallium. He likewise added to the understanding of the development of speech and of binocular vision in man.

Reference

Walker, A. E.: In Haymaker, W. (Ed): *The Founders of Neurology,* pp. 89–92. Charles C Thomas, Publisher, Springfield, Ill., 1953.

Part Fourteen

Environmental Adjustment

De Morbis Artificum (Diseases of Workers)

BERNARDINI RAMAZZINI, M.D.

Modena, Italy

EXCERPTED FROM THE TRANSLATION BY W. C. WRIGHT, PH.D.,* OF THE
SECOND LATIN EDITION OF 1713

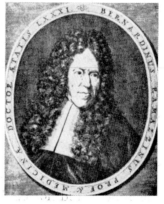

If any new invention is discovered, it appears at first with some roughness, and is afterwards brought to perfection by the industry of others. That this treatise of mine will undergo the like fate, I have reason to believe, particularly because it is something new. It is but reasonable that medicine should contribute to the safety of tradesmen that they may follow trades without injuring their health. The workhouses of tradesmen are the only schools in which we find any satisfactory knowledge of these matters. I have endeavored to suggest such cautions as may serve to prevent and cure the diseases to which tradesmen are subject. Hippocrates informs us that when a physician visits a patient he ought to inquire into many things, to which I would presume to add one interrogation more: namely, what is his trade.

The accident which prompted me to write this treatise is as follows:

In this city which is very populous it is usual to have outhouses cleaned every third year, and while the men were cleaning that at my house, I took note of one who worked with a great deal of anxiety and

* University of Chicago Press, Chicago, 1940.

asked the poor fellow why he did not work more calmly. Upon this the poor wretch lifted up his eyes from the dismal vault and replied, "Above four hours in that place is like being struck blind." After he came out, I took a view of his eyes and found them red and dim. I asked him whether the smell affected the nose or occasioned squeamishness. He answered that the only parts which suffered were the eyes and that if he continued without interruption he should be blind as had happened to others. I am of the opinion that the steams arising from human ordure after three years lying assume a particular nature which injures the eyes only. I have advised them to put transparent bladders over their faces as do those who polish red lead.

Sulfur is employed for many purposes and does serious harm to those who liquefy it or use it in their manufactures. The fumes excite coughing and sore eyes. Martial mentions "the blear eyed vendor of sulfurated wares". Since there is a large amount of sulfur in the composition of iron, it is not surprising that in the process of smelting iron, fine particles of sulfur are given off. These particles attack the eyes and cause acute soreness and ophthalmia. The men should be warned not to gaze at the iron while it bubbles or glows.

Those who separate the flour from the bran with sieves cannot help taking in floating particles of flour with the air they breathe. The eyes also are seriously affected by the particles of flour that stick to them.

There are two kinds of printers, the compositors and the pressmen. Those who work with their hands are threatened with misfortune from having to keep the eyes continually fixed on black letters for they gradually contract weakness of vision and bloodshot eyes. Those who compose will do well to wear spectacles to prevent failure of the tonus of the eyes; also to bathe them in violet-water and the like. I know a Jewess in Modena who used to have extraordinary skill in stringing pearls; she could grade and arrange them in such a way that any blemishes could not be detected, but when she came to be forty and found that no spectacles would fit her, she bade farewell to her trying craft. Once the affection is established, a doctor has no remedy that would restore to the eyes their former strength.

Who would have thought that men who work at a small grindstone sharpening razors or lancets would suffer from impaired vision? These workers have to keep their eyes always steadily on that grindstone which is revolving at high speed, and so inevitably the eyesight becomes dim, just as it does with all who do fine work. If he keeps at work all day long, he often suffers from redness of the eyes. The only precaution that might help is to take a rest from this sort of work.

The Jews are a people whose like is not to be found. These people are pursued by various diseases which result from the trades that they follow and not from some infirmity of the race. Nearly all Jews are employed in work at which they must sit or stand. The women, above all, make their living by needlework. At this they excel and are so expert that they can join and mend garments made of wool, silk or other material so that the seam is quite invisible. This work compels them to apply the eyes closely. Hence they incur all the diseases due to a sedentary life and in time suffer from serious weakness of vision. Besides, the Jews live miserably, shut up in narrow alleys, doing their work by open windows to get what light there is; this causes them to incur headache and sore eyes. We must consider, then, how we can come to the relief of the Jewish people and prevent their suffering so much from their peculiar occupations. For those employed in sewing, I consider that the best thing is bodily exercise. They who sew incessantly should know when to give their eyes a rest, or later their eyes will fail them. My experience shows that in their case venesection is not helpful for their vital force is easily reduced, apart from the fact that they have a deeply rooted conviction, which is not far from the truth, that venesection is the worst possible thing for weak eyes.

Comment: Occupational health is the concern of special committees now in 45 state and 200 county medical societies. The A. M. A. Council on Occupational Health sponsors each year a congress with special exhibits, and occupational health is a major interest of the United States Public Health Service. The 10,000 physicians in the United States who provide in-plant services are represented by the Industrial Medical Association, organized in 1915, and the American Academy of Occupational Medicine. The first state workmen's compensation law was passed in 1890. The evaluation of visual loss is standardized by the section in Ophthalmology of the A.M.A. and the latest revision is available in reprint form on request to the A.M.A. The industrial health movement, as a phase of preventive medicine, was given a tremendous impetus by both world wars. The immense number of ocular hazards that occur in industry has focused attention on means of protection. As Ramazzini noted, the chief hazard is flying particles and the main difficulty lies in persuading workmen to protect themselves. The force of a flying particle depends on its momentum (mass × velocity). A larger mass requires less speed than a smaller one to penetrate the eye. Slivers of steel, 2 to 3 mm. in length, frequently penetrate the eye, but very small particles become impacted usually in the cornea. Hammering and grinding are particularly dangerous; particles of steel or iron broken off by force tend to spin in their flight and so increase their cutting power. An impact perpendicular to the ocular surface is more powerful than one at an acute angle. Distance is also important since the force of a small object is soon spent. Eye protection involves guards fitted appropriately to the machines used, safety lenses in goggles with transparent ventilated sides giving unobstructed side vision and adequate lighting without glare. Each of the three types of safety lenses—laminated, case-hardened, and plastic—is effective in spite of certain deficiencies. Case-hardened and plastic lenses should be checked with both the lensometer and lens measure as not infrequently they will reveal

402

adventitious bitoric curves productive of undesirable meridional magnification though not affecting the lens power. Needless to say, the removal of even surface particles from the eye should be handled by an ophthalmologist.

eferences

Duke-Elder, W. S.: *Textbook of Ophthalmology*, Vol. 6: *Injuries*. The C. V. Mosby Company, St. Louis, 1954.
Kuhn, H. S.: *Industrial Ophthalmology*, Edition 2. The C. V. Mosby Company, St. Louis, 1950.
Resnick, L.: *Eye Hazards in Industry*. Columbia University Press, New York, 1941.

Biographical Notes

Bernardini Ramazzini (1633–1714) was born in Capri, a resort town 30 miles from Modena. He received his Doctor of Medicine at Parma in 1659 and spent the 29 most active years of his life at Modena, where he won the favor of the ducal court of Este. Ramazzini cultivated eagerly friendship with the learned and they paid him equal honor. As the years passed he became a fellow of almost all of the Academies and universities of Europe. Among his regular correspondents were Malpighi, Morgagni and Leibnitz. His two daughters married physicians. He was one of the first to note that the barometer rises when the weather is fair and goes down when the sky is cloudy. He began lecturing on diseases of artisans in 1690 at the University of Modena and 10 years later published the first edition of his treatise, which received immediate acclaim and was translated in all the languages of Europe. The English translation appeared in 1705. In 1700 at the age of 67, he accepted the Chair of Practical Medicine at Padua; succeeding the famed Sanctorius. Toward the end of 1703 he became afflicted with arteriosclerotic headaches and the vision of the right eye deteriorated. Finally he lost his sight, but this did not deter this indefatigable savant from continuing his lectures and publications. In 1709 he was appointed physician to the Duke and made president of the University of Padua. In 1710 he published a treatise on the health of princes that became a best seller, although rejected by his publisher and printed at his own expense. In 1713 he issued an amplified edition of his book on diseases of tradesmen. On his 81st birthday, as he was preparing to lecture, he suffered a sudden stroke and died within 12 hours.

Ramazzini is the recognized father of industrial medicine and occupational hygiene, being the first to explore the vast area of trade diseases. His memory is honored in his birthplace by a marble statue in the public garden, and the Italian journal of occupational hygiene bears the title, *The Ramazzi*. His name accompanies that of Hippocrates and Harvey on the cornice of the facade housing the Department of Health and Sanitation in Foley Square, New York. To dignify the tercentenary of his birth in 1933, the epitaph written by his devoted nephew and amanuensis was carved in stone and placed in the church of St. Francis de Sales where his remains are buried in Padua, and a bronze bust of Ramazzini was unveiled at the Museum of Social Hygiene in Dresden. His 15 Paduan Orations are valuable sources on the status of medicine in his day.

eference

Donoghue, F. D.: Bernardo Ramazzini. New England J. Med., *207:* 695–700, 1932.

On Becoming Blind

LOUIS EMILE JAVAL, M.D.*

Paris, France

EXCERPTS FROM *Entre Aveugles*, 208 PP. MASSON ET CIE., PARIS, 1903†

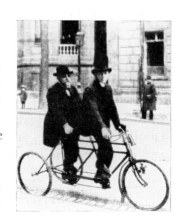

Introduction

Having lost my sight at a relatively late age (I had just entered my sixty-second year), one of my first cares was to inquire what might be done to live with my infirmity. Great was my surprise to find nowhere any collection of advice on this matter.

This sudden and complete loss of sight is a relatively infrequent misfortune. Some soon resign themselves to passing their life in the corner; others, more energetic, continue, as far as possible, their former mode of life with the aid of other's eyes. We have seen Huber, become blind at the age of twenty-seven, assisted by a faithful servant, continue the work of Réaumer on the habits of bees; Augustin Thierry, blind at thirty, not abandon his historical researches; Milton, losing his sight at fifty, dictate to his daughter his celebrated poem of "Paradise Lost"; Fawcett, blinded at twenty-five, change his career of a lawyer for that of a writer, win an election to the House of Commons, and become postmaster-general.

Bondage and Freedom

One of the phases of bondage from which the blind escapes with difficulty is the impossibility of checking by himself the statements of another. If he cannot have absolute veracity in those about him, life becomes intolerable. Never lie to a blind man, be it with the best intent in the world; because, to render him a passing service, you will have killed his confidence, and in consequence his security.

In society the bondage of the blind is almost constant; he does not choose his interlocutor, the other forces himself on him. It is impossible to escape from a bore to join a congenial group.

* The illustration shows the blind Javal taking exercise on a tandem bycicle.
† From the translation by Carroll R. Edson, M.D., Denver.

For most services, paid help is preferable. For example, a paid reader reads what we wish, rereads any passage we wish to remember, skips a chapter which does not interest us. He spares us his comments. If we dictate a letter to him, he does not interrupt to give us his advice.

All efforts should tend to give the blind the maximum of freedom and independence compatible with his condition, by providing him with the means of doing for himself as many things as possible. The more he knows how to do alone, the more he will act for himself and the more content he will be, while less of a care to another.

One kind of thoughtfulness to which the blind is extremely sensitive consists in maintaining around him the most perfect order, so that he is free to find things for himself instead of having to ask for them. He should, as far as possible, sort his papers for himself, so as never to be at the mercy of a particular person when he has need to find them again.

Since the loss of freedom is the worst of the consequences of blindness, when one loses his sight the first thing to do is to hasten to make him familiar with all the procedures which allow him to act for himself; and it is the setting forth of these means which is the object of the present work.

Replacing Sight by the Other Senses

The cane which the blind makes use of may rightly be considered as a prolongation of the tactile sense. This long feeler is much more delicate if the cane is replaced by a light wand. It serves me, so to speak, as an antenna, and saves me from carrying my hands stretched out when I go about. Whether it be in a crowd, as on leaving the theatre, or on a call in an unfamiliar room, I walk with this stick ahead of me, moving it back and forth horizontally, the ferrule near the ground. Its use warns passers of the approach of a blind person and leads them to make room.

Professional Occupation

Since in this little book I ought to dwell upon my own case especially, I will state how much the very idea even of writing the present volume entered into the program about to be expounded. For forty years I have been busied with the physiology of the organs of sense, and yet while following the profession of oculist, I have not allowed myself to be carried away by the practice of this means of making a livelihood, to the point of losing interest in sociologic matters. I have been a Deputy, and a member of many associations for general helpfulnes. All this past seemed to me a useful point of departure from which to make the researches and inquiries which have resulted in this book. I thought that, being no longer able to make optical experiments in the laboratory, I could make others profit by putting together my knowledge.

I have divided among the members of my large family the cares with which they wished to surround me; and since no one is my especial secretary I have reserved to myself the sorting of my papers in portfolios which bear the titles on the back both in ink and in raised points. A faithful friend of very varied learning comes from time to time to keep me in touch with the scientific and literary work of our period. I ask no member of my family to read what can be read by a servant, such as the papers, for instance, or to go with me on my errands; their freedom is respected as well as mine.

My successor at the Sorbonne does me the kindness to tell from time to time what is being done at the laboratory where he was a long time my junior; and if some old patient insists on consulting me, I call in an assistant who for twelve years helped me in my private work and who describes the condition of the invalid and thus gives me the illusion of being still useful as a physician.

Dr. Vosy continues the practice of medicine, either by going as consultant or in attending cases of labor. It appears that for certain young women the blindness of Dr. Vosy is even an additional reason for employing his services. This leads me to recall that in Japan the blind have the monopoly of massage. There is already in Paris a blind masseur who, without being a physician, succeeds in earning his living.

It may be said in general that those who lose their sight late in life, though they may be much less adroit in getting about than those who are born blind, are in a much better position to do well such acts as they are familiar with. Their previous knowledge makes them apt in those duties the learning of which is very hard for the blind from birth.

Helmholtz told me, in 1867, that in the choice of his work he was guided by a kind of inventory which he had made of his mathematical and musical aptitude, of his physiological and anatomical knowledge, and of the means at his disposal in the laboratory at Heidelberg; then he came to the conclusion that he might succeed in making discoveries which had escaped mathematicians, musicians, physiologists and physicians, more eminent than he, each in his own branch.

It is by a process quite analogous that one becoming blind late in life, after having made a review of the means at his disposal, can make a wise choice of a new career.

Psychology of the Blind

Egoism and vanity are the prime motives of human actions; with the blind these faults sometimes assume excessive proportions. The vanity which one often meets in him finds its chief nourishment in the wonder expressed by those who notice every time he does anything alone.

After all is vanity a vice? Is it not rather a motive which often leads to well-doing? "The moralist has said, 'Choke out thy pride.' I say, 'Justify it; it is the secret of all great lives.' "

A characteristic trait of the blind is to reflect much on the past, and to draw logical deductions therefrom; it is not uncommon, then, for a blind man to be a person of good counsel, above all if he has lost sight late.

When a young man first loses his sight, he should be left in an asylum for the blind only for the time absolutely necessary. This very special surrounding is indeed unsuited to the development of the qualities necessary for ordinary life.

Deafness does not wreck a man's career as does blindness; it leaves him free, while the blind man is at the mercy of some one else. The deaf man can let himself be morose; the blind man is obliged to appear amiable. One may say, then, that if the blind is more affable than the deaf man, this is rather the index of the fear he has of being left alone in his darkness.

Those who have never taken thought save of their pleasures and their own affairs are the most unhappy when they lose their sight. Those, on the contrary, who have set before them as the chief aim of life to contribute to the extent of their power to the general progress, find resources in themselves.

Men of science occupy a privileged position; they have, in fact, a whole fund of acquired knowledge which they can make use of. So long as they can still bring their stone, however small it may be, to the building of civilization and progress, they feel that they live.

Comment: With the loss of vision comes a greater dependence on the other senses. The blind can become skilled in interpreting sensations of sound, smell and touch which are of little significance to sighted people. After the frightening shock that comes with blindness, the patient should be encouraged to understand how much of the affairs of life can be carried on without sight. A blind person should be permitted to do everything he can for himself. He learns by doing. A self reliant blind person can be an asset to society. A person can learn to read braille in three months, and with the development of proficiency can read 100 words a minute. Talking books— $33\frac{1}{3}$ speed records—circulate free through the public library. The Readers' Digest is published both on talking book records and in a braille edition.

Most blind people can learn to travel with a cane, but help may be appreciated in crossing busy streets. Never aid a blind person, however, without first asking him if you can be of help; and then let him take your arm as you lead him. No blind person should have a guide dog unless he likes dogs, wants one, has continuous use for it, and can care for it properly. The person with a guide dog almost never needs help at street crossings. Many blind people can work successfully in industry, the professions and in business, once the proper routines are learned. Many blind women do all their housework.

Blindness includes those with no vision at all and those with very limited vision. About 60 per cent of the 230,000 legally blind in the United States have a little sight. Corrected vision limited to 20/200 is considered economic blindness. Half of all blindness comes from cataracts, accidents and glaucoma. The other half results from diabetes, retrolental fibroplasia, trachoma, tuberculosis, meningitis, venereal disease, brain tumors and miscellaneous causes. About 1,500 United States servicemen lost their sight in World War II. The incidence of blindness from retrolental fibroplasia in babies born two months or more prematurely averaged 10 per cent between 1942 and 1953.

More than 50 per cent of blindness could be prevented by proper medical care and precautions against accidents. According to responsible estimates, one person out of 50 past the age of 40 will have glaucoma, which could in most instances be controlled if detected early.

Reference

Some Facts About Blindness. The Chicago Lighthouse, 1954.

Biographical Note

Louis Emile Javal (1839–1907) was not only a world figure in ophthalmology but also a legislator, journalist, educational leader, hygienist and social reformer. In 1806 when the Jews of France were ordered by Napoleon to change their patronymics, Javal's grandfather inscribed on the register his name Jacob, which miscopied by the clerk as Javal became the family name thereafter. Leopold, Javal's father, was an industrial leader and an associate of the financier, Jacques Laffitte. Emile Javal, however, wanted a scientific career and became a mining engineer in the coal mines of his family. His concern about his sister's squint and the discovery of his own astigmatism stimulated some personal investigations on optics which were so well received that he finally embarked on a medical career. After graduation he inaugurated at the University of Paris a laboratory of physiologic optics in the department of physiology in which he was assisted at times by Landolt, Nordenson, Schiøtz and Tscherning. He was the first to attempt functional education in the treatment of squint, particularly as a significant adjuvant to surgical correction, and so founded orthoptics. He also improved the methods of testing astigmatism and with Schiøtz invented the clinical ophthalmometer. His studies on the eye movements in reading, which he was the first to note, and his researches on the ease and speed of reading as affected by variations in light, paper and print foreshadowed the present interest in these subjects. In 1897 an attack of glaucoma was precipitated by the excitement of the Dreyfus trial and three years later Javal was stark blind despite treatment, medical and surgical. He was not to be deterred from further achievement and his book on how the blind can help themselves was very widely circulated. His famous library, donated to the eye clinic of the Hotel Dieu, is the nucleus of its Bibliotheque Javal.

Reference

Lebensohn, J. E.: Louis Emile Javal, a centenary tribute. Arch Ophth., *21:* 650, 1939.